UROLOGY ESSENTIALS

UROLOGY ESSENTIALS

[Book for Surgical Professionals]

DR. PARAG GUPTA

MBBS, MS, MCh Urology (SGPGIMS)

Head, Department of Urology and Renal Transplant

St. Stephen's Hospital

Delhi (INDIA)

PEEPEE

PUBLISHERS AND DISTRIBUTORS (P) LTD.

Urology Essentials

Published by :
Pawaninder P. Vij and Anupam Vij
Peepee Publishers and Distributors (P) Ltd.
Head Office : 160, Shakti Vihar,
Pitam Pura, Delhi-110 034 (India)

Correspondence Address :
7/31, First Floor, Ansari Road, Daryaganj
New Delhi-110 002 (India)
Ph.: 011-65195868, 23246245, 9811156083
e-mail : peepee160@yahoo.co.in www.peepeepub.com

First Edition : 2013
Second Edition : 2015
Reprint : 2017
Reprint : 2018
Reprint : 2020

ISBN : 978-81-8445-182-5

Price : Rs650.. undred Only)

Printed at : Rajasthan Prakashan, Jaipur

To
My parents in recognition of their inspiring guidance !
My wife, Dr. Pratibha, who cooperated with me, first during my MCh preparation and then for preparing this book !
My son Prakhar and daughter Pushti for their unconditional support !

Some books are to be tasted,
Others to be swallowed,
And some few
To be chewed and digested.

–Francis Bacon

PREFACE

There is plethora of material which general surgeon is expected to know.

Obviously it is impossible to summarize urology in 400 pages but our effort is to provide all vital facts of urology through this book.

The Aim of Urology Essentials is to provide Urologists and Surgeons with concise and valuable knowledge. The book is divided into 18 chapters for easy retrieval of information. We have tried to describe various imaging procedures using illustration and intra operative photos without presenting a heavy text book.

This book will also prove helpful for surgeons and postgraduates who are preparing for MCh Urology Entrance Examinations.

I hope readers will find Urology Essentials useful in extending their understanding of exciting speciality of Urology.

I have made all possible attempts to keep the mistakes to minimum but if you find any mistakes or need any clarification you can mail me at drparaggupta1@yahoo.co.in.

Happy reading and good luck to you all !!

–**Dr. Parag Gupta,** MCh

CONTENTS

1. Anatomy.. 1

2. Clinical Decision Making.. 12

3. Basics of Urologic Surgery.. 27

4. Infection and Inflammation 40

5. Molecular and Cellular Biology.. 62

6. Reproductive and Sexual Function.. 68

7. Male Genitalia.. 94

8. Renal Physiology and Pathophysiology.. 119

9. Upper Urinary Tract Obstruction and Trauma...................................... 132

10. Renal Failure and Transplantation.. 144

11. Urinary Lithiasis and Endourology.. 154

12. Neoplasms of Upper Urinary Tract... 173

13. Adrenals... 202

14. Urine Transport, Storage and Emptying.. 209

15. Bladder, Lower Genitourinary Calculi and Trauma................................ 243

16. Prostate... 269

17. Pediatric Urology.. 314

18. Uroimaging...385

Chapter 1
ANATOMY

1. **Boundaries of retroperitoneum-**
    - Posteriorly–abdominal wall (encloses sacrospinalis and quadratus lumborum).
    - Laterally–preperitoneal fat (transversus abdominis).
    - Anteriorly–peritoneum.
2. **Layers of posterior abdominal wall from anterior to posterior**
    - Retroperitoneum
    - Anterior layer of lumbodorsal fascia (LDF)
    - Quadratus lumborum
    - Middle layer of LDF
    - Sacrospinalis
    - Posterior layer of LDF
3. **Sacrospinalis and quadratus lumborum**–comprise the posterior abdominal wall.
4. **External oblique**–originates from lower 8 ribs and inserts into lateral lip of iliac crest.
5. **Internal oblique**–originates from iliac crest and inserts into lower 4 ribs.
6. **Iliopsoas**–inserts into lesser trochanter of femur and helps in flexion of hip.
7. **Dorsal lumbotomy**–allows entrance to the retroperitoneum without muscle cutting.
8. **Limits of pleura**–8th rib anteriorly, 10th rib in midaxillary line, and 12th rib posteriorly.
9. **The aorta**–enters the abdomen via the aortic hiatus at T12 vertebrae.
10. **Arteries arising from abdominal aorta from above downwards**
    - Paired inferior phrenic arteries- first to arise
    - Celiac trunk

- Adrenal arteries
- Superior mesenteric artery
- Renal artery (at L2 vertebrae)
- Gonadal artery
- Inferior mesenteric artery
- Middle sacral artery- final branch
- Bifurcation at L4 vertebrae

11. **The right gonadal artery**–crosses anterior to IVC and then crosses over the ureter (water flows under the bridge).
12. **Confluence of the iliac veins**–posterior and to the right of the aortic bifurcation.
13. **Arteries which can be sacrificed without ill effect because there is collateral circulation are-**
    - Gonadal artery
    - Inferior mesenteric artery
    - Lumbar artery
    - Inferior epieigastric artery
14. **Renal veins**–anterior to the accompanying renal artery.
15. **Right renal vein**–shorter and without branches.
16. **Left renal vein**–longer than the right and receives a lumbar vein posteriorly, the left gonadal vein inferiorly, and the adrenal vein superiorly.
17. **Lymphatic flow**–cranially, laterally and predominantly from the right to the left.
18. **Lymphatic metastases from the right testis drain primarily into** the interaortocaval nodes with drainage to the right paracaval nodes and left para-aortic nodes also.

    Lymphatic metastases from left testis drains primarily to the left para-aortic nodes with drainage to the inter-aortocaval nodes. There is essentially no drainage to the right paracaval nodes from left-sided tumors.
19. **Sympathetic preganglionic fibers**–begins in thoracic and lumbar portions of spinal column.

Parasympathetic preganglionic fibers–begins in the cranial and sacral spinal column segments.

20. **Superior hypogastric plexus**
    - **Autonomic input to the pelvic urinary organs and genital tract travels through this plexus.**
    - This plexus lies on the aorta anterior to its bifurcation and extends inferiorly on the anterior surface of the L5 vertebrae.
    - This plexus is contiguous bilaterally with inferior hypogastric plexuses.
    - **Disruption of the sympathetic nerve fibers that travel through these plexuses during retroperitoneam result in retrograde ejaculation.**
21. **Subcostal, iliohypogastric and ilioinguinal nerves** cross the anterior or inner surface of the quadratus lumborum muscle before piercing the transversus abdominis muscle and continuing their course between transversus abdominis and the internal oblique muscle.
22. **Genital branch of the genitofemoral nerve supplies** the cremaster and dartos muscles in the scrotum.
23. **The genitofemoral nerve**–lies directly on top of psoas muscle through its retroperitoneal course.
24. **Femoral nerve** may be compressed by retractor blades placed inferolaterally against the inguinal ligament in lower abdominal incisions, producing a significant motor palsy that **prevents active extension of the knee.**

    During psoas hitch–sutures placed in the direction of the nerve to avoid nerve damage or entrapment.
25. **The second (descending portion) is of most importance to the urologist** because it lies immediately anterior to the right renal hilum and pelvis.
26. **Right adrenal gland is**–superiorly located in the retroperitoneum and is pyramidal in shape.
27. **Left adrenal gland is**–medial to the upper pole of the left kidney and crescenteric in shape.
28. **Adrenal cortex is**–mesodermal in origin and makes up 90% of the adrenal mass.

29. **Adrenal medulla is**–composed of chromaffin cells derived from neural crest origin.

30. **Adrenal cortex composed of three layers, from external to internal:**
    - Glomerulosa produces mineralocorticoids (e.g., aldosterone)
    - Fasciculata produces glucocorticoids (e.g., cortisol)
    - Reticularis produces sex steroids (androgens).

31. **Adrenal artery**
    - Superior–branch of inferior phrenic artery.
    - Middle–branch of aorta.
    - Inferior–branch of renal artery.

32. **Each kidney weighs** 150 g in the male and 135 g in the female.

    Kidneys measure 10 to 12 cm vertically, 5 to 7 cm transversely, and 3 cm in the anteroposterior dimension.

33. **Fetal lobations**–present at birth and generally disappear by the first year of life.

34. **Columns of Bertin**–the extensions of cortex between the renal pyramids.

35. **Dromedary hump**
    - Normal variation without pathologic significance.
    - Left>right.
    - Caused by downward pressure from the spleen or liver.

36. **Axis of kidney-**

    Lower pole of the kidney–laterally and anteriorly relative to the upper pole.

    Medial aspect of kidney–rotated anteriorly.

    Medially the lower two thirds of the **kidney lie against** the psoas muscle, and laterally against the quadratus lumborum and aponeurosis of the transversus abdominis muscle.

37. **Gerota's fascia**
    - This fascial layer encompasses the perirenal fat and kidney and encloses the kidney on three sides: superiorly, medially, and laterally.

- Medially it extends across the midline to fuse with the contralateral side.
- Fascia is not closed inferiorly.

38. **Anterior to posterior in hilum**–renal vein, renal artery and renal pelvis.

39. **The progression of arterial supply to the kidney**–renal artery →segmental artery →interlobar artery →arcuate artery →interlobular artery →afferent artery.

40. **Ureteropelvic junction obstruction** caused by a crossing vessel Occur when the posterior segmental branch passes anterior to the ureter causing occlusion.

41. **Unlike arterial supply**–occlusion of segmental venous branch has little effect on venous outflow.

42. **Anatomic variations in the renal vasculature**–25% to 40% of kidneys.

    - **The most common variation** is supernumerary renal arteries.

43. **On the left kidney, primary lymphatic drainage**–into the left lateral para-aortic LN.

    On the right kidney, primary lymphatic drainage–into the right interaortocaval and paracaval LN.

44. **Renal pyramid**□papilla□minor calyces□major calyces□renal pelvis.

    Renal papillae–are the at tip of a medullary pyramid.

    - Constitute the **first gross structure** of the renal collecting system.
    - There are 7 to 9 papillae per kidney.

45. The 2 million glomeruli within each kidney represent the core of the renal filtration process.

46. **Ureter begins**–posterior to the renal artery and then passes posterior to gonadal vessels and then anterior to iliac vessels.

47. **Ureter length- 22-30 cm**

    Layers of ureter from inner to outer is-

    - **Transitional epithelium**
    - **Lamina propria**
    - **Muscular - inner longitudinal**

      - outer circular

- **Adventitia-** it encompasses the blood vessels and lymphatics that travel along the ureter.

48. **Three distinct narrowings of ureter**–UPJ, crossing of the iliac vessels, and UVJ.

    True physical restriction of ureter is at- UV junction

49. **Nomenclature-**

    - **Abdominal ureter -** renal pelvis to the iliac vessels
    - **Pelvic ureter -** iliac vessels to the bladder.
    - **Upper ureter -** renal pelvis to the upper border of the sacrum.
    - **Middle ureter -** upper to the lower border of the sacrum.
    - **Lower ureter -** lower border of the sacrum to the bladder.

50. **Ureteral blood supply** is from renal, gonadal, aorta, common iliac, internal iliac, superior vesical, inferior vesical, vaginal, uterine and middle rectal arteries.

51. **Normal ureteral peristalsis** does not require outside autonomic input but, rather, propagates from intrinsic smooth muscle pacemaker sites located in the minor calyces.

52. **Mechanism of renal pain**

    - Pain fibers are stimulated by distention in the renal collecting system.
    - Direct mucosal irritation in the upper urinary tract stimulate nociceptors.
    - Signals travel with the sympathetic nerves and result in a visceral-type pain to the sympathetic distribution of the kidney and ureter (T8 to L2).
    - Pain and reflex muscle spasm are produced over the distributions of the subcostal, iliohypogastric, ilioinguinal, and genitofemoral nerves.

53. At the pelvic inlet, **true and false pelvis are separated by** the arcuate line, which extends from the sacral promontory to the pectineal line of the pubis.

54. **Palpable landmarks**

    - **Anterior and posterior iliac spines**
    - **Iliac crests**

- **Pubic tubercles**
- **Ischial tuberosities**

55. **Sacrospinous ligament separates**–greater and lesser sciatic foramina.

57. **Branch from the femoral vessels to run in Camper's layer** are superficial circumflex iliac, superficial external pudendal, and superficial inferior epigastric vessels.

58. **Superiorly and laterally**–scarpa blends with Camper's fascia.

    Inferiorly–fuses with the deep fascia of the thigh.

    Medially–continuous with Colles' fascia of the perineum.

    After urethral injury blood and urine can accumulate:

    - In the **scrotum** and **penis**.
    - In the **perineum**, (butterfly shaped hematoma).
    - In the **anterior abdominal wall to the clavicles** and around the flank to the back.
    - They will not extend down the leg or into the buttock

59. **Colles' fascia attaches to**–the posterior edge of the UGD and the inferior ischiopubic rami.

    It is continuous with the dartos fascia of the penis and scrotum.

60. **The inguinal canal transmits**

    - **Spermatic cord in the male**
    - **Round ligament in the female**
    - **Ilioinguinal nerve in both sexes**
    - **Anterior wall and floor-** formed by the external oblique muscle
    - **Posterior wall-** formed by the transversalis fascia

61. **The internal inguinal ring** lies midway between the anterior superior iliac spine and the pubic tubercle, above the inguinal ligament, and 4 cm lateral to the external ring.

62. **During transperitoneal laparoscopic pelvic LND**, the obturator packet is accessed by incising the peritoneum lateral to the obliterated umbilical artery.

    During transperitoneal laparoscopic radical prostatectomy, the medial umbilical folds are used as landmarks to guide the dissection of the bladder to expose the space of Retzius.

63. **Median umbilical fold**–overlies the urachus.

Medial umbilical fold (contains obliterated umbilical artery)- important landmark as it can be traced to its origin from the internal iliac artery (IIA) to locate the ureter, which lies on its medial side.

Lateral umbilical fold contains the inferior epigastric vessels.

64. **Inferior epigastric artery**

- Arises from external iliac artery.
- Gives off a cremasteric branch which joins the spermatic cord at the internal inguinal ring.
- In 25%, an accessory obturator artery arises from the inferior epigastric artery.

65. **The superior vesical artery**

- Arises from the proximal portion of the obliterated umbilical artery.
- Gives off a vesiculodeferential branch which supplies seminal vesicles and vas deferens.

66. **Posterior branches from IIA**–lateral sacral, superior gluteal and ascending lumbar.

67. **Iliohypogastric nerve (L1)**–supplies and travel between internal oblique and transversus muscles.

Ilionguinal nerve (L1)–passes through internal oblique and enter inguinal canal laterally.

Genitofemoral nerve (L1, L2)–pierces psoas muscle to reach retroperitoneum.

68. **Sensation on anterior scrotum from**–L2, genital branch of genitofemoral nerve.

Sensation on posterior scrotum from–S2,3,4, posterior femoral cutaneous nerve.

69. **Pelvic plexus**

- **Rectangular** and is 4 to 5 cm long. Its midpoint is at the tips of the seminal vesicles.
- Injury can lead to postoperative impotence.
- **Oriented in sagittal plane** on either side of rectum.
- Pierced by vessels going to and from rectum, bladder and prostate.

- **Communicates behind** rectum and anterior and posterior to bladder neck.

70. **Prostatic capsular** vessels serve as a **surgical landmark for the course of cavernosal nerves** (the neurovascular bundle of Walsh).
71. **During radical prostatectomy (RP)**–nerves are most vulnerable at the apex of the prostate, where they are at the 5 and 7 o'clock positions.
72. **Ureter passes in front of vagina**–and it crosses 1.5 cm anterior and lateral to the uterine cervix.
73. **Blood supply to the pelvic ureter**–laterally.

    Blood supply to abdominal ureter–medially.
74. **The pelvic ureter**
    - High preponderance of plexiform vessels.
    - More susceptible to ischemia and less suitable for ureteroureterotomy.
    - Rich adrenergic and cholinergic autonomic innervation derived from the pelvic plexus.
75. **Layers of bladder from inner to outer is-**
    - **Transitional epithelium**
    - **Lamina propria**
    - **Muscular**
        - **inner longitudinal**
        - **middle circular(preprostatic sphincter** responsible for continence at bladder neck)
        - **outer longitudinal**
76. **In females**
    - **Middle circular layer** of bladder does not appear to be as robust as that of the male.
    - Possess little **adrenergic innervations.**
77. **The muscle of trigone forms three distinct layers**
    - **Superficial layer,** continues from the longitudinal muscle of the ureter and insert at the verumontanum.
    - **Deep layer,** continues from Waldeyer sheath and inserts at the bladder neck.

- **Detrusor layer,** formed by the outer longitudinal and middle circular smooth muscle layers of the bladder wall.

78. **Bulk of bladder lymphatic drainage**- external iliac lymph nodes.
79. **The prostate**–composed of 70% glandular elements and 30% fibromuscular stroma.
80. **Most common zone for prostatic cancers and chronic prostatitis**– peripheral zone.

    Most common zone for BPH–transitional zone.
81. **Arterial supply to the prostate**–inferior vesical artery.(urethral and capsular arteries).

    Minor branches from middle hemorrhoidal and pudendal vessels.
82. **The urethral arteries**
    - Penetrate the prostatovesical junction posterolaterally
    - Approach the bladder neck in the 1 to 5-o'clock and 7 to 11-o'clock positions
    - Supply periurethral glands, and the transition zone.
    - In BPH, these arteries provide the principal blood supply of the adenoma (Flocks artery).
    - During resection of BPH, the most significant bleeding is encountered at the bladder neck, particularly at the 4 and 8-o'clock positions.

    The capsular artery
    - Pass anteriorly to ramify on the prostatic capsule.
    - Runs posterolateral to the prostate with the cavernous nerves (neurovascular bundles).
    - Pierce the prostate at right angles and follow the reticular bands of stroma to supply the glandular tissues.
83. **Membranous urethra average length**–2.0 to 2.5 cm.
84. **Vas deferens**
    - Termir al end is dilated and tortuous.
    - Capable of storing spermatozoa.
    - Outer longitudinal and inner circular smooth muscle.
    - Lined by stratified columnar epithelium.
    - Nonmotile stereocilia.

85. Seminal vesicle

- Lateral outpouching of vas.
- Length is 5 cm. and 3 to 5 cm in diameter with a volume capacity of 13 cm, although they decrease in size with aging.
- Tubules are 15 cm long coiled and convoluted.
- Seminal vesicle secretions are alkaline with capacity3 to 4 ml.
- Does not store sperm.
- Contributes largest (50% to 80%) to ejaculate.
- **These secretions are found in later fractions of the ejaculate.**
- Lies posterior to bladder.
- Normally not palpable on DRE
- Ureter enters bladder medial to tip of seminal vesicle.
- **Begin as bilateral dorsolateral bulbous dilations of distal mesonephric duct at 12 weeks of gestation.**
- Blood supply from vesiculodeferential artery (branch of superior vesicle artery).
- The lymphatic drainage is through the internal iliac lymph nodes.
- Innervated through sympathetic nerves from the superior lumbar and hypogastric nerves. Parasympathetic innervation occurs through the pelvic plexus.

86. The anterior urethra is narrowest at the external meatus.

87. Fournier's gangrene–does not involve testis.

88. The scrotal lymphatics–do not cross the median raphe, while penile lymphatics crosses.

89. Epididymis attaches at–posterolateral aspect of the testis.

Chapter 2
CLINICAL DECISION MAKING

1. **Pain due to inflammation**–steady.

   Pain due to obstruction–fluctuates.

2. **Inflammation of renal parenchyma, prostate and epididymis**-produces pain.

   Inflammation of the mucosa of bladder or urethra- produces discomfort, but not severe pain.

   Pain associated with GU malignancies- late manifestation.

3. Renal pain may be confused with **pain resulting from irritation of the costal nerves,** most commonly T_{10}–T_{12}.

4. **Pain in the flaccid penis** is due to inflammation in the bladder or urethra.

5. **Pain in the erect penis** is due to Peyronie's disease or priapism.

6. **Hematuria** >3RBC/HPF is significant.

7. **Initial hematuria**–arises from the urethra.

   Total hematuria–arises from the bladder or upper urinary tracts.

   Terminal hematuria–arises from bladder neck or prostatic urethra.

8. **Painful hematuria**–upper urinary tract hematuria with obstruction of the ureters with clots.

   Painless hematuria–lower urinary tract hematuria (bladder tumour).

9. **Most common cause of gross hematuria** in patients with >50 years–bladder cancer.

10. **Normal adult voids**–six times per day, with a volume of approximately 300 mL with each void.

    Arise no more than twice at night to void.

11. **Frequency during the day without nocturia**–psychogenic origin and related to anxiety.

    Nocturia without frequency–in CHF and geriatric patient.

12. **Postvoid dribbling**–early symptom of BPH and seldom necessitates treatment.

13. Men with BPH **more commonly present with irritative than obstructive symptoms.**

    Most common presenting symptom–nocturia.

14. **The original AUA symptom score** is based on seven questions.

    - Frequency, urgency, nocturia (FUN), weak urinary stream, hesitancy, intermittency and incomplete bladder emptying.

15. **I-PSS includes**–above seven questions + global quality of life question.

16. **Total symptom score–0 to 35.**

    - Score 0 to 7–mild LUTS.
    - Score 8 to 19–moderate LUTS.
    - Score 20 to 35–severe LUTS.

17. **In ectopic ureter male patients**–never produce urinary incontinence because ureter enters the bladder neck or prostatic urethra proximal to the external urethral sphincter.

18. **Continuos urinary incontinence**–vesicovaginal fistula secondary to surgery, radiation, or obstetric trauma.

    Patient that void most of their urine normally but have a continuous amount of small urinary leakage–ectopic ureter that enters either the urethra or the female genital tract.

19. **Stress urinary incontinence (SUI)** - treated surgically.

    Urge urinary incontinence (UUI)- treated with pharmacologic agents.

20. **Overflow incontinence** (paradoxical incontinence)–can be cured by relief of BOO.

21. **Enuresis-**

    - Urinary incontinence that occurs during sleep.
    - It occurs normally in children up to 3 years of age.
    - Persists in about 15% of children at age 5.
    - Persist in 1% of children at age 15.

22. **All children >6 years with enuresis**–should undergo a urologic evaluation.

23. **If semen volume is normal**–unlikely that endocrine factors are responsible for loss of libido.

24. **Impotence**- inability to achieve and maintain an erection sufficient for intercourse.

25. Causes of an ejaculation-

- Androgen deficiency
- Sympathetic denervation (RPLND)
- Pharmacologic agents (α adrenergic antagonists)
- Bladder neck and prostatic surgery (TURP)

26. Hematospermia

- Results from nonspecific inflammation of the prostate and/or seminal vesicles.
- Resolves spontaneously, within several weeks.
- Can occurs after a prolonged period of sexual abstinence,
- Investigation
  - o Genital examination and DRE (to exclude the presence of tuberculosis).
  - o PSA (to exclude prostatic carcinoma).
  - o Urinary cytology (to exclude TCC of the prostate).

27. Urethral discharge-

- Purulent discharge that is thick, profuse, and yellow to gray- **gonococcal urethritis.**
- Scant and watery discharge- **nonspecific urethritis.**
- Bloody discharge- **carcinoma of the urethra.**

28. **In males <4 years old**–normal for the foreskin to be unretractable and early forceful retraction of foreskin is not recommended.

29. **A firm or hard area within the testis**–considered malignant until proved otherwise.

30. **Most masses arising from the testis**–malignant.

    Most masses arising from the spermatic cord structures–benign.

31. **Age is the most useful criterion**–distinguishing torsion from epididymitis.

    Torsion usually occurs around puberty whereas **epididymitis** occur at > 20 years.

32. Testicular tumors presenting as hydrocele–10%.

33. Suspicion of retroperitoneal neoplasm

- Sudden onset of a varicocele.
- Right-sided varicocele.
- Varicocele that does not reduce in size in the supine position.

34. Men with early prostate cancer–30% will have a normal serum PSA test.

35. BCR–tested by:

- Placing a finger in the rectum and then squeezing the glans penis or clitoris.
- Gently pulling on the Foley catheter.

The BCR tests the integrity of the spinal cord mediated reflex arc involving S2-S4.

36. To evaluate for infection

- In female, a catheterized urine sample should be obtained.
- In male, a midstream urine sample should be obtained.

37. All urine samples should be examined within 1 hour of collection.

Specimen of choice- first morning sample.

Urine samples should be refrigerated at 5°C.

Urine should be cultured within 24 hours of refrigeration.

38. Abnormal colour of urine

Red	Hematuria, hemoglobinuria, phenothiazines and rifampicin
Orange	Dehydration, pyridium
Green blue	Methylene blue, biliverdin
Brown	Urobilinogen, porphyria, nitrofurantoin, metronidazole
Brown-black	Alcaptonuria, melanin, tyrosinosis

39. Cloudy urine most commonly due to–phosphaturia.

40. Specific gravity of urine varies from 1.001 to 1.035.

Specific gravity of 1.010 is a sign of renal insufficiency.

41. Conditions that decrease specific gravity include

(1) increased fluid intake
(2) diuretics
(3) decreased renal concentrating ability
(4) diabetes insipidus.

Conditions that increase specific gravity include

(1) decreased fluid intake
(2) dehydration owing to fever, sweating, vomiting, and diarrhea;
(3) diabetes mellitus (glucosuria)
(4) inappropriate secretion of antidiuretic hormone.
(5) after intravenous injection of iodinated contrast and in patients taking dextran.

42. False-positive result-

Examining urine of high specific gravity such as the first morning voided specimen.

Dehydation and exercise, can increase the number of erythrocytes in the urine.

False negative results-

Glucose and bilirubin seen in the presence of elevated ascorbic acid concentrations in the urine.

43. Osmolality varies from–50 and 1200 mOsm/L.

44. Average urine pH varies from –5.5 and 6.5.

45. In general, the urinary pH reflects the pH in the serum.

In patients with metabolic or respiratory acidosis, the urine is usually acidic.

In patients with metabolic or respiratory alkalosis, the urine is alkaline.

Renal tubular acidosis (RTA) presents an exception to this rule.

Diagnostic of RTA.- inability to acidify the urine below a pH of 5.5 after administration of an acid load.

46. The chemical detection of blood in the urine is based on - peroxidise like activity of hemoglobin.

47. Hematuria can be distinguished from hemoglobinuria and myoglobinuria by microscopic examination of the centrifuged urine.

Presence of a large number of RBC establishes the diagnosis of hematuria.

If RBC are absent, examination of the serum will distinguish hemoglobinuria and myoglobinuria.

Hemoglobinuria, the supernatant will be pink.

Myoglobinuria, the serum remains clear.

48. **Dipstick v/s microscopy**

The sensitivity of urinary dipsticks in identifying hematuria, compared with microscopy, is higher than 90%.

Conversely, the specificity of the dipstick for hematuria compared with microscopy is lower.

49. **Erythrocytes arising from tubulointerstitial (TIN) renal disease-** "ghost cells".

50. **Most common cause of glomerular hematuria**–IgA nephropathy (berger's disease).

Renal biopsy reveals mesangial deposits IgA, IgG, and globulin.

51. **Hematuria**

- **Glomerular hematuria**- dysmorphic erythrocytes, RBC casts and proteinuria.
- **Nonglomerular medical hematuria**–circular erythrocytes, absence of RBC casts and significant proteinuria.
- **Nonglomerular surgical hematuria**–circular erythrocytes, absence of RBC casts and absence of significant proteinuria.

52. **(AUA) Best Practice Policy Panel on Microscopic hematuria** includes:

- Voided urinary cytology.
- Cystoscopy.
- Urinary tract imaging (USG, CT and/or IVU).

53. **Normally adults excrete**- 80 to 150 mg of protein in the urine daily.

The urine protein concentration- seldom exceeds 20 mg/dL.

Normally, urine proteins is about 30% albumin, 30% serum globulins, and 40% tissue proteins, of which the major component is Tamm- Horsfall protein.

54. Proteinuria

- **Glomerular proteinuria**–(most common type of proteinuria) results from increased glomerular capillary permeability to protein, especially albumin.
- **Tubular proteinuria** results from failure to reabsorb normally filtered proteins of LMW such as immunoglobulins.
- **Overflow proteinuria** results from increased plasma concentration of abnormal immunoglobulins and other LMW.

55. Transient proteinuria–results from fever, exercise, emotional stress or CHF.

56. Protein electrophoresis–helpful in distinguishing glomerular from tubular proteinuria.

Immunoassay–for detecting specific proteins such as Bence Jones protein in multiple myeloma.

57. Renal threshold for glucose–< 180 mg/dL; above this level will be detected in urine.

58. Glucose detection with the urinary dipstick is based on a **double oxidative reaction**.

It is specific for glucose, and there is no cross-reactivity with other sugars.

59. **Conjugated bilirubin** does not appear in the urine except in pathologic conditions.

Unconjugated bilirubin does not appear in the urine even in pathologic conditions.

60. Leukocyte esterase activity indicates–presence of WBC in urine.

Nitrites indicates–presence of bacteriuria.

- These tests are used to screen patients for UTIs.
- Leukocyte esterase is produced by neutrophils.
- Major cause of false-positive of these tests is specimen contamination.
- Nitrites are not normally found in the urine.

61. Normal leukocytes/HPF

- In men 1-2
- In women- 5

62. **Glitter cell-** In fresh leukocytes cytoplasm, granules demonstrate glitter-like movement.

63. **Renal tubular cells**–least commonly observed epithelial cells in the urine.

    Most significant (presence in the urine is always indicative of renal pathology).

64. **Casts**

Casts	Significance
Tamm- Horsfall mucoprotein	Basic matrix of all renal casts Originates from tubular epithelial cells.Always present in the urine
Hyaline casts	May not have any pathologic significance.
RBC casts	AGN
WBC casts	AGN, APN ,TIN
Sloughed renal tubular epithelial	Nonspecific renal damage
Granular and waxy casts	Degeneration of cellular elements
Fatty casts	Nephrotic syndrome Lipiduria, Hypothyroidism.

65. **Crystals precipitated in acidic urine**–calcium oxalate, uric acid and cystine.

    Crystals precipitated in an alkaline urine–calcium phosphate and triple-phosphate (struvite).

66. **Five bacteria/HPF reflects colony counts**–100,000/ml.

67. **SI unit of effective dose of radiation exposure is- sievert.**

68. The recommended occupational exposure limit to medical personnel is- **50 mSv per year.**

    ALARA, which stands for- **As Low As Reasonably Achievable.**

69.

Adult effective dose	Examination
USG, MRI	0
CXR	< 0.1 msv
Pelvic radiographs	0.1-1.0 msv
Bone scan	1-10 msv
Abdominal CT, PET scan	10-30 msv

70. **LOCM**–do not ionize in solution, the relative osmotic load is half that of HOCM.

71. **Contrast medium**

Iso osmolar	Nonionic	Dimer	Iodixanol
	Nonionic	Dimer	Iotrolan
Low osmolar	Ionic	Dimer	Meglumine ioxaglate
	Non-ionic	Monomer	Iopamidol
	Non-ionic	Monomer	Iohexol
	Non-ionic	Monomer	Ioversol
	Nonionic	Monomer	Iopromide
High osmolar	Ionic	Monomer	Meglumine diatrizoate

72. **Factors predisposing patient to contrast reaction**

• Infants and >60 years
• Females > males
• Asthma, heart disease, dehydration, renal disease, diabetes
• Myelomas, sickle cell disease, polycythemia
• NSAIDs, IL-2, β-blockers, biguanides
• >20 mg iodine, faster injection rate, intra arterial, previous contrast reactions

73. **Adverse drug reactions associated with intravenous contrast media is divided into two broad categories:**

Idiosyncratic anaphylactoid (IA)

- Potentially fatal and can occur without predisposing factors.
- Not from a true IgE antibody immunologic reaction to the contrast media.
- IA reactions are not dose dependent.

Non idiosyncratic (NI) reactions

- Dose dependent and related to the osmolality, concentration, volume, and injection rate.
- Patients with iodine deficiency are at risk for increased intake of iodine during contrast imaging.

74. **Management of severe life threatening reaction to intravascular radiologic contrast medium (IRCM).**

- Rapid administration of epinephrine is the treatment of choice.
- Immediate delivery of 0.5 mg of 1 : 1000 concentration of epinephrine, injected IM in the lateral thigh.

75. **Contrast-induced nephropathy (CIN)**

- Rise in serum creatinine > 25%, or >0.5 mg/dL within 3 days following exposure to contrast.
- Impair renal function for 3 to 5 days.
- Due to be a combination of tubular injury and renal ischemia.
- Highest risk for developing CIN-are in diabetes and preexisting renal insufficiency.
- Cut off value for performing contrast studies in patients with no risk factors- 1.78 mg/dl. Threshold values are lower in diabetics (mean 1.68 mg/dL).

76. **Nephrogenic systemic fibrosis (NSF)**

- Onset varies from 2 days to 3 months.
- Due to gadolinium contrast.
- Present with pruritus.
- Patients with GFR <30 are at significant risk of NSF.

77. **Prone images**–useful in distending and imaging the ureter.

    Upright images–useful in renal ptosis or layering of contrast media in severely HDN systems.

    Postvoid images–useful in evaluating BOO, diverticula or filling defects within the bladder.

78. **To differentiate ureteric stone from phleboliths.** Phleboliths are:

- Steered to either side of the pelvis and arranged in the distribution of pelvic veins.

- Round and fairly opaque.
- Commonly measure 2 to 6 mm in diameter.

79. **For RGP commonly employed ureteral catheter**- bulb-tip, cone-tip, or wedge tip catheter.

80. **MCU**–to evaluate posterior urethra.

    For evaluating reflux, urethral valves, ureterocele and dysfunctional voiding patterns.

81. **RUG**–to evaluate anterior and posterior urethra.

    For evaluating urethral stricture and urethral trauma.

82. **Transducers of 6 to 10 MHz**- used to image structures near the surface of the body (e.g., testis, pediatric kidney) with excellent resolution.

    Transducers of 3.5 to 5 MHz- used to image deeper structures of the body (e.g .right kidney, bladder) with poorer resolution.

83. **Power Doppler ultrasonography**
    - Provides the amplitude of frequency change to a color map.
    - Does not permit evaluation of velocity or direction of flow.
    - More sensitive mode than color Doppler for detecting blood flow.

84. **For description of ultrasound images**

    The liver is used as a benchmark for echogenicity :
    - Hypoechoic = darker and black
    - Hyperechoic = brighter and white (AML)
    - Anechoic = black, without echoes

85. **Renal parenchyma**- measured from the central band of echoes to the renal capsule (should be >15mm).

    Renal cortex -measured from the outer margin of medullary pyramid to the renal capsule (should be >7 mm).

86. **Koff formula**–evaluation of bladder volume in mL is (age [years] + 2) × 30.

87. **Renal medullary pyramids**–less echogenic than the cortex.

    Adrenal medulla more echogenic than adrenal cortex.

88. **The normal bladder wall**–≤ 6 mm thick.

89. ^{99m}**Tc–MAG3**–cleared by tubular secretion and no glomerular filtration occurs.

^{99m}**Tc–DTPA**–cleared by glomerular filtration.

^{99m}**Tc–DMSA**–cleared by both filtration and secretion.

90. Radionuclide imaging

Free from allergic reactions.

DMSA–useful as a renal cortical imaging agent to evaluate for cortical scars or pyelonephritis.

DTPA–useful for evaluation of obstruction and renal function.

MAG–useful for evaluation of renal function and diuretic scintigraphy.

- Excellent tracer to evaluate renal plasma flow.
- Agent of choice in patients with renal insufficiency and urinary obstruction.

91. PET has better diagnostic accuracy than CT–for staging and restaging in the assessment of a residual mass following chemotherapy for seminoma.

92. Multi detectors CT offers the advantages

- Faster scanning
- Fewer motion artifacts
- Thinner imaging sections
- Precise diagnostic accuracy
- Increased concentration of contrast material
- Shorter scanning time
- Significant increase in anatomic coverage with a single scan

93. The HU scale or attenuation value

- **Air is −1000 HU**
- **Dense bone is +1000 HU.**
- **Water is 0 HU.**

94. Unenhanced CT is imaging modality of choice for evaluation of urolithiasis.

95. **Diagnostic for solid enhancing mass, (renal cancer)** - an increase in HU by 15 to 20.

    Diagnostic for angiomyolipoma -the presence of fat, which enhance< 10 HU.

96. **Phases of CT scan**

    At 0 second- unenhanced scan.

    At 30 to 70 seconds- corticomedullary phase.

    At 85 to 120 seconds- nephrogenic phase.

    At 3 to 5 minutes- excretory phase.

97. **If the density of an adrenal mass is <0 HU** on unenhanced CT–adenoma.

98. **Investigation of choice for evaluation of pheochromocytoma is**–MRI.

99. **CT angiography**–oral administration of contrast agent is usually avoided.

100. **On T1weighted images**–fluid is dark and fat is bright.

     On T2weighted images–fluid is bright and fat is dark.

101. **Investigation of choice in determining the extent of tumor thrombus in the IVC**–MRI.

102. Using MRI artifact referred to as **chemical shift,** MRI can define benign lipid-containing adenomas.

103. **Consistent with renal cancer-** on MRI if the lesion is brighter on the postcontrast image and increases in signal intensity by >15%, it is declared enhancing.

104. **Erectile Dysfunction scales**

     - International Index of Erectile Function (IIEF)
     - Self-Esteem and Relationship Questionnaire (SEAR)
     - Male Sexual Health Questionnaire (MSHQ)
     - Brief Sexual Function Inventory (BSFI)
     - Erectile Dysfunction Inventory of Treatment Satisfaction Questionnaire (EDITS)
     - Erection Distress Scale (EDS)

105. Karnofsky Performance Status Scale Definitions Rating (%) Criteria

- 100%–normal, no complaints, no signs of disease.
- 90%–capable of normal activity, few symptoms or signs of disease.
- 80%–normal activity with some difficulty, some symptoms or signs.
- 70%–caring for self, not capable of normal activity or work.
- 60%–requiring some help, can take care of most personal requirements.
- 50%–requires help often, requires frequent medical care.
- 40%–disabled, requires special care and help.
- 30%–severely disabled, hospital admission indicated but no risk of death.
- 20%–very ill, urgently requiring admission, requires treatment.
- 10%–moribund, rapidly progressive fatal disease processes.
- 0%–death.

106. Lansky scoring system for children

- 100 fully active, normal.
- 90 minor restrictions in strenuous physical activity.
- 80 active, but gets tired more quickly.
- 70 greater restriction of play and less time spent in play activity.
- 60 up and around, but active play minimal; keeps busy by being involved in quieter activities.
- 50 lying around much of the day, but gets dressed; no active playing participates in all quiet play and activities.
- 40 mainly in bed; participates in quiet activities.
- 30 bedbound; needing assistance even for quiet play.
- 20 sleeping often; play entirely limited to very passive activities.
- 10 doesn't play; does not get out of bed.
- 0 unresponsive.

107.

ECOG PERFORMANCE STATUS	
Grade	**ECOG**
0	Fully active, able to carry on all pre-disease performance without restriction
1	Restricted in physically strenuous activity but ambulatory and able to carry out work of a light or sedentary nature, e.g., light house work, office work
2	Ambulatory and capable of all selfcare but unable to carry out any work activities. Up and about more than 50% of waking hours
3	Capable of only limited selfcare, confined to bed or chair more than 50% of waking hours
4	Completely disabled. Cannot carry on any selfcare. Totally confined to bed or chair
5	Dead

108. A translation between the Zubrod and Karnofsky scales that works especially well for healthy patients has been validated as

- Zubrod 0-1 equals Karnofsky 80-100
- Zubrod 2 equals Karnofsky 60-70
- Zubrod 3-4 equals Karnofsky 10-50.

❑❑

Chapter 3
BASICS OF UROLOGIC SURGERY

1. **American society of anesthesiologists**

ASA Class 1	Normal healthy patient
ASA Class II	Patient with mild systemic disease
ASA Class III	Patient with severe systemic disease that limits activity but is not incapacitating
ASA Class IV	Patients who have incapacitating disease that is a constant threat to life
ASA Class V	Moribund patient not expected to survive 24 hours with or without an operation
ASA Class VI	A declared brain-dead patient whose organs are being removed for donor purposes

ASA Class E–Emergent nature of surgery

2. **The Child classification assesses perioperative morbidity and mortality and is based on**
    - bilirubin,
    - albumin,
    - prothrombin time
    - encephalopathy
    - ascites
3. **Noninsulin diabetics patients**
    - Discontinue long-acting hypoglycemics before surgery because of risk of intraoperative hypoglycemia.
    - Shorter-acting agents or sliding scale insulin regimens are generally preferable.
4. **Safest time to perform surgery in pregnancy**–second trimester because organ system differentiation has occurred and there is

almost no risk for anesthetic-induced malformation or spontaneous abortion.

5. **Surgical wound classification**

Clean	Uninfected wound without inflammation or entry into the genital, urinary, or alimentary tract
	Primary wound closure closed drainage
Clean contaminated	Uninfected wound with controlled entry into the genital, urinary, or alimentary tract
	Primary wound closure closed drainage
Contaminated	Uninfected wound with major break in sterile technique (gross spillage from gastrointestinal tract or nonpurulent inflammation)
	Open fresh accidental wounds
Dirty infected	Wound with preexisting clinical infection or perforated viscera
	Old traumatic wounds with devitalized Tissue

6. **Administration of antibiotics**

- Antibiotics is given within 30 minutes of incision
- The duration of antibiotic prophylaxis should not be more than 24 hours in a patient without an established infection.
- There is level 1 evidence for the use of fluoroquinolones as prophylaxis for urologic endoscopic procedures

7. **Mechanical bowel preparation**

By polyethylene glycol solution (GoLytely) and sodium phosphate solution (Fleet's Phospho-soda) **Both regimens are suitable for most patients; however, polyethylene glycol is preferred in**

- Elderly
- Patients with renal insufficiency
- Congestive heart failure
- Electrolyte disturbances
- Cirrhosis

8. **Prophylactic antibiotics is not indicated in all the cases of**
   - Removal of external urethral catheter
   - Cystography
   - Urodynamic study
   - Simple cystoscopy
   - Open/lap without entering GU tract
9. **Anticoagulant therapy**
   - Cessation of warfarin 5 days before surgery to ensure an INR less than 1.5
   - Aspirin and clopidogrel need to be stopped 7 to 10 days before surgery
   - In cases in which surgery cannot be delayed, aspirin and clopidogrel can be given during the perioperative period
10. **Nitrous oxide (NO)**
    - Most commonly used agents due to its propensity of rapid induction and emergence
    - Low potency.
    - Use contraindicated in small bowel obstruction and pneumothorax.
11. **Halothane**
    - Significant cardiac effects and can precipitate failure in patients with left ventricular dysfunction.
    - It sensitizes the myocardium to the effects of catecholamines.
    - Incidence of fulminant hepatitis
12. **Isoflurane**
    - Less expensive
    - Low risk for cardiac depression, less myocardial sensitization to catecholamines, and minimal metabolism.
    - Unique toxicity is variable response tachycardia.

Sevoflurane

- Rapid induction and emergence
- Decreased incidence of postoperative nausea (important in outpatient surgery)

- Minimal cardiac toxicity.
- Preferred agent for difficult airways requiring mask induction and in patients with severe bronchospastic disease.

13. Ketamine

- It is a preferred choice for procedures that are brief and superficial because of its profound amnesia and somatic analgesia.
- It is advantageous during induction for hypovolemic and asthmatic patients

14. Propofol

- Most commonly used anesthetic agents, especially in outpatient surgery.
- It has a rapid onset, produces excellent bronchodilation in patients with reactive airway disease, and, is associated with smooth, nausea-free emergence from anesthesia.
- Primary adverse effect is significant blood pressure reduction

15. Midazolam,

- Never used as a single agent
- Produces profound amnesia and anxiolysis
- Have rapid onset/short duration and produces minimal cardiac side effects.

16. Fentanyl

- Synthetic opioid
- Widely used because of its potency (100 to 150 times that of morphine)
- Rapid onset, and short duration of action.

17. Succinylcholine

- Rapid onset
- Short duration (5 minutes), and rapid metabolism.
- Its use is limited due to the risk of malignant hyperthermia, hyperkalemia, and bradycardia in children

18. Whereas the hematocrit in whole blood is 40%, it is 70% in PRBC units

19. Platelet transfusion is rarely indicated empirically except in patients with

Sgnificant thrombocytopenia (<50,000/mm3) and planned surgical procedure

Moderate thrombocytopenia (50,000-100,000/ mm3) and either high-risk procedure or evidence of platelet dysfunction.

20. The current indications for FFP transfusion are

- Immediate reversal of warfarin-induced coagulopathy
- Replacement in patients with specific clotting factor deficiencies
- Bleeding and INR > 1.5
- Patients with massive transfusion and no INR readily available, FFP should be given after replacement of 1 blood volume.

21. Risk of HIV and hepatitis C transmission is 1 in 20,00,000 cases

Risk of hepatitis B is 1 in 2,00,000

22. Wound healing can be divided broadly into three stages :

- **The reactive phase-** occurs immediately with the two primary responses of hemostasis and inflammation
- **The proliferative phase-** results in the formation of granulation tissue
- **Maturation stage-** occurs with further deposition of collagen and wound contraction.

23. The scar regains strength

- 3% after 1 week,
- 20% after 3 weeks
- 80% after 3 months

24. Blood product transfusion should be advocated for **hematocrit < 21%** in most patients unless there are specific cardiopulmonary risk factors.

25. Sutures and there properties

Suture	**Absorption**	**Tensile strength**	**Configuration**
Vicryl	Absorbable	65% at 2 weeks 40% at 4 weeks	Braided
Monocryl	Absorbable	30% at 2 weeks	Monofilament
PDS	Absorbable	75% at 2 weeks 50% at 4 weeks 25% at 6 weeks	Monofilament

Chromic gut	Absorbable	0% at 3 weeks	Monofilament
Nylon	Non absorbable	50% at 1-2 years	Monofilament
Silk	Non absorbable	No significant loss over time	Braided
Prolene	Non absorbable	Degrades over time	Monofilament

26. **Closure with continuous, slowly absorbing suture**- results in the lowest risk of incision-related complication

28. **1Fr=0.33 mm** in diameter.

29. **Catheter sizes refer to** outside circumference of the catheter.

30. **Silicone catheters**

- For patients requiring a longer period of indwelling time.
- Relatively inert, causing less tissue reaction, and is associated with less bacterial adherence
- Lower incidence of urinary tract infections compared with those made of latex

31. **Coudé tip** - patients with a high bladder neck or prominent median prostate lobe,

    Councill catheter- when catheterization over a guidewire is required

32. **Urethral catheters**

    Catheter with no self retaining mechanism- Robinson, Nelaton and Jaques

    Catheter with self retaining mechanism-Foley, Madduri, Malecot and Pezzer

    Curved catheters- Coude

    End hole catheters- Councill and whistle

33. **The cone tip catheter**–designed to occlude the ureteral orifice, thus filling the ureter and renal collecting system at the same time

34. **An inability to deflate a Foley balloon can be managed by**

- Place another 1 to 2 mL of fluid in the balloon to ensure normal balloon contour
- Cut the inflation port.
- Insert a stiff end of a 0.035-inch hydrophilic-coated guidewire through the valve inflation lumen

- USG-guided needle puncture can be conducted using either a transrectal, transvaginal, or suprapubic probe

Maneuver to be avoided

- Overinflation of the balloon
- Use of chemical instillations such as ether or toluene

35. **Double J and pigtail stents** invented by Finney, Hepperlen and colleagues

    Fernström and Johansson established a percutaneous tract for the removal of kidney calculi

36. First plastic polymer used in stent- **polyethylene**

    Most biocompatible material tested to date **silicone**

    Shares characteristics common to both silicon and polyethylene, making a good overall stent material- **polyurethane**

37. **Percutaneous lithotripsy techniques do not require routine stenting.** Exceptions to this include

    - Extensive perforation of the collecting system,
    - Significant stone burden remains with the need for subsequent shock wave lithotripsy (SWL)
    - Ureteral obstruction due to edema
    - Concurrent ureteropelvic obstruction
    - Stone fragment migration into the ureter
    - Supracostal access
    - Persistent urinary fistula after nephrostomy tube removal.

    Indications for pre-SWL stenting are

    Stone burden > 2 cm

38. **Stent morbidity can be significant.**

    - LUTS such as frequency, urgency, dysuria, and pain (flank or suprapubic) occur in almost 100%
    - More than 80% of patients experience stent-related pain affecting daily activities

39. **The duration of stent insertion is a significant risk factor for**

    6.8% develop UTI and 20.5% developing stent colonization at 30 days

    28.6% develop UTI and 64.9% stent colonization after 90 days.

Predisposing factors include chronic renal failure, diabetes, and female gender

40. Rigid endoscope VS flexible endoscope

Rigid endoscope	Flexible endoscope
Improved image quality	Improved patient comfort
Larger working channel	Increased options for patient positioning
Better visualization	Ease in passage over an elevated bladder neck or median lobe
Easier to manipulate and orient during endoscopy	Ability to deflect the endoscope tip in any direction, permitting full inspection of the bladder
Easier to stabilize with one hand	

41. **A 0 degree lens**–for urethroscopy.

    A 30 degree lens–for visualization of the base and anterolateral aspect of the bladder.

    A 70 to 90 degree lens–for viewing the bladder dome.

    A 120 degree lens–for visualization of anterior bladder neck.

42. **Semirigid ureteroscopy** is used for diagnosis and treatment of pathologic processes below the iliac vessels.

    Flexible ureteroscopy is used for the diagnosis and treatment of pathologic processes above the level of the iliac vessels.

43. **Guidewire diameters and lengths** range from 0.018 to 0.038 inch and 145 to 280 cm, respectively

44. **Balloon dilators** exert radial force and can exert pressures up to 20 atm

45. **Ureteral access sheaths**

    - Reduce renal pressures during ureteroscopy
    - Function as an open conduit into to the kidney, allowing fluid to enter through the endoscope and exit through the sheath
    - Shorter operative times
    - Reduced cost

- Provides direct visualization of ureteroscope insertion and simple reentry
- Decrease endoscope damage
- Incidence of stricture after ureteroscopy same as that with ureteroscopy alone

46. Stone migration devices

- Stone cone
- NTrap
- Accordion
- Urojel

47. Surgeons who are noble prize winners

- Emil Theodore Kocher
- Allvar Gullstrand
- Alexis Carrel
- Robert Bárány
- Frederick Banting
- Alexander Fleming
- Walter Hess
- Werner Forssmann (urologist)
- Charles B. Huggins (urologist)
- Joseph Murray (urologist)

48. Consent

It is essential that the consent is taken regarding inherent risk with all minimally invasive procedures such that the procedure may need to be converted to open surgery owing to hemorrhage, bowel injury, failure to progress

49. Contraindications to laparoscopic surgery include

- Uncorrectable coagulopathy
- Intestinal obstruction
- Significant abdominal wall infection
- Massive hemoperitoneum
- Generalized peritonitis
- Malignant ascites

50. In the lateral position, the bottom leg is flexed approximately 45 degrees while the upper leg is kept straight; to prevent undue stretch on the **sciatic nerve.**

51. Hand assisted devices-

- The first generation of hand port devices–Handport, Intromit, and Pneumosleeve
- Second generation of devices–Gelport. Omniport, and the LapDisc

52. William osler- "father of modern medicine,"

Hopkins–introduced large, rod-shaped quartz lenses to transmit light.

Veress–introduced a needle for closed insufflation of the abdomen.

Semm–"father" of modern-day laparoscopy.

Clayman–performed the first clinical laparoscopic nephrectomy.

53. Hemostatic and tissue sealants

Agent	Ingredient	Properties	Time to set up
Fibrin based-Tisseel	Fibrinogen, CaCl, thrombin, aprotinin	Topical hemostatic Tissue glue	20 minutes
- Cross seal	Fibrinogen, CaCl, thrombin, aprotinin	Topical hemostatic Tissue glue	Immediately
Nonfibrin based-Floseal	Gelatin granules Thrombin	Topical hemostatic	2 minutes
Chemical based sealants- Bioglue	Albumin + glutaraldehyde	Tissue sealant	Immediately
Coseal	Polyethylene glycol polymers	Tissue sealant	Immediately

54. Pneumoperitoneum

- **Most common gas used as insufflant**–CO_2.
- **In severe COPD**–helium as an alternative insufflant.
- **Room air, O_2, NO**–not used (risk of air embolus and intra abdominal explosion).
- **Xe, Ar, Kr**–not used (high cost and poor solubility in blood).

55. Insufflation

Overall, the most commonly selected pressure for performing laparoscopy is 15 mm Hg

Beginning–pressure set at 15 mmHg with rate of gas flow of 1 liter/min.

Once safe entry achieved–pressure can be raised to 20-25 mm Hg and flow rate by veress needle can be increased to maximum of 2 liter/min.

56. **With increasing pneumoperitoneum pressure**

Parameter which increases is-

Mean arterial pressure, end tidal CO_2, Pco_2

Parameter which decreases is-

Heart rate, venous return, cardiac output, GFR, urine output and arterial pH

57. **Hormones noted to increase** during laparoscopic surgery as a response to tissue manipulation, intraoperative trauma, and postoperative pain- (e.g., β-endorphin, cortisol, prolactin, epinephrine, norepinephrine, dopamine)

58. **Balloon dilation** in posterior pararenal space facilitates creation of working space for retroperitoneoscopy.

59. **Color coding of staple load cartridge :**

2.0-mm staples (gray)

2.5-mm staples (white) are preferred for vascular (renal vein or renal artery) stapling,

3.8-mm (blue)

4.8-mm (green) staples are used in thicker tissues (ureter, bowel, bladder).

60. **The first sign of intravascular insufflation** is acute cardiovascular collapse (Hypotension and associated tachycardia).

The diagnosis is usually made by the anaesthesiologist based on an abrupt increase of end-tidal CO2 accompanied by a sudden decline in oxygen saturation and then a marked decrease in end-tidal CO2

61. **Bowel injury**

In the case of a one-wall injury of the bowel

- Leave the trocar in place and pass a second trocar in another location using an open access technique. At this time, the surgeon may elect to open and repair the bowel or, if skilled in laparoscopy, may close the bowel using laparoscopic suturing or stapling techniques.

When the injury to the bowel is a through-and-through

- Safest path is to open and proceed with repair

62. **If blood is coming through the trocar,** then the trocar should be closed and left in place. An emergency laparotomy is performed, and the trocar is followed to its point of entry into the vessel
63. **Occurrence of inadvertent peritoneotomy during retroperitoneoscopy** does not interfere with subsequent steps of procedure and conversion to transperitoneal laparoscopic technique is not mandatory.
64. **The first commercially available robotic system**–RoboDoc.

    The first commercial robotic system used specifically for **laparoscopic applications** was the Automated Endoscopic System for Optimal Positioning (AESOP).
65. **Electrosurgically induced thermal injury** may occur because of one of four mechanisms:
    - Inappropriate direct activation
    - Coupling to another instrument
    - Capacitive coupling
    - Insulation failure
66. **Minor postoperative thermal injuries of the bowel,**
    - If discovered >5 to 7 days postoperatively ,can be managed conservatively, aided by administration of antibiotics and an elemental diet.
        - o A closed fistula may develop that will heal with this approach.
        - o If the patient does not respond rapidly or develops peritonitis, open surgical exploration is mandatory
67. **Lymphocele**
    - Most commonly associated with pelvic lymph node dissection or with renal transplantation.
    - May take weeks to develop and may occur despite a transperitoneal approach.
    - Presentation may be by a mass effect, which can lead to local compression causing lower extremity edema, and in rare cases, venous thrombosis and pulmonary embolism.

- Diagnosed by CT.
- Treatment is immediate percutaneous drainage.
- Sclerosant therapy can be used to treat the lymphocele
- If both the above are unsuccessful, then a transperitoneal laparoscopic marsupialization procedure is usually successful

68. **In retroperitoneoscopy** (In compansion to transperitoneal approach)
    - The risks of inadvertent bowel injury and postoperative ileus are minimized.
    - More rapid postoperative recovery.
    - Rapid and direct access to the renal hilum
    - If a partial nephrectomy is planned, it may be more effective to approach a posterior tumor from the retroperitoneal approach

❑❑

Chapter 4
INFECTION AND INFLAMMATION

1. **Bacteriuria without pyuria**–indicative of bacterial colonization.

   Pyuria without bacteriuria–indicative of tuberculosis, stones or cancer.

2. **Acute pyelonephritis**–syndrome of chills, fever, and flank pain that is accompanied by bacteriuria and pyuria

   Chronic pyelonephritis- shrunken, scarred kidney, diagnosed by morphologic, radiologic, or functional evidence of renal disease

3. **Pyelonephritic atrophy caused by UTI-** produces irregular cortical scarring. All the calyces extend to the capsule with irregular, intervening areas of cortex.

   Pyelonephritic atrophy caused by obstruction- uniform, regular atrophy of the renal cortex that suggests reflux of bacteria simultaneously into virtually all nephrons.

4. **Uncomplicated infection**

   - Infection in a healthy patient with a structurally and functionally normal urinary tract.
   - The majority of these patients are women

   Complicated infection

   - Associated with factors that increase the chance of acquiring bacteria and decrease the efficacy of therapy.
   - Urinary tract is structurally or functionally abnormal, the host is compromised, and the bacteria have increased virulence or antimicrobial resistance.
   - The majority of these patients are men.

5. **Nomenclature**

   - **First or isolated infection**–occurs in an individual who has never had a UTI
   - **Unresolved infection**–infection that has not responded to antimicrobial therapy.

- **Recurrent infection** is one that occurs after documented, successful resolution of an antecedent infection.
  - o **Reinfection-** new event associated with reintroduction of bacteria into the urinary tract from outside.
  - o **Bacterial persistence-** recurrent UTI caused by the same bacteria reemerging from a focus within the urinary tract.

6. **Risk of recurrent bacteriuria remains the same-** whether a patient receives no treatment at all or short-term, long-term, or prophylactic antimicrobial treatment.

   Prophylactic antimicrobial therapy reduces reinfections but does not alter the underlying predisposition to recurring infection

7. **There is no association** between recurrent infections and renal scarring, hypertension, or progressive renal azotemia.

8. **Most episodes of pyelonephritis are caused by** -retrograde ascent of bacteria from the bladder through the ureter to the renal pelvis and parenchyma.

   Reflux of urine is not required for ascending infections

9. **The prevalence of bacteriuria**
   - <1 year–male > female.
   - Young women–30 times more common than in men.
   - > 65 years women–2 times more common than in men.

10. **Most reinfections occurred after 2 weeks**

11. Kidney is occasionally secondarily infected by **hematogenous route** in patients with Staphylococcus aureus bacteremia or with Candida fungemia

12. **Most UTIs are caused by facultative anaerobes originating from the bowel flora.**

    E. coli- accounts for 85% of community-acquired and 50% of hospital-acquired infections

    S. saprophyticus causes 10% of symptomatic lower UTIs in young, sexually active female.

13. **Types of pilli**

	Type 1 pilli	**P pilli**
Expressed on	Nonpathogenic and pathogenic E. coli	Pyelonephritogenic strains of UPEC

Hemagglutination of	Guinea pig	Human erythrocytes
Mannose	Sensitive (MSHA)	Resistant (MRHA)

14. **Phase variation**
    - **Can occur in both in vivo and in vitro.**
    - **Type 1 pilli may be advantageous** to bacteria for adhering and colonising bladder mucosa.
    - **Can be disadvantageous** as it can enhance phagocytosis.
15. **First demonstrable biologic difference in women susceptible to UTI**-increased adherence of pathogenic bacteria to vaginal epithelial cells
16. **Initial step leading to UTIs-** fimH-mediated binding to the bladder epithelium.

    FimH binds mannosylated residues on the uroplakin molecules covering bladder superficial epithelial cells
17. **Normal flora of periurethral area, and the urethra-** lactobacilli, coagulase-negative staphylococci, corynebacteria, and streptococci
18. **Biofilms**
    - Shield bacteria from environmental challenges such as antimicrobial agents and the host immune response
    - Increase protection include the slower growth rate of the bacteria and the inability of the antimicrobial agent to penetrate the biofilm matrix
    - The biofilm also protects the bacteria from neutrophils because they are unable to effectively penetrate the intracellular bacterial communities and engulf the bacteria.
19. **Most inhibitory factors for UTI-** the osmolality, urea concentration, organic acid concentration, and pH
20. **In adults, the presence of reflux** does not appear to decrease renal function unless there is stasis and concurrent UTIs.
21. **Conditions associated with renal papillary necrosis** are (POSTCARDS):
    - Pyelonephritis, Obstruction of urogenital tract, Sickle cell disease, Tuber Cirrhosis of liver, Analgesic, alchol abuse, Renal transplant rejection, DM and Systemic Vasculitis.
22. **The prevalence of bacteriuria in pregnant women-**4% to 7%

    The prevalence of pyelonephritis in pregnant women-1% to 4%

The prevalence of pyelonephritis in pregnant women with bacteriuria- 20% to 40%

23. **The easiest way to prevent catheter-induced infections is**–single dose of an oral trimethoprim–sulfamethoxazole.

24. **In dysuric patients threshold value for defining significant bacteriuria is**–10^2 cfu/ml.

25. **Most accurate assessment status of bladder urine**–suprapubic aspiration of bladder urine.

26. **Catheterization of a male patient for urine culture is**–not indicated.

    In females catheterization should be performed and a mid catheterized specimen collected.

27. **Efficacy of the antimicrobial therapy dependent on**- antimicrobial levels in the urine and the duration that this level remains above the minimal inhibitory concentration of the infecting organism

28. **Bacterial resistance**
    - Inherited chromosomal-mediated resistance
    - Acquired chromosomal
    - Acquired extrachromosomal (plasmid)

29. **Extra chromosomal-mediated resistance**
    - Called R-factor resistance
    - Occurs in the bowel flora
    - All antimicrobial classes are capable of causing plasmid mediated resistance.
    - For fluoroquinolones resistance is rarely transmitted by plasmids
    - For nitrofurantoin plasmid-mediated resistance has not been reported

30. **TMP-SMX**
    - Effective against common uropathogens
    - Not effective against Enterococcus and Pseudomonas species.
    - Inexpensive
    - Minimal adverse effects on the bowel flora.

31. **Nitrofurantoin**
    - Effective against common uropathogens
    - Not effective against Pseudomonas andProteus species

- It is rapidly excreted from the urine but does not attain therapeutic levels in most body tissues
- Not useful for upper tract and complicated infections
- Minimal effects on the resident bowel and vaginal flora and is effective in prophylactic regimens

32. Cephalosporins

- First generation- active against gram-positive organisms as well as E. coli and Klebsiella pneumoniae
- Second generation- active against anaerobes.
- Third-generation- active against community-acquired and nosocomial gram-negative organisms
- They are safe for use during pregnancy.

33. Aminoglycosides

When combined with TMP-SMX or ampicillin, aminoglycosides are the first drugs of choice for febrile UTIs.

34. Aztreonam

- Not nephrotoxic (no dose reduction in renal failure)
- Spectrum of activity is less broad than the third-generation cephalosporins.
- It should be used primarily in patients who have penicillin allergies.

35. Fluoroquinolones

- Inhibit DNA gyrase, a bacterial enzyme integral to replication.
- Ideal for the empirical treatment of UTIs.
- Effective against Enterobacteriaceae as well as P. aeruginosa.
- Effective against S. aureus and S. saprophyticus, but, antistreptococcal coverage is marginal

36. Antimicrobial prophylaxis is indicated in

All patients undergoing-

- Cystourethroscopy with manipulation
- Transrectal prostate biopsy
- ESWL, PCNL and URSL
- Open or laparoscopic surgery involving genitourinary tract.

38. **In uncomplicated cystitis**

- Three-day therapy in women
- Seven-day therapy in men

39. **Screening and treatment of asymptomatic bacteriuria** is required only in

- Pregnant women
- Patients undergoing urological intervention.

40. **Most common cause of unresolved bacteriuria-** bacterial resistance to the drug selected for treatment

41. **Fluoroquinolones are ideal for self-start therapy**

They have a spectrum of activity broader than any of the other oral agents and are superior to many parenteral antimicrobials.

42. **Treatment of acute pyelonephritis**

- Ambulatory patients- fluoroquinolone for 7 days
- Complicated pyelonephritis and positive blood cultures-parenteral therapy until clinically stable followed by 10-14 days of oral antibiotic therapy
- In patients with fever lasting >72 hours, CT is most helpful for ruling out obstruction and identifying renal and perirenal infections.
- Patients who experience relapse usually are cured by a second 14-day course of therapy

43. **Emphysematous pyelonephritis (EPN)**

- High tissue glucose levels produce CO_2.
- All cases occur in adults.
- Classic triad of fever, vomiting and flank pain.
- E. coli is most commonly identified organism.
- CT is the investigation of choice.

44. **Types of EPN**

- Type 1–streaky or mottled gas with 50% to 60% mortality rate.
- Type 2–bubbly or loculated gas with <20% mortality rate.

45. **Huang classification for EPN**

- **Class 1:** gas in the collecting system only.

- **Class 2**: gas in the renal parenchyma without extension to extrarenal space.
- **Class 3A**: extension of gas or abscess to perinephric space.
- **Class 3B**: extension of gas or abscess to pararenal space.
- **Class 4**: bilateral EPN or solitary kidney with EPN.

Prognostic parameters (4)

- Thrombocytopenia, acute renal function impairment, disturbance of consciousness or shock.
- **For localized EPN** (classes 1 and 2)–Percutaneous drainage (PCD) + antibiotics.
- **In extensive EPN** (classes 3 and 4), with >2 risk factors–higher failure rate on conservative management than those with no or only 1 risk factors (92% vs 15%).

46. **Ring sign**–increased vascularity of the abscess wall.
47. **Management of renal abscesses (carbuncle)**
    - CT is the investigation of choice
    - **<3 cm abscesses**–IV antibiotics.
    - **3 to 5 cm abscesses and smaller abscesses in immuno-compromised hosts those that do not respond to antimicrobial therapy**–percutaneous drainage.
    - **>5 cm abscesses**–surgical drainage.
48. **Pyonephrosis**–infected hydronephrosis + destruction of the parenchyma of the kidney.
49. **Phenomena of renal thyroidisation**–chronic pyelonephritis.
50. **Xanthogranulomatous pyelonephritis (XGPN)**
    - **Unilateral.**
    - Non-functioning, enlarged kidney with obstructive uropathy secondary to **nephrolithiasis.**
    - The kidney is usually massively enlarged but has a **normal contour.**
    - Xanthogranulomatous cells are **not specific** to XGPN.
    - **Proteus**–most common organism involved.
    - CT–investigation of choice.
    - Associated with RCC, papillary TCC of the pelvis or bladder, and

infiltrating squamous cell carcinoma of the pelvis

- The **"bear paw" sign** with areas of low-attenuation nonenhancing dilated calyces and abscesses within areas of high-attenuation enhancing renal parenchyma may be present

51. Malacoplakia (soft plaque)

- Large histiocytes, known as **von Hansemann cells.**
- Basophilic, extracytoplasmic, or intracytoplasmic calculospherules are called **Michaelis-Gutmann bodies.**
- **Michaelis-Gutmann bodies** are pathognomonic but may be absent in early malacoplakia and are not necessary for the diagnosis.
- Immunohistochemical staining for **α1-antitrypsin** may be a useful test
- Most patients are >50 years.
- The F:M ratio in urinary tract is 4:1

52. Echinococcosis

- **Produced** by larval form of the tapeworm.
- **Definitive host**–intestine of dog
- **Principal intermediate host**–sheep.
- Hydatid cyst develops at a rate of 1 cm/yr.
- Albendazole, 400 mg twice daily for 1 to 6 months, is the recommended medical therapy.
- **Surgery–mainstay of treatment.**
- Praziquantel and albendazole have been recommended preoperatively for 7 to 10 days to minimize or prevent secondary seeding by daughter cysts if they accidentally contaminate the operative field

53. Layers of hydatid cyst

- **Adventitial layer**-- a peripheral zone of fibroblasts derived from tissues of the host
- **Intermediate laminated layer**- becomes hyalinised
- **Inner germinal layer**- composed of nucleated epithelium. Gives rise to brood capsules that increase in number, become vacuolated, and remain attached to the germinal membrane by a pedicle.

54. **Earliest metabolic change in septicemia is** - respiratory alkalosis.

55. **The prime initiator of gram negative bacterial septic shock-** endotoxin, an LPS component of the bacterial outer membrane

    TNF is regarded as a **central mediator** of pathophysiologic changes associated with sepsis

56. **SIRS**

    General

    - Temperature extremes (>38° C [100.4° F] or <36° C [96.8° F])
    - Tachycardia (heart rate >90 beats per minute)
    - Tachypnea
    - Altered mental status
    - Significant edema or positive fluid balance (20 mL/kg/24 hr)
    - Hyperglycemia (plasma glucose >120 mg/dL or 7.7 mol/L) in the absence of diabetes

    Inflammatory

    - Leukocytosis (WBC count >12,000/dl)
    - Leukopenia (WBC count <4000/dl)
    - Normal WBC count with >10% immature forms

    Organ Dysfunction

    - Arterial hypoxemia (PaO2/FIO2 >300)
    - Acute oliguria (urine output 0.5 mL/kg in 1 hr for at least 2 hr)
    - Creatinine increase of 0.5 mg/dL
    - Coagulation abnormalities (INR 1.5 or aPTT >60 sec)
    - Ileus (absent bowel sounds)
    - Thrombocytopenia (platelet count <100,000/µL)
    - Hyperbilirubinemia (plasma total bilirubin >4 mg/dL or 70 mmol/L)

    Tissue Perfusion

    - Hyperlactatemia (>1 mmol/L)
    - Decreased capillary refill or mottling

57. **Bedside findings differentiating septic shock from other types of shock include**

    - Warm patient

- Brisk capillary refill
- Bounding pulse reflecting pyrexia
- Peripheral vasodilation
- Decreased systemic vascular resistance

58. Pregnancy

- Renal **length increases**–1 cm.
- The collecting system–**decreased peristalsis.**
- **Hydroureter**–due to the muscle-relaxing effects of increased progesterone and to mechanical obstruction of the ureters.
- Uterus displaces the bladder–**superiorly and anteriorly.**
- **Glomerular filtration increases**–30% to 50%.
- **Serum creatinine** levels >0.8 mg/dL–further evaluation of renal function is required.
- **Urinary protein** is not considered abnormal until >300 mg of protein in 24 hours is excreted

59. Agents considered safe in pregnancy

- Ampicillin
- Amoxicillin
- Cephalexin
- Cefaclor
- Nitrofurantoin (may be used during the first two trimesters)
- Sulfasoxazole (may cause kernicterus in the newborn; also may cause hemolytic anemia when G6PD deficiency is present; especially avoid in last few weeks of gestation)

Agents that should be avoided in pregnancy

- Fluoroquinolones- Possible damage to immature cartilage
- Chloramphenicol- Associated with "gray baby" syndrome
- Trimethoprim- May cause megaloblastic anemia because of antifolic acid action
- Erythromycin- Associated with maternal cholestatic jaundice
- Tetracyclines

60. The development of bacteriuria-10% per day of catheterization.

61. Fournier's gangrene

- Idiopathic gangrene of the scrotum, streptococcal scrotal gangrene, perineal phlegmon, and spontaneous fulminant gangrene of the scrotum
- In cases originating in the genitalia the infecting bacteria probably pass through the **Buck fascia** of the penis and spread along the **dartos fascia** of the scrotum and penis, the **Colles fascia** of the perineum, and the **Scarpa fascia** of the anterior abdominal wall
- Wound cultures generally yield multiple organisms, implicating anaerobic-aerobic synergy
- Orchiectomy is almost never required.
- The mortality rate averages approximately 20%

62. **Most common urological diagnosis in men < 50 years**–prostatitis.

63. **Most common urological diagnosis in men > 50 years** (1) BPH (2) prostate cancer (3) prostatitis.

64. **Most common pattern of inflammation is** a lymphocytic infiltrate in the stroma immediately adjacent to the prostatic acini

65. **Acute bacterial prostatitis-** generalized infection of the prostate gland and is associated with both lower UTI and generalized sepsis.

    Chronic bacterial prostatitis- associated with recurrent lower UTIs secondary to areas of focal uropathogenic bacteria residing in the prostate gland.

66. **Most common organism of bacterial prostatitis** is- Escherichia coli

67. PSA levels can be markedly elevated during an acute episode of bacterial prostatitis and slowly resolve to normal levels over the course of **6 weeks**

68. **NIH chronic prostatitis index score (CPSI)** consist of 3 domains and 9 questions.

69. **Meares and Stamey**–described classic four-glass urine collection technique.

70.

	Acute pain	EPS/VB3 (WBC)	EPS/VB3 (bacteria)
Acute bacterial prostatitis (1)	+	+	+
Chronic bacterial prostatitis (2)	–	+	+
CPPS (chronic nonbacterial prostatitis) (3a)	Pain during ejaculation	+	–
CPPS (prostatodynia) (3b)	–	–	–

71. **For prostatitis**

- **Mandatory tests**–history, physical examination, urinalysis, urine culture.
- **Recommended tests**–LUT localisation test, NIHCPSI, Qmax, PVR, urine cytology.

72. **U POINT classification for CPPS**–domains are Urinary, Psychosocial, Organ specific, Infection, Neurologic and Tenderness.

73. **Treatment of prostatitis**

Category 1- antibiotics

Category 2- antibiotics + α blockers + prostatic massage

Category 3- antibiotics + α blockers + anti-inflammatory + phytotherapy/ pentosan polysulfate/ finasteride

74. **Prostate abscess**

- Best detected with TRUS or CT
- Patients who fail to respond quickly to antibiotics is optimally drained by the transurethral incision route
- Transperineal incision is used when the abscess has penetrated beyond the prostatic capsule or penetrated through the levator ani muscle.
- Percutaneous drainage of the abscess is the most effective and less morbid procedure

75. **Chronic orchitis**–inflammation and pain in the testis, persisting for more than 6 weeks.

76. **Epididymitis**

- **In pediatric and elderly**-most common organism is E coli.
- **<35 years in sexually active** most common organism–N gonorrhoeae.
- **Homosexual men practising anal intercourse**–most common organism is E coli, H influenza.

77. **Guidelines for the treatment of infectious epididymitis includes**

- Ceftriaxone or doxycycline for men younger than age 35 years
- Levofloxacin or ofloxacin for men older than age 35

78. **(NIDDK) Diagnostic Criteria for Interstitial Cystitis (IC)**

- Either glomerulations or Hunner ulcer.
- Either pain associated with the bladder or urinary urgency.
- The glomerulations must be diffusely present in $\geq$ three quadrants of the bladder and there must be $\geq$ 10 glomerulations per quadrant.
- Glomerulations are not specific for IC.
- All the following should be excluded:
  - o Bladder capacity >350 ml, absence of urge to void at 150 ml, symptoms < 9 months, age < 18 years, frequency < 8 times/day.

79. **Salient features of IC**

- Female-to-male- 5 : 1
- Symptoms tend to fluctuate, with no long-term deterioration.
- No deleterious effect on pregnancy outcomes.
- Men are diagnosed at an older age and have a higher prevalence of a Hunner lesion.
- Not a premalignant lesion.
- Allergies are the most common association
- 50% incidence of temporary remission unrelated to therapy, with a mean duration of 8 months

80. **Pathognomonic marker in IC is**–mast cells.

81. IC is due to **defect in the epithelial permeability barrier** of the bladder surface GAGs

82. **Most sensitive and specific marker of PBS/IC**–urine antiproliferative factor.

83. **Tests for diagnosis of IC**

Mandatory tests- clinical history, physical examination and urinalysis

Recommended tests- urine culture, cytology, IPSS, frequency volume chart, PVR, PSA, CPE and hydrodistention

84. **Drug of choice for IC**–amitriptyline.

Three major pharmacologic actions:

(1) central and peripheral anticholinergic actions

(2) block the active transport system in the presynaptic nerve ending that is responsible for the reuptake of the released amine neurotransmitters serotonin and norepinephrine,

(3) sedatives, an action related to their antihistaminic properties

85. **Oral drugs with level 1 evidence in the treatment of IC is-** hydroxyzine, L-arginine, nalmefene and sodium pentosan polysulfate.

Intravesical drugs with level 1 evidence in the treatment of IC is- hyaluronic acid, capsaicin and BCG.

86. **Bladder cocktail**–50 mL of 50% DMSO + 10 mg of triamcinolone +40,000 units of heparin + 44 mEq of sodium bicarbonate.

87. **BPS/IC symptom questionnaires are-**

- The University of Wisconsin–IC Scale
- The O'Leary-Sant IC Symptom Index and IC Problem Index
- Pelvic Pain and Urgency/ Frequency–(PUF) Scale

88. **Patients with genital, perianal, or anal ulcers should undergo (CDC recommendation)**

(1) serology and either darkfield examination or direct immunofluorescence for Treponema pallidum

(2) culture or PCR test for HSV

(3) serologic testing for type-specific HSV antibody

89.

Disease	Lesion	Pain at lesion	Site	Pain in LN	Treatment	organism
Primary syphilis	Indurated clean base single	–	B/L	–	Benzthiazide penicillin G 2.4 MU IM	T. pallidum
Genital herpes	Shallow multiple	+	B/L	+	Acyclovir 400 mg tid for 7–10 days	Herpes simplex
Chancroid	Undermined purulent Suppurative	+	U/L	+	Azithromycin, 1g	H ducreyi
LGV	Small ulcer	–	Matted	+	Doxy 100 mg bid × 3 weeks	Chlamydia

90. **Pathognomonic for HSV-** group of vesicles on an erythematous base that does not follow a neural distribution.

91. **Primary syphilis-** ulcer occurring at the site of inoculation that appears about 3 weeks after inoculation and persists for 4 to 6 weeks.

Secondary syphilis- begins 4 to 10 weeks after the appearance of the ulcer but may present as long as 24 months after the initial infection. It manifests with mucocutaneous, constitutional, and parenchymal signs and symptoms

Tertiary syphilis- one third of untreated patients will develop. It is a systemic disease that can affect almost any organ or system, especially the cardiovascular, skeletal, and central nervous systems, and skin.

92. **In C. trachomatis and N. gonorrhoeae-** vaginal epithelium is resistant to infection but cervix is not.

93.

	Vaginal discharge	Treatment	Dose
Candida	Thick,curdy	Fluconazole	150 mg
Trichomoniasis	Frothy strawberry vulva	Metronidazole	2.0 gm
Gonococcus	Mucopurulent	Ceftriaxone intramuscularly	125 mg IM

94. **Types 6 and 11 HPV** are low risk for conversion to invasive carcinoma of the external genitalia.

Types 16, 18, 31, 33, 35, 39, 45, and 51 HPV have been associated with cervical dysplasia and neoplasm in women and squamous intraepithelial neoplasia in men

Cervical cancers and anal cancers are associated, **most commonly HPV 16 and 18**

95. **The first AIDS case was described in 1981.**

96.

Route of exposure	Risk of HIV
Contaminated blood	85-100%
IV drug use	0.8%
Needle stick	0.28%-0.33%
Insertive vaginal intercourse	0.03-0.09%
Receptive vaginal intercourse	0.005-0.02%

97. **HIV transmission**
    - Circumcised men are at lower risk for HIV infection.
    - Men are more likely to transmit HIV to their female partners.
98. **HIV2** = Less cases, less virulent, less readily transmitted (in comparision with HIV1).
99. **HIV infection**
    - Initially attaches to the CD4 receptor on susceptible host cells.
    - After entry, viral RNA is converted into DNA.
    - This process of reverse transcription occurs within 4 to 6 hours of infection.
100. **In the absence of therapy**
    - 60% to 70% of HIV-infected patients median time between infection and the development of AIDS is 10 to 11 years.
    - Ten to 20 percent of HIV infected people are "rapid progressors".
    - Five to 15% of HIV-infected people are "slow progressors".
    - AIDS usually leads to death in 2 to 3 years.
101. **HIV can be detected in the draining lymphoid tissue**-within 2 days of infection.

     The time from mucosal infection and initial plasma viremia ranges from 4 to 11 days.
102. **HIV RNA**
    - After acute infection HIV RNA detected from day 12.
    - Sensitivity 100% and specificity 97%.
    - First antibodies can be detected on day 21.

- Powerful predictor of disease progression and death at all stages of disease.
- The nadir in plasma HIV RNA levels is a marker for the duration of virus suppression
- Increasing levels suggest treatment failure

103. **Sanctuaries** are defined as cells and organs where the HIV can be sheltered

 Tissue sanctuaries include the lymphoid tissue, mucosa associated lymphoid tissue, the genital organs, and the CNS.

 Concentrations of antiviral drugs (especially protease inhibitors) may be suboptimal.

104. **Testing of HIV is recommended in all STD patients.**

105. **HIV ELISA**
 - Sensitivity and specificity approaches 100%.
 - Low positive predictive value.

106. **To exclude false positive results of ELISA,** western blot is done as confirmatory test (more specific).

107. Urinary retention is the **most common voiding dysfunction** (54%) in HIV infected patients.

108. **Kaposi sarcoma**
 - KS is the most common vascular neoplasm
 - Virus involved- human herpesvirus 8.

 NHL is the most common lymphoreticular neoplasm.

109. **Post exposure prophylaxis in severe disease**–three-drug regimen (zidovudine, lamivudine and one additional agent).

110. **Indinavir causes**–Renal stones.
 - Incidence–12% to 24%.
 - Stones–nonopaque and not detected on NCCT.
 - Conservative treatment in most cases (hydration, analgesics and temporary cessation).
 - Indinavir crystals develop at pH 7.0 and can be dissolved when the pH is <4.0.
 - After 2 weeks, indinavir crystalluria remains constant at 25%.

- HIV-infected patients on protease inhibitors also form stones that do not contain protease inhibitors

111. HIV–associated nephropathy (HIVAN)

- Occurs in patients with low CD4 counts, but overt AIDS is not a prerequisite.
- Presents as nephritic range proteinuria and renal insufficiency.
- Renal ultrasound evaluation shows echogenic kidneys with preserved or enlarged size despite severe renal insufficiency.
- Diagnosis of HIVAN is based on a renal biopsy specimen showing characteristic focal segmental glomerulosclerosis with collapsing features.
- Antiretroviral therapy appears to delay progression of HIVAN to end-stage renal disease.

112. Primary cutaneous lesion

Macule	–	Flat
Papule	–	Elevated < 0.5 cm
Nodule	–	Elevated > 0.5 cm
Plaque	–	Elevated > 0.5 cm superficial
Vesicle	–	Collection of fluid < 0.5 cm
Bulla	–	Collection of fluid > 0.5 cm

113. Secondary cutaneous lesion includes- Scale, crust, erosion, ulcer, fissure, atrophy and scar

114. Cutaneous disease

- **Erythema multiforme**–target lesion.
- **Psoriasis**–erythematous plaque with silvery-white scales.
- **Reiter's syndrome**–urethritis, arthritis, ocular findings, oral ulcers and skin lesions.Associated with the HLA-B27.
- **Lichen planus**–lesion is a small, polygonal, violaceous, flat-topped papule.
- The late stage of **lichen sclerosus** is called balanitis xerotica obliterans (BXO).
- **Behcet syndrome**–Mucocutaneous lesions oral cavity +genitalia+ ocular involvement (uveitis). Genital lesions are larger and more painful than the oral lesions.
- **Pemphigus-** autoimmune blistering diseases characterized by intraepidermal blisters.

- **Bullous pemphigoid-** subepidermal blistering disease.

115. March 24th is "**World Tuberculosis Day.**"
April 7th is "**World Health Day.**"

116. **Extrapulmonary sites account for** 10% of tuberculosis cases.

Genitourinary TB accounts for 30% to 40% of all extrapulmonary TB

117. **TB unlikely in** –< 5 years.

118. **The probability that an HIV-infected person who was previously infected with M. tuberculosis will develop active TB is** 10% per year.

Normal host without HIV infection will have–5% to 10% lifetime probability of developing active TB.

119. **In TB-genital tract**, epididymis and fallopian tubes are primary landing sites for hematogenous spread of TB.

120. **Renal tuberculosis-**

- The kidneys are the primary site of hematogenous spread of TB.
- Mycobacteria lodge in the renal capillaries causing microscopic foci near the glomeruli
- Renal cortex is the favoured site

121. Tuberculosis causes necrosis of the **adrenal gland**, which manifests as Addison disease.

122. **Tuberculous ureteritis** extension from the kidney. Most commcn site affected is–UVJ.

123. **Bladder lesions** secondary to renal TB.

Earliest affected is–ureteral orifice.

124. **Tuberculous epididymitis** Tubercle bacilli reach the epididymis by hematogenous spread

Painful, inflamed scrotal swelling.

Most common site globus minor.

125. **TB of the testis**–secondary to epididymis via direct extension.

126. **Humans are the only reservoir** for M. tuberculosis.

127. **Positive montoux**

- $\geq$ 5 mm of induration–HIV patients, recent contact with TB.
- $\geq$ 10 mm of induration–IV drug abusers.
- $\geq$ 15 mm of induration–patients with no risk of TB.

128. **M. tuberculosis is slow growing**–doubling time of 15 to 20 hours.

129. **In tuberculosis**–calcification is intraluminal and appears as a cast of the ureter, which is thickened and not dilated.

In schistosomiasis–calcification is mural and the ureter is generally dilated and tortuous.

130. **At least three, but preferably five,** consecutive early morning specimens of urine should be cultured.

Urine cultures are sensitive in 80% to 90% of cases and have a specificity of nearly 100%.

131. **For TB evaluation**

IVU has traditionally been the gold standard tool.

- Early signs include the moth-eaten appearance of calyceal erosion and papillary irregularity.
- Scarring and angulation of the ureteropelvic junction (UPJ) may also occur, the so-called "**Kerr's kink**".
- Tuberculosis of the ureter is commonly seen as a rigid, straightened "**pipe-stem**" ureter. A beaded, corkscrew appearance is also seen.

CT has become more widely available and has arguably replaced **IVU as the investigation of choice.**

A "**golf-hole**" ureteric orifice is suggestive of tuberculosis, and, when found, upper tract imaging or endoscopy should be done.

132. **Drugs used in management of tuberculosis**

Drug	**Bactericidal or bacteristatic**	**Active against**	**Action**	**Dose modification in renal failure**	**Pregnancy**
Isoniazid	Bactericidal	Extracellular and intracellular	Inhibit the synthesis of mycolic acid	Not required	Not contraindicated
Rifampicin	Bactericidal	Extracellular and intracellular	Inhibits bacterial RNA	Not required	Not contraindicated (add vitamin k)
Streptomycin	Bactericidal	Intracellular	Inhibit protein synthesis	Avoid usage	Contraindicated

Pyrizinamide	Bateriostatic	Intracellular	Inhibition of fatty acid synthesis	Required only if GFR <10ml/min	Not contraindicated
Ethambutol	Bacteriostatic		Inhibit mycobacterium cell wall synthesis	Avoid usage	Not contraindicated

133. **Duration of therapy**. The first 2 months involve three to four drugs: (Rifampicin, isoniazid, and pyrazinamide are administered daily; ethambutol is added if drug resistance to isoniazid is suspected).

    Next 4 months of rifampicin and isoniazid daily

134. **Indications for partial nephrectomy**

    Lesion containing calcification that has failed to respond after 6 weeks of chemotherapy.

    Area of calcification that is slowly increasing.

135. **S. mansoni and S. japonicum**–mesenteric veins.

    S.haematobium–perivesical venous plexus and cause urinary schistosomiasis.

136. **S. haematobium** eggs are terminally spined, S. **mansoni** eggs are laterally spined.

137. **S. haematobium**–early onset and a high frequency of squamous cell carcinomas.

138. **Drug of choice for all schistosoma species**–praziquantel.

139. **Human lymphatic filariasis**–Wuchereria bancrofti. (No animal reservoir)

140. **Non-lymphatic filariasis**–Onchocerca volvulus (African river blindness).

    Cause "hanging groin", and scrotal elephantiasis.

141. The presence of microfilariae in peripheral blood, chylous urine, or hydrocele fluid is diagnostic. Blood samples must be taken when **peak microfilaremia occurs (midnight)**

142. **Filarial infection**–DEC, 6 mg/kg/day in three divided doses for 2 weeks.

143. **Vulvovaginal candidiasis**–oral fluconazole (a single 150-mg dose) is as effective as topical intravaginal therapy.

144. **Itraconazole**–effective in the treatment of infections caused by Aspergillus, Blastomyces, Coccidioides and Histoplasma **not candida.**

145. **Triazoles** (fluconazole, itraconazole, voriconazole).

- Similar in chemical structure to the imidazoles.
- Greater affinity for fungal cytochrome P450 enzymes than the imidazole.

146. **Incubation period**

Scabies 2-6 weeks
LGV 3-30 days
Gonorrhea 3-14 days
Trichomoniasis 4-28 days

❑❑

Chapter 5

MOLECULAR AND CELLULAR BIOLOGY

1.

	Complement
Phagocytosis	C3b
Most critical component	C3
Membrane attack complex	C5b+ C6 - 9
Anaphylatoxins	C3a ,C5a
Chemoattractant	C5a

2. **A primary immune response**–has a lag period.
   A secondary response–more rapid and more vigorous.

3.

	Membrane component
CD 3	Pan T cell marker
CD 4	Receptor for MHC class II and HIV virus
CD 8	Receptor for MHC class I
CD 16	Fc receptor, phagocytosis, and ADCC
CD 19	Pan B cell marker
CD 25	IL 2 receptor (Tac)

4. **Antigen presenting cell (APC)**

   Dendritic cells are commonly referred as "professional APC".

   Macrophages, monocytes, some B cells, Langerhans cells of the skin, dendritic reticulum cells and vascular endothelium are APC

5. Monocytes usually occupy perivascular areas and can be called– **Kupffer cells in the liver, alveolar macrophages in the lung, and histiocytes in connective tissue, brain microglia, or kidney glomerular mesangial cells.**

6. **NK cells**

   - These are large granular lymphocytes
   - Can destroy various nucleated cells including tumors and virus-infected cells.
   - Do not require prior contact with antigen, nor are they MHC-restricted.

- They release cytotoxic factors such as perforin, serine proteases called granzymes, and TNF-β
- They can trigger apoptosis in their targets.
- They also participate in antibody-dependent cell mediated cytotoxicity (ADCC), by the binding of their cell surface Fc receptor (CD16) to the Fc portion of antibody-coated cells.

7. **The primary lymphoid organs are-**
   - Thymus, responsible for the selection and education of T cells
   - Bone marrow, responsible for the education of B cells.

   Secondary or peripheral lymphoid tissue-

   Spleen, lymph nodes, and unencapsulated tissues lining the alimentary, respiratory, and urogenital tract.

8. **MHC**–located on chromosome 6.
9. **HLA class I antigens**–expressed by all nucleated cells.

   HLA class II antigens–expressed by B cells, monocytes macrophages, and APCs.
   - Each individual inherits two class I and one class II antigen from each parent, so six HLA antigens constitute an individual's tissue type (three from each parent).
10. **The immunoglobulin molecule consists of-** two identical heavy (H) and two light (L) chains held together by disulfide bonds
11. **Jak3**
    - Mutations result in severe combined immunodeficiency (SCID).
    - Jak3 activation is necessary for normal development and survival of T and B cells but not for dendritic cells
12. **Type 1 cytokines** include IFN-γ and TNF-β (also called lymphotoxin) and are critical components of cell mediated immune responses, particularly responses to intracellular parasites and tuberculin delayed-type hypersensitivity

    Type 2 cytokines include IL-4, IL-5, IL-6, IL-9, and IL-10 and are critical components of allergic responses and immune responses to extracellular parasites such as helminths
13. **The immunosuppressive drugs cyclosporine and tacrolimus function by** blocking the NFAT pathway

14. **Caspase**
    - **Caspase-8 and 10** are the initiator caspases for extrinsic pathway
    - **Caspase-9** is the initiator for the intrinsic pathway (mitochondrial pathway).
    - **Caspases-3, -6 and -7** function to carry out the final steps of the committed apoptotic program
15. **Neutrophils and macrophages–first line of defense** of the innate immune system by killing bacteria and fungi.
16. **DNA**–Base + sugar (in of DNA called 2dioxyribose, for RNA called ribose) + phosphate.
    - The two strands are held together by the **hydrogen bonds.**
17. **Adenine (A) binds to** thymine (T). **In the RNA molecule, adenine binds** to uracil (U).

    Guanine (G) binds to cytosine (C).
18. **Types of RNA**
    - Translation of **mRNA** into protein occurs in the cytoplasm where ribosomes are located.
    - **Transfer RNA** is a small adapter molecule that is covalently linked to a single amino acid at one end and an anticodon in the middle of the chain.
    - **Ribosomal RNA** comprises 80% of the RNA within a cell and makes up part of the ribosome that is responsible for protein synthesis
19. **Tumor suppressor genes** are the retinoblastoma gene (*RB*) and *TP53*

    Oncogenes that are over expressed in a variety of cancers include c-MYC and c-MET
20. **Mechanisms by which a proto-oncogene can be converted to an oncogene are by**

    (1) Mutation of the protooncogene
    (2) Gene amplification
    (3) Chromosomal rearrangement.
21. **STOP codons**–UAA, UAG and UGA, do not encode for any amino acids.
22. **First and rate-limiting, step of translation**–initiation.

23. **Philadelphia chromosome** of CML–exchange between the long arms of chromosomes 9 and 22.

24. **DNA methylation occurs exclusively on**–dinucleotide sequence CG.

25. **Disease with their associated chromosomes**

Syndrome	**Chromosome**
Wilms' tumor	11p13
Beckwith-Wiedemann	11p15
Von-Hippel-Lindau	3p25
Hereditary papillary renal cell carcinoma	7q31
Birt-Hogg-Dubé	17p11.2
MEN type II	10q11

26. **G_1** cell prepares to duplicate its DNA.

S phase is when the cell duplicates its DNA.

G_2 is when the cell prepares to divide.

M phase is when the cell divides.

The two main points of control–G_1S and G_2M checkpoints.

27. **TP53 is most common** mutated gene in human tumors, including genitourinary malignancies (50%).

TP53 mediates both G1S and G2M arrest, and has critical role in preserving genomic integrity.

Cyclin D expression is critical at–G_1S checkpoint.

28.

Cytokine	Major activities
IL 1	Activation of macrophage and T cells
IL 2	T cell growth factor
IL 4	T cell growth factor, B cell growth factor
IL 6	Stimulation of acute phase protein
IL 10	Immunosuppression
TGF β	Immunosuppression

29. **G_1S checkpoint**–responds to variety of extracellular signals in addition to DNA damage.

G_2M checkpoint–responds only to DNA damage.

30. **Most frequent somatic genome alteration reported in prostate cancer**–Aberrant methylation of the CpG island at the glutathione-S-transferase Pi (*GSTP1*) locus

- Methylation of *GSTP1* has been detected in 90% of prostate carcinomas and approximately 70% of PIN lesions, but is not present in normal prostate tissue or BPH

31.

Nucleotide excision repair	Repairs DNA damage caused by UV radiation and chemical exposure
Base excision repair	Repairs damage caused by spontaneous deamination of bases, radiation, oxidative stress (ROS), alkylating agents or replication errors
Mismatch repair	Repairs nucleotides mispaired by DNA polymerases
Double stranded repairs	Repairs damage arising from ionizing radiation or X-rays, free radicals, chemicals, and during replication of a single-strand break

32. **In testicular GCT,** gain of chromosome 12p is universal finding, with the exception of spermatocytic seminoma subtype

33. **Most common chromosomal abnormality found in advanced prostate cancer is-** 8q gain

34. **Apoptosis**–controlled cell death via caspases.

35. **BAX**–best studied pro-apoptotic BCL2 family member.

    BCL2–best studied anti-apoptotic BCL2 family member.

36. **Initiation phase of apoptosis** involve integration of signals to trigger cell death via **caspases.**

37. **Earliest and most common genetic abnormality in prostate cancer**–LOH on chromosome 8 p.

    LOH of chromosome 10q also occurs in prostate cancer.

38. **TGF-α**

- Positive regulator of stromal cell growth.
- Stimulates ECM production.
- Induces cell cycle arrest in epithelial and hematopoietic cell populations.

- Potent immunosuppressant.

39. **Death receptor is CD95, or FAS,** play an important role in cancer immunosurveillance

40. **Most potent endogenous vasoconstrictor**–endothelin-1.

41. **Integrins**–bridges gap between the ECM and the cytoskeleton.

    Cadherins–responsible for cell-cell adhesion and tissue integrity.

    Caveolins–involved in transport mechanisms for many proteins and cell signalling.

42. **Angiogenesis activators**–FGF/ VEGF.

    Angiogenesis inhibitors–Bleomycin, vincristine, linomide, fumagillin, endostatin, INF, thrombospondin.

43. **Three classes of biomaterials have been used for engineering of genitourinary tissues:**

    - Collagen and alginate.
    - Acellular tissue matrices–bladder submucosa and small-intestinal submucosa.
    - Synthetic polymers–polyglycolic acid (PGA), polylactic acid (PLA), and polylactic-co-glycolic acid (PLGA).

44.

Stem cell	Advantages	Disadvantages
Human embryonic	Pluripotent	Transdifferentiate to malignant phenotype
		Require immuno-suppression
		Ethical issues
Adult	No ethical issues	Not pluripotent
	Do not transdifferentiate	
Fetal	No ethical issues	
	Do not transdifferentiate	
	Multipotent	

❑❑

Chapter 6
REPRODUCTIVE AND SEXUAL FUNCTION

1. **Peptide hormones**
   - Small, secretory proteins that act through cell surface receptors.
   - Examples of peptide hormones are LH and FSH.

   Steroid hormones
   - Derived from cholesterol.
   - They are not stored in secretory granules.
   - In plasma, these hormones are usually bound to carrier proteins
   - Steroid hormones are cell membrane–permeable.
   - Examples of steroid hormones are testosterone and estradiol.
2. **Pituitary gland**
   - It has two lobes: **posterior and anterior.**
   - **Posterior lobe, or neurohypophysis**
     - Formed during development as a ventral outpocket of the hypothalamus.
     - **Oxytocin and vasopressin**, are secreted by posterior pituitary.
     - Neurohypophysial hormones are regulated by **neural stimuli**
   - **Anterior pituitary or adenohypophysis**
     - Glandular structure regulated by **bloodborne factors.**
     - **ACTH, TSH,PRL GH, LH and FSH** are secreted by anterior pituitary.
3. **Substances that inhibit GnRH secretion- opiods, peptide hormones and sex steroids**
4. **Testosterone**
   - **Normal testosterone production in men is approximately 5 g/day**

- Testosterone is metabolized into two major active metabolites in target tissue:
  (1) **DHT** through the action of 5α-reductase
  (2) **estradiol** through the action of aromatases.
- DHT is a much more potent androgen than is testosterone.
- In the testis and skeletal muscle, conversion to DHT is not essential for hormonal activity.

5. **FSH–Primary site of action is on Sertoli cells within seminiferous tubules.**

   Through FSH-mediated factors,

   - Seminiferous tubule growth is stimulated
   - Sperm production is initiated during puberty.
   - Stimulate quantitatively normal levels of spermatogenesis.

6. **Testosterone feedback occurs mainly at the hypothalamus**

   Estrogens feedback occurs mainly at the pituitary

7. Testosterone is the primary regulator of LH secretion

   Estradiol is the predominant regulator of FSH secretion

8. **Testosterone** induces development of the **internal genitalia**

   DHT masculinizes the genital anlage to form the **external genitalia**

9. **Sertoli cells** within the developing testis synthesize MIS,that prevents the müllerian duct from developing into uterus and fallopian tubes

10. **A critical gene for sex determination** is *SRY* (sex-determining region Y gene) on the short arm of the Y chromosome.

11. **The hypothalamic capacity to generate GnRH pulses arises** at, 12th year.

    Puberty is likely initiated by kisspeptin, melatonin, and leptin

12. **"Antitestis" genes-** WNT4 and DAX1

13. **The first identifiable step separating the ovarian and testicular pathways of differentiation is :**

    - Movement of primordial germ cells into the medullary cords.
    - Occurs at **7 weeks** after conception.

14. **FSH stimulates**–sertoli cells (promote spermatogenesis).

    LH stimulates–leydig cells (secrete testosterone).

15. **The testicular parenchyma is surrounded by:**
    - Outer visceral layer of the tunica vaginalis.
    - Middle layer of tunica albuginea.
    - Innermost layer of the tunica vasculosa.

16. **Major testicular artery branches**–inferior pole of the testis.
    - **Testicular biopsy done from**–upper pole.
    - **Kidney biopsy done from**–lower pole.

17. **Seminiferous tubules** (250 m) connects to **rete testis.**
    - The rete testis forms 6 to 12 **ductuli efferentes**, connect to **caput epididymis.**
    - **Individual seminiferous tubules** harbor developing germ cells and interstitial tissue.
    - **Interstitial tissue**
      - Composed of Leydig cells, mast cells and macrophages
      - Comprises 20% to 30% of total testicular volume

18. **The testis has no known somatic innervation.**

    It receives autonomic innervation primarily from the intermesenteric nerves and renal plexus

    The innervation of the penis is both autonomic and somatic

    Arterial supply to the human testis and epididymis:
    - Internal spermatic testicular artery (abdominal aorta).
    - Deferential vasal artery (internal iliac artery).
    - External spermatic or cremasteric artery (inferior epigastric artery).

19. **Peaks of testosterone**
    - **The fetal peak** occurs between 12 and 18 weeks of gestation.
    - **The neonatal peak** occurs at approximately 2 months of age.
    - **The pubertal peak** in testosterone occurs between 12 and 17 years of age.

    The most important regulator of testosterone production is LH

20. Blood testis barrier is formed by:

- Tight junction of sertoli cells.
- At the level of endothelial cells in capillaries.
- At the level of peritubular myoid cells.

Functionally develop at the onset of spermatogenesis.

Germ cells are not necessary for barrier.

21. Outside the blood-testis barrier in the basal compartment–spermatogonia and young spermatocytes.

Above the barrier in the adluminal compartment–mature spermatocytes and spermatids.

22. Spermatogenic process in humans requires–64 days.

Human sperm production is–1200 sperms per second

23. Differences in mitosis and meiosis

MITOSIS	MEIOSIS
Occurs in somatic cells	Occurs in sexual cells
1 cell division, 2 daughter cells	2 cell divisions, 4 daughter cells
Chromosome number maintained	Chromosome number halved
No pairing, chromosome homologs	Synapse of homologs, prophase I
No crossovers	>1 crossover per homolog pair
Identical daughter genotype	Genetic variation in daughter Cells

24. Spermiogenesis

During this maturation sequence, cell division does not occur

Changes include

- loss of cytoplasm
- migration of cytoplasmic organelles
- formation of the acrosome from the Golgi apparatus
- formation of the flagellum from the centriole
- nuclear compaction to about 10% of former size
- reorganization of mitochondria around the sperm midpiece

25. DAZ-gene localized on–long arm of Y chromosome in a region referred to as AZFc.

SRY gene is located on–short arm of Y chromosome.

26. **With fluoresence in-situ hybridization technology (FISH),** subtle paternal-age effects on sperm aneuploidy can be detected

27. **Sperm transport through the human epididymis** takes 2 to 12 days
    - **Most common site for epididymal spermatozoa storage is**–caudal region.
    - **Maximum mature motility pattern seen in**–caudal region.
    - **Sperm fertility maturation is at**–distal corpus or proximal cauda epididymis.

28. **The human spermatozoon is approximately 60 μm**
    - **Sperm head**–4.5 μm long and 3 μm wide, nucleus (chromatin material, acrosome).
    - **Acrosome**–helps in penetration.
    - **Sperm middle piece**–mitochondria surrounding a set of outer dense fibers and the characteristic 9 + 2 microtubular structure of the sperm axoneme.
    - **The outer dense fibers, rich in disulfide bonds**–provide the sperm tail with the rigidity necessary for progressive motility.

29. **Ductus deferens**

    Layers
    - Outer adventitial connective tissue (contains blood vessels and small nerves)
    - Muscular coat that consists of a middle circular layer surrounded by inner and outer longitudinal muscle layers
    - Inner mucosal layer with an epithelial lining
    - Lined by pseudostratified epithelium
    - 30 to 35 cm in length.

30. **Greatest muscle-lumen ratio** (10:1) of any hollow viscus in human body–ductus deferens.

31. **Normal couple conceives**–20% to 25% per month, 75% by 6 months and 90% by 1 year.
    - Male factor–20% of infertility.
    - Male and female factors–30% to 40% of infertility.
    - Infertile couples without treatment–25% to 35% will conceive at some time by intercourse.

32. **Conception may occur when sexual relation**–5 days before ovulation to 1 day after ovulation.

    Recommendation is intercourse frequency every 2 days near the time of ovulation

33. **Spermatogenesis may be impaired for**–3 months after febrile illness.

34. **CBAVD/ Ejaculatory duct obstruction**

    Seman analysis-low volume, azoospermic, acidic, fructose-negative semen that does not coagulate.

35. **WHO 2010**

Parameter	**Lowest Reference**	**Range**
Semen volume (ml)	1.5 ml	1.4-1.7
Total sperm number (per ejaculate)	39 million	33-46
Sperm concentration (per ml)	15 million	12-16
Total motility (PR + NP, %)	40	38-42
Progressive motility (PR, %)	32	31-34
Vitality (live spermatozoa, %)	58	55-63
Sperm morphology (normal forms, %)	>30%	
pH	7.8	
Viscosity	4 mm threading	
Coagulation	<20 minutes	
Color	Whitish grey	

36. **Primary hormone etiology**–3% of males with infertility.

    Antisperm antibodies–10% of males with infertility.

    Microdeletions of Yq chromosome–13% of azoospermic men.

    CBAVD–6% of men with obstructive azoospermia

37. **Secondary testicular failure (paratesticular causes)**, are endocrine in nature and relate to either congenital (Kallman syndrome) or acquired hypogonadotropic hypogonadism

    Primary testicular failure(testicular causes), are intrinsic disorders of spermatogenesis

38.

DIAGNOSIS	FSH (mIU/mL)	LH (mIU/mL)	TESTOSTERONE (ng/dL)
Hypospermatogenesis	High	Normal or high	Normal or low
Germinal cell aplasia	Very high	High	Low
Maturation arrest	Normal	Normal	Normal
Klinefelter syndrome	Very high	High	Low
Hypogonadotropic Hypogonadism	Low	Low	Low

39. **Factors that increase sex hormone binding globulins**–estrogen, hyperthyroidism, cirrhosis, aging and anticonvulsants

Factors that decrease sex hormone binding globulins–obesity, hypothyroidism, acromegaly, nephritic syndrome and insulin.

40. **Testicular biopsy**

- Azoospermic patients with normal testicular size, palpable vas deferens, and normal serum FSH levels require a diagnostic testicular biopsy
- FSH levels, greater than two times normal, are indicative of primary testicular failure, and diagnostic testicular biopsy is not required
- A normal testicular biopsy is pathognomonic for genital tract obstruction.

41. **The most common complication after testis biopsy**–bleeding.

The most serious complication after testis biopsy is– inadvertent biopsy of the epididymis.

42. **Oligospermia**

- Sperm density of < 20 million/ mL.
- Endocrinopathies are rarely observed in patients with concentrations > 10 million/mL
- Endocrine screening with serum testosterone and FSH levels are reserved for counts < 10 million/ml

43. **Most common cause of ejaculatory failure is**–spinal cord injury (SCI)

44. Drugs used in treatment of retrograde ejaculation

- Phenylpropanolamine
- Ephedrine
- Pseudoephedrine
- Imipramine

45. The best candidates for penile vibratory stimulus are patients with complete SCI who have an intact ejaculatory reflex system: Specifically, patients with complete UMN lesions above T10

46. After vasectomy–60% of men develop antisperm antibodies (ASA)

With CBAVD–1/3 are found to have ASA.

47. Ipsilateral renal anomalies (Most common–renal agenesis) are present in–80% of men with unilateral absence of the vas deferens.

48. Kallmann syndrome–congenital hypogonadotropic hypogonadism (HH), anosmia and midline facial defects.

49. For induction of spermatogenesis in the HH patient

- First-line therapy for HH–hCG
- When testicular volume and serum testosterone levels are stable without significant further improvement, FSH stimulation is added
- FSH may be administered in the form of human menopausal gonadotropin (hMG)

50. Most common cause of endogenous androgen excess–CAH.

Most common of the five enzyme defects responsible for CAH–deficiency of 21-hydroxylase.

51. Genetic hallmark of Klinefelter's syndrome–presence of an extra X chromosome.

- A phenotypic male with small firm testes, gynecomastia, azoospermia and elevated gonadotropins.
- Increased risk of breast cancer, non-Hodgkin lymphoma and extragonadal mediastinal germ cell tumors
- Sperm retrieved is associated with high fertilization rates with ICSI

52. Kartagener syndrome includes chronic sinusitis and bronchiectasis, situs inversus, and infertility (low or absent sperm motility).

53. **Most common correctable cause of male infertility**–varicocele.
    - 90% varicoceles–left sided.
    - 10% of varicoceles–bilateral.
    - 15%–normal population.
    - 40%–male infertility.
    - 70%–secondary infertility.

54. **Grade of varicocele**
    - Grade I varicoceles–detectable only during the Valsalva maneuver;
    - Grade II varicoceles–palpated without Valsalva
    - Grade III varicoceles–visible through the scrotal skin and classically described as feeling like a "bag of worms."

55. **Results of varicocele repair**
    - **Improvement in seminal parameters in**–70% of patients after varicocele repair.
    - **Motility**–most common (70%) improved parameter.
    - **Improvement in conception rates**–40% to 50% with pregnancies occurring after 8 months.
    - **Larger the varicocele**– the more the improvement on correction.

56. **Bilateral complete ejaculatory duct obstruction**

    Acidic, fructose negative, low volume ejaculate azoospermia with palpable vas

    Main DD-**CBAVD**–diagnosed by absence of vas on physical examination

57. **The absolute indications for vasography are as follows:**
    1. Azoospermia +
    2. Complete spermatogenesis with many mature spermatids on testis biopsy +
    3. At least one palpable vas

58. **If the testis biopsy reveals many sperm, consider the following:**
    1. **Absence of sperm in vasal fluid indicates** epididymal obstruction.
    2. **Copious vasal fluid containing many sperm indicates** vasal or ejaculatory duct obstruction.

3. **Copious thick white fluid without sperm in a dilated vas indicates** secondary epididymal obstruction in addition to a potential vasal or ejaculatory duct obstruction.

59. Vasography

- **Should be performed** only at the time of definitive repair of obstruction
- **Always sample vasal fluid first to allow cryopreservation of motile sperm if found.**
- **Use indigo carmine instead of methylene blue to confirm patency**

60. Ultrasound examination consistent with the diagnosis of a varicocele is veins >3.5 mm in diameter, with reversal of venous flow after the Valsalva maneuver.

61. Causes of vasal calcification

Diabetes mellitus- most common

Normal ageing

Tuberculosis, syphilis, gonorrhea,schistosomisis, chronic UTI

62. Candidate for a varicocele repair:

- Couple has known infertility +
- Female partner has normal fertility +
- Varicocele is palpable on physical examination +
- Male partner has an abnormal semen analysis.

63. Complication and recurrence with varicocele repairs

	Artery preserved	**Hydrocele (%)**	**Recurrence (%)**
Conventional	No	3-39 (Max)	9-16 (Max)
Microscopic	Yes	0 (Min)	<2 (Min)
Laparoscopic	Yes	5-8	<2 (Min)
Radiographic	Yes	0 (Min)	4-11
Retroperitoneal	No	7	11-15

Lymphatic obstruction is a more likely than venous obstruction as cause of hydrocele formation.

64. Vasvasostomy if there are sperm or sperm parts (sperm heads, sperm with partial tails) in large numbers or the fluid is clear and copious with no visible sperm.

Vasoepididymostomy–if the fluid is thick, pasty and devoid of sperm or contains only a few sperm heads (fluid from the testicular end of vas).

65. Comparision of techniques for vasoepididymostomy

TECHNIQUES	ADVANTAGES	DISADVANTAGES
Intussusception	2-3 sutures placed in the epididymal tubule provide 4 and 6 points of fixation.	Cannot assess tubular fluid for sperm before anastomosis setup.
	Virtually bloodless anastomosis.	
End-Side	Virtually bloodless anastomosis.	Difficult suture placement to a collapsed tubule
	Epididymal fluid can be examined before anastomosis	
End-End	Epididymal fluid can be examined before anastomosis.	Difficult hemostasis on transacted epididymis.
	Easy and rapid identification of the level of obstruction in the epididymis.	Difficult to identify tubule for anastomosis.
		Difficult outer-layer closure.
	Allows upward mobilization of epididymis to bridge a large vasal gap.	Vasal blood supply from inferior epididymal artery is sacrificed.

66. Most common known causes of epididymal obstruction–vasectomy.

67. In **obstructive azoospermia**, no significant difference in open vs percutaneous in sperm extraction (however open technique retrieves more sperm).

In non-obstructive azoospermia–open surgical testicular sperm extraction only.

68. Techniques for sperm retrival

Techniques	Advantages	Disadvantages
MESA (microsurgical epididymal sperm aspiration)	Lower complication rate.	Requires anesthesia and microsurgical skills
	Sperm has better motility	
	Large number of sperm can be harvested	
PESA (percutaneous epididymal sperm aspiration)	No microsurgical skill required.	Hematoma, pain, and vascular injury to testes and epididymis.
	Local anesthesia.	
	Sperm has better motility	Smaller quantity of sperm obtained
TESA (testicular sperm aspiration)	No microsurgical skill required.	Hematoma, pain, and vascular injury to testes and epididymis
	Local anesthesia.	Small quantity of sperm obtained.
		Immature or immotile testicular sperm.
TESE (testicular sperm extraction)	Low complication rate if performed microsurgically.	Requires anesthesia and microsurgical skills.
	Preferred technique for nonobstructive azoospermia.	

69. Varicocele repair has been demonstrated to be more cost effective than–IVF with ICSI.

Patients after vasectomy, vasectomy reversal is more cost effective than–IVF with ICSI.

Patients who have failed one vasectomy reversal, a repeat vasectomy reversal has been found more cost effective than–IVF with ICSI.

Patients with epididymal obstruction, vasoepididymostomy has been more cost effective than–IVF with ICSI.

IUI as an initial treatment for infertile couples is more cost effective than–IVF.

70. Corpora cavernosa is a bilayered structure

- Inner-layer bundles support and contain the cavernous tissue and are oriented circularly.
- Outer-layer bundles are oriented longitudinally.
- Between the 5 and 7 o'clock positions outer layer is absent (most prostheses tend to extrude fromventral groove)

Corpus spongiosum lacks an outer layer or intracorporeal struts.

71.

	Corpus spongiosum	Glans
Tunica albuginea	Thin (lack outer layer)	Absent
Compression by muscle	Yes	Absent
Venous occlusion during errection	Absent	Absent

72. Internal iliac artery →internal pudendal artery→common penile artery →

1. Dorsal artery–engorgement of glans during erection.
2. Bulbourethral artery–supplies the bulb and corpus spongiosum.
3. Cavernous artery–tumescence of the corpus cavernosum.

73. Sexual stimulation leading to erection includes:

1. Dilation of arterioles.
2. Trapping of blood by expanding sinusoids.
3. Compression of venules.
4. Stretching of tunica further occluding venous outflow.
5. Increase in PaO_2
6. Further increase in pressure with contraction of ischiocavernous muscle.

74. The sympathetic pathway originates from–T11 to L2 spinal segments and passes through the white rami to the sympathetic chain ganglia.

The parasympathetic pathway arises from–intermediolateral cell columns of the **S234** spinal cord segments.

75. During rigid-erection production in normal men, cerebral impulses travel as follows:

- Inhibiting the sympathetic pathway and thus decreasing norepinephrine release

- Stimulate parasympathetic, pathway thus releasing NO and acetylcholine
- Stimulate somatic pathway releasing acetylcholine.

76. **Center of somatomotor penile innervation**–Onuf's nucleus in S234 spinal segments.
77. **Contraction of the ischiocavernosus muscles**–produces the rigid-erection phase.

    Contraction (rhythmic) of the bulbocavernosus muscle–necessary for ejaculation.
78. **Hippocampus**–Involved in penile erection

    Right insula and inferior frontal cortex–Visually evoked sexual stimulation

    Hypothalamus (paraventricular nucleus)–Facilitates penile erection

    Hypothalamus (Medial preoptic area)–Ability to recognize a sexual partner
79. **Norepinephrine**–principal neurotransmitter for penile flaccidity and detumescence.
80. - **NO released from nonadrenergic/noncholinergic (NANC) neurotransmission and from the endothelium** are principal neurotransmitter mediating penile erection.
    - NO increases the production of cGMP, which in turn relaxes the cavernous smooth muscle.
81. **Dopaminergic and adrenergic receptors**–promote sexual function.
82. **5-HT1 A receptor agonists**–inhibit erectile activity but facilitate ejaculation.

    5-HT2 C receptor agonists–enhanes erection.
83. **Norepinephrine** from nerve endings **and (endothelins and $PGF_2\alpha$) from endothelium** → ↑ IP_3 and DAG, → release of Ca^{2+}, → Ca^{2+} binds to calmodulin →catalyzes phosphorylation of myosin light chains →activates myosin ATPase, which hydrolyzes ATP to provide energy for muscle contraction.
84. GTP $\xrightarrow{\textbf{(guanyl cyclase)}}$ c GMP $\xrightarrow{\textbf{(PDE5)}}$ 5GMP.
85. **NO stimulates guanyl cyclase**–increases c GMP.

    PDE inhibitors–prevent degradation of c GMP.

86. Larginine and oxygen $\xrightarrow{\text{(NOS)}}$ Lcitrulline and NO.

		Ca^{2+} dependent	NADPH dependent
n NOS	Neurons	Yes	Yes
e NOS	Endothelial cells	Yes	Yes
i NOS	All cells	No	Yes

87. With the exception of PDE6–which is specifically expressed in photo-receptor cells, all PDEs have been identified in the corpus cavernosum.

88. Reflexogenic erection is preserved in 95% of patients with complete upper-cord lesions but in only about 25% of those with complete lower-cord lesions

89. Testosterone

- Enhances sexual interest
- Increases the frequency of sexual acts
- Increases the frequency of nocturnal erection
- **Little or no effect on fantasy-induced or visually stimulated erections.**

90. Antihypertensive causing ED–diuretics, β blocker (nonselective), α_2 blocker

91. Most common self-administered questionnaires (SAQs) include:

- International Index of Erectile Function **(IIEF).**
- Brief Male Sexual Function Inventory **(BMSFI).**
- Dysfunction Inventory for Treatment Satisfaction **(EDITS).**

92. The IIEF is the most widely used SAQ.

- **Its 15 items** address and quantify **five domains**: erectile function, orgasmic function, sexual desire, intercourse satisfaction and overall satisfaction.

93. Differentiation between Psychogenic and Organic ED

Characteristic	Organic	Psychogenic
Onset	Gradual	Acute
Circumstances	Global	Situational
Course	Constant	Varying
Noncoital erection	Poor	Rigid

Psychosexual problem	Secondary	Long history
Partner problem	Secondary	At onset
Anxiety and fear	Secondary	Primary

94. The metabolic syndrome includes glucose intolerance, insulin resistance, obesity, dyslipidemia, and hypertension and higher prevalence of ED

95. Most common performed diagnostic procedure for ED

Intracavernosal injection of vasodilator combined with genital or audiovisual sexual stimulation (CIS)

- It bypass–**neurologic and hormonal influences.**
- Evaluate the **vascular status** of the penis directly and objectively.

96. CIS and blood flow measurement by duplex ultrasound (7 to 10 MHz)

- Most reliable and least invasive evidence-based assessment of ED.
- Best tool available for the diagnosis of high-flow priapism.
- For localization of a ruptured artery.

97. RI; PSV–EDV ÷ PSV (Resistive index; peak systolic velocity- end diastolic velocity ÷ peak systolic velocity)

98. PSV >35 cm/s–associated with normal arteriography and defines normal cavernous arterial inflow.

RI > 0.9–normal penile vascular function

99. Rigiscan

- It is an automated, portable device used for **(nocturnal penile tumescence and rigidity)** NPTR
- Monitors radial rigidity, tumescence, number, and duration of erectile events

100. Recommended criteria for normal NPTR include

- Four to five erectile episodes per night
- Mean duration longer than 30 minutes
- Increase in circumference of more than 3 cm at the base and more than 2 cm at the tip

- Maximal rigidity above 70% at both base and tip

101. **In measuring serum testosterone** blood should be drawn–**between 8:00 AM and 11:00 AM.**
    - The typical reference range for the total testosterone measurement is 280 to 1000 ng/dL

102. **Indications for pituitary imaging:**
    - Severe central hypogonadism (testosterone <150ng/dL)
    - Panhypopituitarism,
    - Persistent hyperprolactinemia
    - Symptoms of tumor mass effect

103. **Testosterone preperations are-**
    - Intramuscular, subcutaneous, buccal, oral, transdermal and in pellets form

104. **Potential adverse effects of androgen therapy**
    - Erythrocytosis
    - Sleep apnea
    - Urinary symptoms
    - Prostate cancer progression risk
    - Gynecomastia
    - Acne

    On oral androgen therapy

    (hepatitis,cholestatic jaundice, hepatomas, hemorrhagic liver cysts, and hepatocellular carcinoma)

105. **PDE inhibitors**

	Sildenafil	**Vardenafil**	**Tadalafil**
Half-life	3-5 hr	4-5 hr	17.5 hr
Fatty food	Reduced absorption	Reduced absorption	No effect
Bachache	Rare	Rare	Yes
Blurred/blue vision	Yes	Rare	Rare
Precaution with antiarrhythmics	No	Yes	No

106. PDE inhibitors therapy

Nitrate use in any form is an absolute contraindication
Side effects observed

- Headache (**Most common-**15% to 16%)
- Dyspepsia (4% to 10%) and flushing (4% to 10%)
- Myalgia/back pain (0% to 3%),
- Nasal congestion (3% to 4%)
- Visual disturbances (0% to 3%).

107. Common intracavernous agents

Drug	Advantages	Disadvantages/Side effects
Papaverine	Low cost Stable at room temp	Fibrosis, priapism Elevation of liver enzymes
Papaverine + phentolamine	More potent than papaverine alone	Fibrosis, priapism
Alprostadil	Priapism rare	Painful erection Requires refrigeration Relatively expensive
Papaverine + phentolamine alprostadil	**Most potent**	Requires refrigeration

108. Papaverine–nonspecific PDE inhibitor, which prevents the degradation of cAMP and cGMP

Phentolamine methylate–is a competitive α-adrenoceptor antagonist with equal affinity for α_1- and α_2- adrenergic receptors.

PGE_1–causes smooth muscle relaxation, vasodilation, and inhibition of platelet aggregation through elevation of intracellular cyclic AMP.

109. MUSE (Medicated Urethral System for Erection)

- This technique relies on the absorption of medication through the mucosal lining into the surrounding corpus spongiosum
- Synthetic formulation of prostaglandin E1
- Response rate is approximately 50%
- Most common side effect–local urogenital pain (approximately one third of patients) and minor urethral bleeding (5%)

110. **Priapism**–full or partial erection that continues >4 hours beyond sexual stimulation and orgasm or is unrelated to sexual stimulation

111. **Stuttering priapism** described as recurrent unwanted and painful erections in men with sickle cell disease (SCD)

112. **Classification of priapism**

	Ischemic	**Nonischemic**
Priapism	Veno-occlusive or low-flow	Arterial or high-flow
Corpora cavernosa	Rigid and tender to palpation	Not fully rigid or painful
Blood gas analysis	Hypoxia, hypercapnia and acidosis	Do not reveal hypoxia or acidosis
Cavernosal artery	Minimal or absent blood flow	Normal or high flow
First line treatment	Evacuation of blood and irrigation with phenylephrine	Observation
Next line treatment	Distal shunt	Selective artery embolisation
Perineal trauma	Seldom	Usually
Hematologic abnormalities	Usually	Seldom

113. **PDE type 5 inhibitor with increased risk for priapism:**
- Sickle cell disease
- Spinal cord injury
- Men who used PDE5 inhibitor recreationally
- Men who used PDE5 inhibitor in combination with ICI
- Men with history of penile trauma
- Men on psychotropic medications
- Men abusing narcotic

114. **Causes of priapism**
- **α-Adrenergic Receptor Antagonists** (tamsulosin)
- **Antianxiety Agents** (Hydroxyzine)

- **Anticoagulants** (Heparin, warfarin)
- **Antidepressants and Antipsychotics** (trazodone, lithium, sertaline)
- **Antihypertensives** (Hydralazine, guanethidine, propanolol)
- Alcohol, cocaine
- Straddle injury, coital injury, pelvic trauma
- Sickle cell disease, thalassemia, leukemia, multiple myeloma, G6PD deficiency)
- Gonadotropin-releasing hormone, testosterone
- Scorpion sting, spider bite, rabies, malaria
- Amyloidosis, Fabry disease, gout
- **Neoplastic** (Prostate, urethra, testis, bladder, rectum, lung, kidney)
- Papaverine, phentolamine, prostaglandin E1, oral PDE type 5 inhibitors

115. Role of penile imaging in priapism

Color doppler ultrasound is an adjunct to the corporal aspirate in differentiating ischemic from nonischemic priapism

MRI has three possible roles:

- Imaging of a well-established arteriolar-sinusoidal fistula
- Identifying corporal thrombus
- Identifying corporal metastasis

116. Treatment of ischemic priapism

Initial treatment of ischemic priapism is the decompression of the corpora cavernosa by aspiration

- 19-gauge needle should be inserted at the peno-scrotal junction at 3 or 9 o'clock
- Compress the penile shaft between the thumb and first digit
- Aspirate the shaft until it is soft.
- Leaving the needle in place, the shaft is permitted to refill.
- Compression is reapplied and aspiration repeated.
- Aspiration should be repeated until no more dark blood can be seen coming out from the corpora

Corporal aspiration, if unsuccessful, should be followed by ICI of α-adrenergic injection or irrigation.

- Phenylephrine can be concentrated as 200 μg/ml in saline and administered intermittently as 0.5 mL to 1.0 mL, every 5 to 10 minutes to a maximum dosage of 1 mg.

117. Treatment of stuttering priapism

A trial of daily oral α-adrenergic, daily oral PDE5 inhibitor, baclofen and gonadotropin-releasing hormone (GnRH) agonists or antiandrogens may be used

118. Shunt procedures are subdivided on the basis of anatomic location on the penis

- Percutaneous distal shunts–Ebbehoj , Winter, or T-shunt
- Open distal shunt–Al-Ghorab
- Open proximal shunt–Quackles or Sacher
- Saphenous vein–Grayhack
- Deep dorsal vein shunt–Barry

119. Erectile function outcomes decline significantly when ischemic priapism has lasted >24 hours and that complete ED is anticipated if it persists for >36 hours

120. First choice–distal cavernoglanular shunt

- **Winter shunt**–placement of a large biopsy needle.
- **Ebbehoj shunt**–a scalpel percutaneously through the glans.
- **El-Ghorab shunt**–excision of the tunica albuginea at the tip of the corpus cavernosum (**most effective distal shunt,** although it is more invasive).

Proximal shunting by:

- **Quackels or Sacher shunt**–creation of a window between the corpus cavernosum and corpus spongiosum.
- **Grayhack shunt**–anastomosis of the saphenous vein to one of the corpora cavernosa.

121. Penile prosthesis implantation in the acute management of ischemic priapism should be considered early as there is preservation of penile length and technically easier implant insertion.

Delayed placement of penile prosthesis is technically challenging due to corporal fibrosis

122. Treatment of nonischemic priapism

- Cavernous aspiration has only a diagnostic role in high-flow priapism.
- Repeated aspirations, injection and irrigation with intracavernous sympathomimetics have no role
- Patients demanding immediate relief can be offered selective arterial embolization
- Where angio-embolization fails or is contraindicated, surgical ligation is reasonable.

123. Ejaculation is a reflex, which requires a complex interplay among somatic, sympathetic, and parasympathetic pathways involving dopaminergic and serotonergic neurons

In antegrade ejaculation, two basic phases are involved: emission and expulsion.

- **Emission-** first phase of ejaculation,and defined as the deposition of seminal fluid into the posterior urethra.
- **Expulsion-** due to the combined action of sympathetic and somatic pathways

Orgasm- pleasurable sensation resulting from cerebral processing of the increased pressure in the posterior urethra and contraction of the bulbar urethra bulb and accessory sexual organs.

124. Ejaculate

- First portion is provided by the bulbourethral glands followed by some fluid from the prostate.
- Second portion includes the bulk of the spermatozoa and is contributed by the epididymis and vas deferens, along with prostate and seminal vesicle contributions

125. Responsible for the expulsion phase of the ejaculate–somatic nervous system (represented by the pudendal nerve)

126. 5HT2C and 5HT1A receptor–former to delay and the latter to facilitate ejaculation.

127. Premature ejaculation as having three components:

(1) ejaculation that nearly always occurs within about 1 minute of vaginal penetration

(2) the inability to delay ejaculation on all or nearly all vaginal penetrations

(3) negative personal consequences such as distress, bother, frustration, and/or the avoidance of sexual intimacy.

128. **Paroxetine** exerts the strongest ejaculation delay.

129. **Dapoxetine**

- Time to maximum serum concentration (Tmax) of 1.3 hours
- Half-life (T1/2) of 1.5 hours

130. **Therapy for ED**

- First-line therapy- PDE5 inhibitors
- Second-line therapy- VCDs, IUD
- Third-line therapy- Intracavernous injections
- Fourth-line therapy- Penile prosthesis Implantation

131. **Malleable devices**

- Advantage of low mechanical failure rates and ease of use.
- Disadvantages include constant penile rigidity and an increased risk of erosion

Positionable penile prosthesis is a semirigid device

- Better able to maintain its upward and downward positions

Two-piece inflatable prosthesis

- Advantage–ease of implantation because there is no third piece (abdominal fluid reservoir).
- Disadvantage–compared with malleable devices is the increased risk of mechanical failure.

132. **All three-piece devices** provide penile girth expansion and rigidity similar to that of a normal erection. AMS 700 LGX–Inflatable penile prosthesis that also provides length expansion

133. **Comparison of Infrapubic and Penoscrotal Implant Approaches**

	Infrapubic Approach	**Penoscrotal Approach**
Advantages	Reservoir placement under vision	Better corporeal exposure
		No dorsal nerve injury
		Pump fixation possible
Disadvantages	Limited corporeal exposure	Blind reservoir placement
	Possible dorsal nerve injury	
	Inability to anchor pump	

134. When penile prosthesis gets infected

All components of the prosthesis should be removed.

Prosthesis reimplantation is done-

As soon as possible after device removal for infection to minimize loss of penile size and to facilitate corporeal dilation

135. If urethral perforation occurs during implantation of prosthesis

Implant procedure should be abandoned and a urethral catheter should be left in for 7 to 10 days.

Prosthesis reimplantation may be done at a later date

136. In the case of erosion of one cylinder of an inflatable device into the meatus or through the glans

- This cylinder should be removed as soon as possible
- Implantable plug is placed in the pump tubing that led to that cylinder.
- Later procedure to reimplant the second cylinder is not always necessary.

137. The symptomatic incidence of Peyronie's disease–1%.

- **Average age at onset of Peyronie's disease**–53 years.
- **Asymptomatic prevalence**–0.4% to 1.0%.

138. Thirty percent to 40% of men with Peyronie's disease will also have **Dupuytren disease**

139. In Peyronie's disease there are two phases.

- **Active phase,** associated with painful erections and changing deformity of the penis.
- **Secondary phase,** characterized by stabilization of the deformity, with disappearance of painful erection.

One third of patients, present with sudden development of painless deformity

140. Cause of Peyronie's disease.

- α-adrenergic blockers
- Phenytoin
- Urethral instrumentation
- Buckling trauma to the penis
- Paget disease of the bone

141. **Plaque of Peyronie's disease can be demonstrated on** USG, X-RAY and MRI (no role of CT)

142. Most patients with Peyronie's disease demonstrate lesions–**dorsally**

143. **Agents tried as medical management in peyronie's disease**

- Vitamin E
- Potassium aminobenzoate
- Terfenadine
- Tamoxifen
- Colchicine
- Carnitine
- Collagenase
- intralesional corticosteroid
- intralesional verapamil
- intralesional interferon
- Extracorporeal shockwave therapy

Radiation therapy should be avoided because of potential risk of malignant change and ED.

144. **The most common donor artery for penile revascularization**–inferior epigastric artery (usually connected to the dorsal artery of the penis by microvascular surgery).

- An end-to-end anastomosis from the arterial donor site to the recipient vessel is the **most physiologic choice.**

145. **With testosterone therapy**–fat mass decreases, bone and muscle mass increases (reverses the effect of aging).

146. **Three questionnaires have been developed to detect hypogonadism in adult men :**

(1) St. Louis University's ADAM
(2) Aging Male Survey (AMS)
(3) MMAS.

147. **The most widely accepted test is serum total Testosterone (T) levels.**

- >12 nmol/L (350 ng/dL) do not require substitution.

- <8 nmol/L (230 ng/dL) usually benefit from T treatment.
- If the levels are between 8 to 12 nmol/L, repeating total T once or twice may be helpful.

148. Equilibrium dialysis is the gold standard for free T measurement.

149. T treatment is contraindicated in men with prostate or breast cancer

T is relatively contraindicated in men at high risk of developing carcinoma of the prostate (family history).

Men should not be treated with T-

- Significant erythrocytosis
- Untreated obstructive sleep apnea
- Untreated severe congestive heart failure

(**Age–Not a contraindication** to initiate testosterone treatment).

Chapter 7
MALE GENITALIA

1. **Testicular cancer is the most common malignancy** among men aged 20 to 40 years and the second most common malignancy in males aged 15 to 19 years
2. The incidence of **bilateral germ cell tumor** (GCT) is approximately 2%
3. **Localized seminoma** is the most common presentation of GCT, representing 50%

   Regional or distant metastasis at diagnosis is present in approximately two thirds of NSGCTs and 15% of pure seminomas
4. **Risk factors for testicular cancer:**
   - Cryptorchidism,
   - Family history of testicular cancer,
   - Personal history of testicular cancer
   - Intratubular germ cell neoplasia (ITGCN).
5. **Males with undescended testes (UDT)**
   - Four to 6 times more likely to be diagnosed with testicular cancer
   - Relative risk (RR) falls to 2 to 3 if orchidopexy is performed before puberty
   - Contralateral descended testis is also at slightly increased RR of 1.74
6. **Patients with testicular cancer**

   Cumulative **risk of developing a GCT in the contralateral testis** was found to be 5.2%

   It is similar to the prevalence of **CIS in the contralateral testis.**
7. **Risk factors for the development of testicular CIS**
   - History of testicular carcinoma (5% to 6%).
   - EGCT (40%).
   - Cryptorchidism (3%).

- Contralateral testis with unilateral testicular cancer (5% to 6%).
- Atrophic contralateral testis with unilateral testicular cancer (30%).
- **Somatosexual ambiguity (25% to 100%).**
- Infertility (0.4% to 1.1%).

8. **In GCT 70% have an extra copy of chromosome 12 in the form of an isochromosome 12p**
9. **Primary mediastinal nonseminomatous (NSGCT) differ from those originating in the testis or retroperitoneum.**
   - Less sensitive to chemotherapy
   - Poor prognosis with a 5-year overall survival of about 45%.
   - More likely to have yolk sac tumor components and thus elevations in AFP.
   - Associated with Kleinfelter syndrome
   - Associated with hematologic malignancies that carry extra copies of the 12p
   - (Mediastinal seminomas carry a similar prognosis to testicular seminomas).
10. **GCTs are composed of five basic cell types**–seminoma, embryonal cell carcinoma, yolk sac tumor, teratoma and choriocarcinoma.
11. **Seminoma**
    - **Typical**–Most common in thirties, Syncytiotrophoblastic elements (α-hCG) occur in 10% to 15%.
    - **Anaplastic**
      - o More aggressive and more lethal.
      - o Greater mitotic activity.
      - o Higher rate of local invasion.
      - o Increased rate of metastatic spread.
      - o Higher β-hCG production.
    - **Spermatocytic**
      - o Prognosis is favorable.
      - o No documented cases of metastatic disease
      - o Not associated with a history of cryptorchidism or bilaterality,
      - o Does not express PLAP or i(12p)

- o Does not occur as part of mixed GCTs
- o Almost always cured with orchiectomy
- o Does not arise from CIS

12. Embryonal carcinoma

- Exhibits large areas of hemorrhage and necrosis.
- Is an aggressive tumor associated with a high rate of metastasis, often with normal serum tumor markers.
- It is the most undifferentiated cell type of NSGCT, with totipotential capacity to differentiate to other NSGCT cell types (including teratoma)

13. Choriocarcinoma

- Rare and aggressive tumor that presents as elevated serum hCG levels and disseminated disease.
- Common sites of metastases include lungs and brain.
- Prone to hemorrhage, sometimes both spontaneously and immediately after chemotherapy is initiated
- Choriocarcinoma has a propensity for hematogenous dissemination.

14. Yolk sac tumor

- **Most common testis tumor of infants and children.**
- Endodermal sinus tumor, adenocarcinoma of the infantile testis, juvenile embryonal carcinoma, and orchioblastoma are all used synonymously.
- **Schiller-Duval bodies** are present.

15. Teratomas

- Contain well-differentiated or incompletely differentiated elements of at least two of the three germ cell layers of endoderm, mesoderm, and ectoderm.
- Resistant to chemotherapy
- Teratomas may grow uncontrollably, invade surrounding structures, and become unresectable (known as growing teratoma syndrome)
- Teratoma may transform into a somatic malignancy such as rhabdomyosarcoma, adenocarcinoma, or primitive neuroectodermal tumor

- Unresected teratoma in patients with advanced NSGCT may result in late relapse

16. **Tumor markers**

Seminoma	AFP (0), HCG (10%)
Yolk sac tumor	AFP (90%), HCG (0)
Embryonal carcinoma	AFP (rare), HCG (rare)
Teratoma	AFP (25%)
Choriocarcinoma	AFP (0%), HCG (99%)

17. **Seminoma express–PLAP, CD 117**

    Embryonal tumor express–Keratin , CD 30.

18.

	AFP	**HCG**
Glycoprotein	Single chain	α and β polypeptide chains
M.W.	70,000	38,000
Half life	5-7 days	24-36 hours

19. **AFP levels may also be raised in patients with**
    - Cancers of the liver, stomach, pancreas, biliary tract, and lung.
    - Patients with nonmalignant liver disease (infectious, drug induced, alcohol-induced, autoimmune)
    - Ataxic telangiectasia and hereditary tyrosinemia.
20. **hCG levels may be elevated in**
    - Cancers of the liver, biliary tract, pancreas, stomach, lung, breast, kidney, and bladder.
    - Primary hypogonadism
    - Marijuana
21. **LDH**
    - Levels are elevated in approximately 20% of low stage GCTs and 20% to 60% of advanced GCTs.
    - LDH is expressed in smooth, cardiac, and skeletal muscle.
    - Lymphoma may also cause elevated LDH levels.
    - LDH-1 is the most frequently elevated isoenzyme in GCT.

- The magnitude of LDH elevation correlates with the bulk of disease.
- Main use is in the prognostic assessment of GCT at diagnosis.
- The serum half-life of LDH is 24 hours.

22. **Most common presentation** of testicular cancer is a painless testicular mass
23. **Testis-sparing surgery (or partial orchiectomy)**
    - May be considered for organ confined tumors of <2 cm in patients with synchronous bilateral tumors or tumor in a solitary testis with sufficient testicular androgen production
    - Adjuvant radiotherapy to the residual testis using doses of 20 Gy is sufficient to prevent the development of a GCT
24. **EAU 2012 guidelines**
    - Testicular ultrasound is mandatory assessment.
    - Orchidectomy and pathological examination of the testis are necessary to confirm the diagnosis and to define the local extension.
    - AFP, hCG and LDH must be performed before and after orchidectomy for staging and prognostic reasons.
    - The state of the retroperitoneal, mediastinal and supraclavicular nodes and viscera must be assessed in testicular cancer (chest and abdomino-pelvic CT).
25. **CT is the optimal modality for staging the retroperitoneum**

    False-negative results occur in 25% to 35% and 14% to 20% of patients with CS I NSGCT and seminoma, respectively, when a 1-cm cutoff is used
26. **Chest CT should be performed in**
    - Patients with elevated postorchiectomy levels of serum tumor markers
    - Evidence of metastatic disease by physical examination or abdominopelvic CT
    - Abnormal or equivocal findings on chest radiography.
27. **Scrotal ultrasonography** is extremely accurate in identifying solid intratesticular lesions with greater than 95% sensitivity and specificity.

28. Carcinoma-in-situ (CIS)

- Preinvasive precursor of all testicular GCTs except spermatocytic seminoma.
- 50% of men in whom CIS was found on biopsy developed "invasive" disease within 5 years if left untreated.
- Biopsy of the contralateral testis is not indicated in patients with GCT, owing to the protracted course of CIS.
- In patients with an atrophic testis, history of UDT, or age < 40 years, the risk of intratubular germ cell neoplasia (ITGCN) in the contralateral testis has been reported in up to 36%
- Open inguinal biopsy of the contralateral testis may be considered in patients with risk factors for ITGCN
- Radical orchiectomy and low-dose (20 Gy) radiation therapy are effective treatment options for ITGCN

29. With the exception of seminoma, the growth rate among GCTs tends to be high.

- **Doubling times range from 10 to 30 days.**

30. Ferility issues after chemotherapy and radiotherapy

- Virtually all patients will become azoospermic after chemotherapy
- 50% of patients with normal semen parameters at diagnosis will return to these levels within 2years and 80% within 5 years
- After two or four cycles of platinum-based chemotherapy a nadir in spermatogenesis is reached in 10 to 14 months.
- Recovery of spermatogenesis after radiation therapy for seminoma may take 2 to 3 years or more
- Despite defects in spermatogenesis and exposure to cytotoxic therapy, the incidence of birth defects is not increased in children conceived after treatment of testicular cancer
- Sperm cryopreservation should be offered to all patients before RPLND, chemotherapy, or radiation therapy owing to the potential effects of these treatments on fertility

31. TNM (UICC 2009)

pT1 Tumor limited to the testis and epididymis and no vascular/lymphatic invasion

pT2 Tumor limited to the testis and epididymis with vascular/ lymphatic invasion or tumor extending through the tunica albuginea with involvement of tunica vaginalis

pT3 Tumor invades the spermatic cord

pT4 Tumor invades the scrotum

N1 Lymph node mass <2 cm

N2 Lymph node mass, >2 cm but <5 cm

N3 Lymph node mass >5 cm

M1 Non-regional nodal or pulmonary metastases

M2 Non-pulmonary visceral masses

Serum Tumor Markers (S)

	LDH	hCG (mIU/mL)	AFP (ng/mL)
S1	<1.5 × N	<5,000	<1,000
S2	1.5-10 × N	5,000-50,000	1,000-10,000
S3	>10 × N	>50,000	>10,000

32. Among patients with NSGCT

- 50% to 70% have elevated levels of AFP.
- 40% to 60% have elevated levels of hCG.
- If both markers are measured simultaneously, approximately 90% of patients have elevation.
- 10% to 15% of patients can have normal marker level.

33. Seminoma GCT v/s nonseminomatous GCT

	Seminoma	Nonseminoma
Incidence at presentation	Stage 1- 85% Stage 2-10% Stage 3-5%	Stage 1- 33% Stage 2-33% Stage 3-33%
Incidence of occult metastasis	10% to 15%	25% to 35%
Risk of systemic relapse after treatment of retroperitoneum	1% to 4% after RT	10% after RPLND
Radiosensitive and chemosensitive	Yes	No
Poor risk category	No	Yes
Teratoma at metastatic site	No	Yes

34. **The most commonly identified risk factors for occult metastasis are** lymphovascular invasion and a predominant component of embryonal cell component.

35. **Seminoma**

STAGE 1

Stage 1 with no risk factors–tumors <6 cm in diameter, absence of vascular invasion, and normal β-hCG levels–option of surveillance.

Stage 1 with risk factors–radiation–25 Gy to para-aortic nodes only.

- **EAU 2012 guidelines**

Recommended option–Surveillance

Can be recommended–Carboplatin-based chemotherapy

STAGE 2 and 3

Stage IIA–N1 disease–Radiotherapy with 30 Gy (ipsilateral external iliac, the bilateral common iliac, the paracaval, and the paraaortic nodes superiorly)

Stage II B–N2 disease–Radiotherapy with 35 Gy. (>3 cm LN- 3 BEP)

Stage II C and III–3 BEP for good risk and 4 BEP for intermediate risk

- **EAU 2012 guidelines**

II A/B–Radiotherapy (RT)

IIB–Chemotherapy (3 × PEB, in good prognosis) is an alternative to RT

IIC and III–Chemotherapy (CT)

RESIDUAL MASSES

- Patients with discrete, residual masses >3 cm after first-line chemotherapy should undergo further evaluation with FDG-PET.
- Patients with PET-positive residual masses should undergo postchemotherapy surgical resection.
- Residual masses that are PET negative or < 3 cm can be safely observed after chemotherapy.
- (FDG-PET has no role in the assessment of NSGCT patients with residual masses after chemotherapy)

36. NSGCT

STAGE 1

Stage 1 no risk factors–surveillance.

Stage 1 with risk factors–modified RPLND/ 2 BEP (>40% of embryonal carcinoma, stage T2 or greater, presence of vascular or lymphatic invasion).

- **EAU 2012 guidelines**

pT1–If the patient is willing–**surveillance**

Not willing to undergo surveillance–2 BEP/nerve sparing RPLND

(pT2–pT4)–2BEP

Not willing to undergo BEP–surveillance/nerve sparing RPLND

STAGE 2

Stage IIA/B with elevated markers or LN > 3cm–CT

Stage IIA/B without marker elevation and LN < 3cm–RPLND

- **EAU 2012 guidelines**

Stage IIA/B with elevated markers–three or four cycles BEP.

Stage IIA/B without marker elevation–RPLND

Stage IIC with a good prognosis–three cycles of BEP.

Intermediate or poor prognosis–four cycles of BEP.

Surgical resection of residual masses after chemotherapy in NSGCT is indicated in the case of visible residual masses and when serum levels of tumor markers are normal

STAGE 3

Same as stage 2c.

RELAPSE

- The standard approach to patients who experience relapse within 2 years after first-line chemotherapy is conventional dose, second-line chemotherapy with ifosfamide-containing regimens (VIP).
- All patients with residual masses should undergo postchemotherapy resection given the 70% to 80% incidence of residual disease (viable malignancy and teratoma).
- The standard approach to patients who experience relapse 2 years or more after initial therapy is surgical resection of all sites of disease if feasible.

37. BEP×4 has remained the standard regimen for intermediate- and poor-risk GCT.

VIP (etoposide, ifosfamide and cisplatin)×4 resulted in more high-grade hematologic and genitourinary toxicity

38. Prognostic factors

NSGCT	SGCT
Good Prognosis	**Good Prognosis**
Testis or retroperitoneal primary No nonpulmonary visceral metastases S1	Any primary site No nonpulmonary visceral metastases Normal AFP, any LDH and hCG
Intermediate Prognosis Testis or retroperitoneal primary No nonpulmonary visceral metastases S2	**Intermediate Prognosis** Any primary site Nonpulmonary visceral metastases Normal AFP, any LDH and hCG
Poor Prognosis Mediastinal primary Nonpulmonary visceral metastases S3	**Poor Prognosis** No patient

39. Side effects

Bleomycin	Pulmonary fibrosis
Etoposide	Myelosuppression, alopecia, secondary leukemia
Cisplatin	Neurotoxic, nephrotoxic, nausea

40. Most common sites of origin of extragonadal germ cell tumor, in decreasing order of frequency–mediastinum, retroperitoneum, sacro-coccygeal region, and pineal gland.

41. Leydig cell tumor (Interstitial cell tumors)

- Most common of the sex cord–mesenchyma lesions.
- Excessive androgen or estrogen production.
- 10% malignant.
- Pathognomonic cigar-shaped crystals **(Reinke's crystals)** found in 40% of tumors.

- Radical inguinal orchiectomy is the initial treatment of choice.

42. **Most common secondary neoplasms of the testis**–lymphoma.
    - **Most common of all testicular tumors in patients >50 years**–lymphoma.
    - Orchidectomy for primary disease, chemotherapy for secondary lymphoma.
43. **Initial site of relapse in boys with ALL**–testis.
44. **The common primary sources, for carcinoma testis in decreasing order of frequency**–prostate, lung, gastrointestinal tract, melanoma and kidney.
45. **Adenomatoid tumor**
    - **Most common paratesticular tumor.**
    - **Epididymis is most common location.**
    - Within the epididymis the **globus minor is the most common site.**
    - These tumors are benign and managed by inguinal exploration and surgical excision
46. **Paratesticular rhabdomyosarcoma**
    - Most common sarcoma in children and adolescents.
    - Most commonly seen during the first 2 decades of life.
    - In adults liposarcoma is the most common histology in older adults
47. **The first echelon of LN draining the right testis–interaortocaval** area, followed by the precaval and preaortic LN.

    The primary "landing zone" for left-sided tumors–para-aortic and preaortic lymph nodes, followed by the interoartocaval LN.

    - After RPLND–**left para-aortic region is** the most common site of local recurrence prompting reoperation.

    Epididymis drain into–external iliac LN.

    Scrotal involvement by the primary tumor involves–inguinal LN.
48. **Contralateral spread is more common with** right-sided tumors, rare with left-sided tumors.
49. **Recommendations for patients with scrotal violation:**
    1. **Low stage seminoma**–radiation portals should be extended to include the ipsilateral groin and scrotum.

2. **Low-stage NSGCT**–scrotal scar should be widely excised with the spermatic cord remnant at the time of RPLND.

   (These patients are not good candidates for surveillance).

3. Patients treated with full-dose platinum based regimens- should have the cord stump removed at the time of RPLND

50. The rationale for treatment of the RPLND in patients with testicular cancer is based on several factors.

- RPLN spread is usually the first and often the only site of metastatic disease.
- In 15% to 40% of patients their disease is clinically understaged, particularly in retroperitoneum.
- Untreated RPLN metastases are usually fatal
- Most common site of late recurrence of both teratoma and viable GCT is **retroperitoneum**
- Late recurrences are usually chemorefractory, and survival rates are poor

51. Most common site of suprahilar disease is in the retrocrural space

52. Nerve-sparing techniques involve preservation of–sympathetic chains, the postganglionic sympathetic fibers (T12 to L4) and the hypogastric plexus.

53. In an effort to avoid disruption of sympathetic nerves and the hypogastric plexus, modified template goals are:

- Thoroughly resect all interaortocaval and ipsilateral LN between the level of the renal vessels and the bifurcation of the common iliac artery.
- Minimize contralateral dissection, particularly below the level of the IMA.

54. Post-chemotherapy pathologic findings in patients with advanced NSGCT **after induction therapy** are approximately as follows: necrosis, 50%; teratoma, 40%; viable carcinoma, 10%.

55. Post-chemotherapy pathologic findings in patients with advanced NSGCT **after salvage therapy** are approximately as follows: necrosis, 10%; teratoma, 40%; viable carcinoma, 50%.

56. In seminoma if post-chemotherapy residual masses <3 cm they may be observed.

An FDT PET scan should be done only for masses >3 cm (one of the only approved indication of PET scan in urology).

57. **Chylous ascites**

- Present with abdominal distention, prolonged ileus, pleural effusion, or chylous leakage from the incision.
- Ultrasonography or CT with paracentesis is diagnostic and may provide symptomatic relief.
- Chylous fluid has a milky or turbid appearance with a fat content of 4 to 40 g/L and a total protein content >30 g/L.
- Initial management is with diuretics and dietary manipulation (low-fat diet with medium-chain triglycerides) and/or TPN.
- Persistent drainage of chyle that is refractory to conservative measures may require peritoneovenous shunting
- Reoperation to repair lymphatic leakage is associated with a high failure rate and should be avoided.
- Asymptomatic lymphoceles require no treatment
- Percutaneous drainage for infection, hydronephrosis, or bowel obstruction is necessary in 1% to 2% of cases.

58. **Benign lesion**–pearly penile papules, hirsute papillomas and coronal papillae.

59. **Premalignant lesion**–cutaneous horn, psuedoepitheomatous micaceous, keratotic balanitis, BXO and leukoplakia.

60. **Associated with gross condylomata and Low grade dysplasia**–HPV types 6, 11 and 42 to 44.

    Association with malignant disease–HPV types 16, 18, 31, 33, 35 and 39.

61. **Topical treatment of choice for condyloma**–Imiquimod cream (5%).

62. **Condylomata**–regardless of size, always remain superficial and never invade adjacent tissue.

    BuschkeLöwenstein tumor–displaces, invades and destroys adjacent structures by compression.

63. **Carcinoma in situ (Tis) of the penis**

- **Erythroplasia of Queyrat**–involves the glans penis, prepuce,or penile shaft.

- **Bowen's disease**–involves the remainder of the genitalia or perineal region.

Progression to invasive carcinoma may occur in 5% to 33% of cases and metastasis rarely occur.

64. **Most frequently detected HPV type in primary carcinomas**–HPV-16.
65. **The earliest route of dissemination from penile carcinoma is** metastasis to the regional femoral and iliac nodes
66. **Lymphatics of the prepuce**
    - Joins with the lymphatics from the skin of the shaft.
    - These tributaries drain into the superficial inguinal LN (the nodes external to the fascia lata).

    Lymphatics of the glans
    - Join the lymphatics draining the corporal bodies.
    - Form a collar of connecting channels at the base of the penis that drain to superficial nodes.

    The superficial nodes →deep inguinal nodes (those deep to the fascia lata) →pelvic nodes (external iliac, internal iliac and obturator).
67. **In penis lymphatics**–no evidence of "skip" drainage.

    No report of spontaneous remission of carcinoma of the penis is known

    Multiple cross-connections exist at all levels of drainage–penile lymphatic drainage is bilateral to both inguinal areas.
68. **Penile tumors most common site-glans** (48%).
69. **Buck fascia acts as a temporary natural barrier** to local extension of the tumor, protecting the corporeal bodies from invasion.

    Penetration of Buck fascia and the tunica albuginea permits invasion of the vascular corpora and establishes the potential for vascular dissemination.
70. **Most tumors of the penis are squamous cell carcinomas** demonstrating keratinization, epithelial pearl formation, and various degrees of mitotic activity

    The **lower-grade carcinomas** demonstrate keratin, prominent intercellular bridges, and keratin pearls, characteristics that are absent in high-grade tumors.

- Half the tumors originating in the shaft are poorly differentiated tumors
- 10% of tumors located in the prepuce are high-grade tumors

71. Hypercalcemia without detectable osseous metastases has been associated with penile cancer

- Hypercalcemia is a function of the bulk of the disease.
- Associated with inguinal metastases and may resolve after excision of involved inguinal nodes
- Parathyroid hormone and related substances may be produced by both tumor and metastases that activate osteoclastic bone resorption
- Medical treatment of hypercalcemia includes aggressive saline hydration.
- Bisphosphonates (zoledronic acid) is first-line therapy

72. Role of imaging

- Small-volume glanular lesions, imaging studies add virtually no additional information.
- Role in examination of the inguinal region in obese patients or in those who have had prior inguinal surgery and for whom the physical examination may be unreliable

73. 2009 TNM Cancer Staging for Penile Cancer

Ta	Noninvasive verrucous carcinoma
T1a	Tumor invades subepithelial connective tissue without lymphovascular invasion and is not poorly differentiated
T1b	Tumor invades subepithelial connective tissue with lymphovascular invasion and/or poorly differentiated
T2	Tumor invades corpus spongiosum or cavernosum
T3	Tumor invades urethra or prostate
T4	Tumor invades other adjacent structures
N1	Palpable mobile unilateral superficial inguinal LN
N2	Palpable mobile multiple or bilateral superficial inguinal LN
N3	Metastases in deep inguinal or pelvic LN; unilateral or bilateral or fixed LN
M1	Distant metastasis

74. Strong risk factors for penile carcinorna :

- Phimosis.
- Chronic inflammatory conditions, e.g., balanoposthitis, lichen sclerosus and BXO.
- Sporalene and ultraviolet A photochemotherapy.
- Sexual history (multiple partners, early age of first intercourse).
- Condylomata (3-5-fold increased risk of penile cancer).
- Smoking.
- Penile trauma

75. Male early circumcision has been shown to be effective against penile carcinoma and HIV-1 infection.

There was no protective effect of circumcision for herpes simplex virus type 2 infection, syphilis, or gonorrhea.

Adult circumcision does not protect against penile cancer.

76. Most important adverse pathological prognostic factors– perineural invasion, lymphovascular invasion, and high histological grade.

77. Patients with penile primary tumors

- For low risk cohort (stages Tis, Ta, T1; grade 1 and grade 2 tumors)10% incidence of inguinal metastasis (this group is optimal candidates for organ preservation)
- For the high-risk cohort–50% to 70% incidence of inguinal metastasis.

78. EAU guidelines 2012

Tis, Ta, T1a (G1, G2)	Laser/wide excision/MMS
T1b (G3) and T2 (glans only)	Glansectomy
T2 (invasion of the corpora)	Partial amputation
T3 (invasion of urethra)	Total amputation with perineal urethrostomy
T4 (adjacent structures)	Neoadjuvant chemotherapy followed by surgery in responders.

79. 80% 5-year survival–<2LN, unilateral involvement, no evidence of extranodal extension of cancer and absence of pelvic nodal metastases.

80. **Requires combination therapy**–Patient with fixed LN, > 4 cm LN, Pelvic LN involvement.

81. **Prognostic markers of LN status**

HPV, P 53, CDKN2A, TA-4, Ki 67, E- Cadherin and MMP-9

82. **CO2 laser**

- Wavelength-10600
- Superficial depth of penetration (limited to 0.01 mm) makes it less than optimal for the treatment of penile carcinoma in situ or small T1 tumors.
- Local recurrence rates have been shown to be as high as 50%

Nd:YAG laser

- Protein denaturation at a depth of up to 6 mm by emitting at a wavelength of 1060 nm.
- Recurrences is 6.9%

KTP laser

- 532-nm wavelength laser
- Intermediate depth of penetration
- Better hemostasis than the CO2 laser.

83. **Management of LN**

T cis and Ta→

- Nonpalpable LN → observe
- Palpable L → confirm with 4 weeks antibiotics → FNAC
  - o Negative → confirm with excisional biopsy
  - o Positive →complete modified dissection

T1G1→

- Nonpalpable LN→ observe
- Palpable LN →confirm with 4 weeks of antibiotics →
  - o Negative→ observe
  - o Positive→ complete modified dissection

T1G2, 3 and T2 to T4 (minimum is complete modified dissection)

Bilateral nonpalpable → bilateral complete modified dissection
  - o Negative →observe
  - o Positive→deep inguinal+PLND

Unilateral palpable → complete modified on negative side→deep inguinal+PLND on positive side

Bilateral palpable→ consider FNAC →

- o Negative→complete modified dissection
- o Positive→ deep inguinal+PLND

84. Inguinal lymphadenectomy should be bilateral rather than unilateral for patients presenting with unilateral adenopathy at initial presentation of the primary tumor

85. Bilateral inguinal lymphadenectomy should not be performed in patients who present with unilateral lymphadenopathy some time after the initial presentation and treatment of the primary tumor

(Exception- in patients with a bulky unilateral recurrence, a contralateral inguinal staging procedure should be considered)

86. Pelvic lymphadenectomy should be performed in all patients with inguinal metastases

(**Exception-**in patients with only a single small lymph node metastasis discovered at the time of a inguinal dissection with no extracapsular extension, nor high grade)

87. Pelvic lymphadenectomy should include the distal common iliac, external iliac, and obturator nodes.

(No further benefit is gained from proximal iliac or paraaortic dissection)

88. Key aspects of the modified inguinal lymphadenopathy

- Shorter skin incision.
- Limitation of the dissection by excluding the area lateral to the femoral artery and caudal to the fossa ovalis.
- Preservation of the saphenous vein.
- Elimination of the need to transpose the sartorius muscle.
- Indicated for patients at increased risk for inguinal metastasis and clinically negative groins on examination (stage T2 or greater, presence of vascular/ lymphatic invasion, or high grade).

89. The most common sign of penile metastasis–priapism.

90. Chemotherapy for penile cancer

PMB (cisplatin, methotrexate, and bleomycin)

TIP (paclitaxel, ifosfamide, and cisplatin)

91. **Extramammary Paget disease of the penis**

- Disease is identified microscopically by presence of large, round or oval, clear-staining **hydropic cells** with hypochromatic nuclei (i.e., Paget cells).
- The cells stain positively for CK 7 and CEA but are S-100 protein negative
- Slow-growing intraepithelial adenocarcinoma with cells derived from apocrine glands.
- Cells may become invasive with dermal tumor deposits metastasizing to LN via dermal lymphatics
- Penoscrotal extramammary Paget disease may be associated with other malignancies of the genitourinary tract, such as prostate, bladder, and renal malignancies

92. **Bilateral pelvic lymphadenectomy** is best accomplished by an extraperitoneal approach through a lower midline incision.

    For unilateral dissection–modified Gibson incision or an S-shaped ilioinguinal incision

93. **Etiologic factors for urethral malignancies**

    Chronic inflammation due to a history of frequent STD, urethritis, and urethral stricture, and HPV 16 in squamous cell carcinoma of the urethra

94. **Treatment for urethral malignancies**

    Carcinoma of penile urethra-

    - Partial penectomy with a 2-cm negative margin is the treatment of choice
    - Ilioinguinal lymphadenectomy is indicated in the presence of palpable inguinal lymph nodes without evidence of metastatic disease.
    - Prophylactic inguinal lymph node dissection is not indicated

    Carcinoma of bulbomembranous urethra-

    Radical cystoprostatectomy, pelvic lymphadenectomy, and total penectomy are usually required.

95. **Most common site of male urethral tumor**–bulbomembranous urethra (60%)

96. **Most common urethral cancers**–squamous cell carcinoma (80% in male and 50%–70% in female).

97. Urologic malignant neoplasm that is Female > Male–urethral carcinoma.

98. The initial phase, **imbibition**, takes about 48 hours. The second phase, **inosculation**, also requires about 48 hours.

99.

	Split thickness graft	Full thickness graft
Structure	100% epidermis and part of dermis	100% epidermis and dermis and part of fat
Graft endurance	High chance	Lower chance
Confronting to trauma	Less resistance	More resistance
Cosmetic appearance	Poor, more contraction	Good, less contraction
Disadvantage	Poor cosmetic appearance	High risk of graft failure, greater risk for deformation

100. Buccal mucosal graft

- Panlaminar plexus.
- Graft can be thinned somewhat, provided a sufficient amount of deep lamina is carried to preserve the physical characteristics.
- Graft is thought to have optimal vascular characteristics.
- Wet epithelium.

101. Four grafts that have been successfully used for primary urethral reconstruction are

- full-thickness skin graft
- bladder epithelial graft
- oral mucosal graft
- rectal mucosal graft

102. A random flap is a flap without a defined cuticular vascular territory.

The term **axial flap** means that there is a defined vessel in the base of the flap. There are three types of axial flaps:

- **A peninsular flap**–vascular continuity and the cutaneous continuity of the flap base are left intact.
- **An island flap**–vascular continuity is maintained; however, the cuticular continuity is divided.
- **The microvascular free transfer flap**–vascular continuity and the cuticular continuity interrupted.

103. Reiter syndrome

- Classic triad of arthritis, conjunctivitis, and urethritis.
- Can have episode of diarrhea.
- Circinate balanitis, this lesion is diagnostic (10%-20%).
- Urethritis can causes severe inflammation with necrosis of mucosa, producing uncompromising stricture disease.

104. Lichen sclerosus (LS) or balanitis xerotica obliterans (BXO)

- Incidences of LS have been described in people of all ages
- The most common cause of meatal stenosis is LS
- It appears as a whitish plaque that involve the prepuce, glans penis, urethral meatus, and fossa navicularis.
- The combination of topical steroids and antibiotics may help stabilize the inflammatory process
- Retrograde urethrography should be performed before the initiation of therapy.
- Squamous cell carcinoma occurs in patients with a long history of lichen sclerosus

105. The term urethral stricture refers to anterior urethral disease, or a scarring process involving the spongy erectile tissue of the corpus spongiosum (spongiofibrosis)

106. Posterior urethral "strictures" are not included in the common definition of urethral stricture.

- Posterior urethral stricture is an obliterative process in the posterior urethra that has resulted in fibrosis and is generally the effect of **distraction.**

107. Evaluation of urethral stricture

- USG of the bulbous urethra possibly more accurately determines the length of the stricture than contrast studies.
- If the patient is not in steep lateral oblique position for RGU, the length of the stricture will be underestimated.

108. Parts of urethra

- **Fossa navicularis** is lined with stratified squamous epithelium.
- **Pendulous urethra** is lined with simple squamous epithelium.
- **Bulbous urethra** is lined distally with squamous epithelium.

- **Membranous urethra**
  - o Unattached to fixed structures.
  - o Only portion of the male urethra that is not invested by another structure.
  - o Lined with a delicate transitional epithelium.
- **Prostatic urethra** surrounded by the prostatic stromal and glandular tissue.

109. Glands of Littre

- Open into the urethra along its dorsal surface.
- Distributed more numerously distally and less proximally.
- These can form small diverticula called lacunae of Morgagni.

Cowper's glands

- Open into the urethra in the bulb.
- Travel to the glands located in the urogenital membrane adjacent to the membranous urethra.

110. Internal urethrotomy

- **Indicated in**
  - o Strictures of the bulbous urethra
  - o Stricture should be <1.5 cm in length
  - o Sticture should not be associated with deep, dense spongiofibrosis
- **Done by making a single incision at the 12-o'clock position**
- **The most common complication** is recurrence of stricture
- **Failure rate with long-term catheterization** after internal urethrotomy is similar to that seen with 3 to 7 days of catheterization.
- When the catheter is removed, the patient is started on a **self catheterisation** regimen.
- Most regimens require more frequent catheterizations early in the recovery period, with a tapering schedule during the next 3 to 6 months.

111. "Gold standard" form of repair for anterior urethral strictures- excision with primary anastomosis

112. Onlay procedures (graft or flap) are attended with a higher success rate than tubularized grafts or tubularized skin islands.

Tubularized flaps provide better results than tubularized grafts.

113. Pelvic fracture urethral injuries

- They are the result of blunt pelvic trauma and accompany about 10% of pelvic fracture injuries.
- These injuries most commonly involve only the bulbous urethra
- Distraction injuries are for all intents unique to the membranous urethra
- Reconstruction should be considered within 4 to 6 months after trauma

114. Chordee without hypospadias includes– types I, II and III anomaly.

- This term implies that although the meatus is not improperly placed, curvature is due to inappropriate fetal development of the ventral penile structures.
- These patients are not characterized by large erect penises. In contrast, patients with congenital curvature of the penis seem to have exceptionally large erect penises.

Congenital curvature of the penis–type IV anomaly.

Congenital short urethra–type V anomaly.

115. Classification of congenital curvatures

- **In type I,** the urethral meatus is at the tip of the glans. **None** of the surrounding layers are normally formed.
- **In type II**, a dysgenetic band of fibrous tissue thought to be derived from the mesenchyma, which would have produced **Buck's fascia and the dartos fascia,** lies beneath and lateral to the urethra. Urethra is contained within normal corpus spongiosum.
- **In type III,** the urethra, corpus spongiosum and Buck's fascia are all normally developed and ventrally fused but abnormal development of **dartos fascia.**
- **In type IV,** although the urethra, corpus spongiosum and fascial layers are normally developed, there is relative shortness or **inelasticity of one aspect of the tunica albuginea** of the corpora cavernosa.
- **Type V** implies that there has been correct fusion of all elements of the penis (i.e., tunica albuginea, urethral epithelium, corpus spongiosum, Buck's fascia, dartos fascia and ventral skin) but during erection urethra and corpus spongiosum are **not long or compliant** enough to match compliance of other ventral tissue layers.

116. Most common employed method for total phallic construction and penile reconstruction–forearm flaps.

117. Blood supply

TESTIS	EPIDYDIMIS	VAS DEFERENS
Testicular (internal spermatic) artery ← aorta	**Superior epididymal artery**← testicular artery	Seminal vesicle region: **deferential artery**←internal iliac/superior vesicle artery
Deferential artery ←internal iliac/superior vesicle artery	**Inferior epididymal artery**← Deferential artery	Testicular region: **deferential artery**← inferior epididymal artery
Cremasteric (external spermatic) artery ← inferior epigastric artery		

118. No-scalpel vasectomy

- Significantly decreases the rate of hematomas, infections, and pain
- Patient can resume sexual activity sooner after surgery and have a shorter operative time
- Fascial interposition is the technique that has been found to decrease vasectomy recanalization rates the most significantly
- Division of the vas deferens should be performed approximately 3 cm distal to the cauda of the epididymis in the straight portion
- Semen analysis at three months and twenty ejaculations after vasectomy should reveal azoospermia.
- Vasectomy should be repeated if any motile sperm are found in the ejaculate three months after the initial vasectomy
- Hematoma is the most common complication of vasectomy.

119. Chronic orchitis is defined as constant or intermittent scrotal pain lasting at least 3 months or longer, and of unclear cause

High-frequency transducer sonography (7.5 to 10 MHz) is considered the best modality for evaluation of scrotal pathology including orchitis

120. **80% of patients with absence of a seminal vesicle or vas deferens had ipsilateral renal agenesis.**

121. **Seminal vesicle pathology**

- **Ejaculatory duct obstruction or absence of seminal vesicles**–semen analysis revealing a low seminal volume and a lack of liquefaction and fructose.
- **Mainstay imaging** for the diagnostic evaluation of seminal vesicle pathology–high-resolution TRUS
- **Seminal vesicle obstruction may result in** following characteristics
  - Anteroposterior diameter > 15 mm
  - Length > 35 mm
  - Large anechoic areas, which contain sperm when aspirated

122. **Surgical approach to the seminal vesicles**

- **Anterior approach**–for patients with large benign masses or cysts, and for patients with an ectopic ureter draining into a seminal vesicle cyst, so the kidney, ureter, and seminal vesicle can all be approached concomitantly
- **Transperineal approach**–offers minimal blood loss, minimal pain, and early ambulation
- **Transcoccygeal approach**–useful for patients who have had previous suprapubic or perineal surgeries

123. **Tumors of the seminal vesicles** are extremely rare and most common is benign primary tumours

❑❑

Chapter 8
RENAL PHYSIOLOGY AND PATHOPHYSIOLOGY

1. **Renal blood flow**–20% of total cardiac output.

   Flow to the outer cortex is 3 times greater than that to the **inner cortex**, which in turn is 3 times greater than that to the **medulla.**

2. **GFR depends on:**

   - Transglomerular pressure (most significant determinant).
   - Renal plasma flow.
   - Glomerular permeability.
   - Oncotic pressure.

3. **Autoregulation** of intraglomerular capillary pressure (IGP) is effective to a mean arterial pressure (MAP) of about 70 mm Hg

   Tubuloglomerular feedback (TGF)–are monitored by delivery of sodium cations and chloride anions to the distal tubule

4. **Best measure of GFR**–inulin clearance.

   The most widely used estimate of GFR–24-hour creatinine clearance.

   Plasma cystatin C–This test likely will replace PCr as the standard test in GFR assessment.

5. **Creatinine**

   - Creatinine production is constant within an individual from day to day
   - Marked variation in production rates between individuals.
   - The absolute rate depends upon muscle mass, which in turn is influenced by age, sex, and body mass.
   - Every 50% reduction in GFR results in a doubling of PCr.
   - As GFR falls, tubular secretion of creatinine increases; so, PCr may not change noticeably
   - Creatinine clearance may overestimate GFR as renal function slowly declines when measured in the "steady state."

- Creatinine production may increase in states of increased muscle breakdown or increased dietary protein intake
- Creatinine production may decrease with liver cirrhosis

6. **Cockcroft and Gault**–the formula is (140-age) × weight × 0.85 (women)/ P cr × 72.

   MDRD formula–this estimate of GFR depends on four-variable (PCr, age, sex and ethnicity).

7. **Vasoconstrictor of renal artery tone**–angiotensin, norepinephrine, endothelin ,vasopressin, ANP.

8. **Angiotensin** II–pronounced constrictive effect on the efferent than the afferent arteriole.

   - Vasoconstriction, aldosterone release, sodium retention and β adrenergic stimulation is mediated by the AT1 receptor

9. **Norepinephrine** vasoconstricts all the major vascular beds in the kidney, mediated through the α1 receptor

10. **Endothelin is the most potent vasoconstrictor yet identified.**

    The ET1 receptors are subclassified into

    - ET (A) which are purely vasoconstrictive
    - ET (B) receptors may cause either vasodilation (stimulate release of NO from endothelial cells), or vasoconstriction of vascular smooth muscle cells

    Properties of ET-1

    - Aldosterone secretion
    - Produces positive inotropy and chronotropy in the heart
    - Decreases renal blood flow and GFR
    - Releases ANP

11. **Vasopressin** does not directly change RBF at low doses.

    At high doses potentiate the vasoconstrictive effects of norepinephrine and can induce renal ischemia

12. **Atrial natriuretic peptide (ANP)**

    - Increase GFR without a change in renal blood flow (afferent arteriolar VD and efferent arteriolar VC)
    - ANP increases natriuresis through inhibition of sodium

reabsorption in the medullary collecting duct , decreased renin and decreased aldosterone production.

13. **Vasodilators of renal artery tone**–NO, CO, Acetylcholine, PGE2.

14. **Arginine + NADPH + O_2 Citrulline + NADP + H_2O + NO**

15. **Erythropoietin production**–kidney from interstitial fibroblasts (90%) and liver (10%).

16. **Vitamin D_3 requires two hydroxylations to become active.**

    - **The first hydroxylation occurs in**–liver to form 25 hydroxycholecalciferol **(calcidiol).**
    - **A second hydroxylation occurs in**–tubular cell of kidney to form 1,25-dihydroxycholecalciferol **(calcitriol).**
    - Calcitriol is the biologically active form and 100 times more potent than calcidiol.

17. **Calcitriol primary function** is the maintenance of serum calcium and phosphorus levels. Main target organs are

    - Intestine (increases intestinal absorption of calcium, and to a lesser extent, phosphorus)
    - Bones (regulates osteoblast activity, and in combination with PTH, allows for osteoclast activation and bone resorption)
    - Kidney (increases reabsorption of calcium)
    - Parathyroid gland (suppresses PTH release).

18. **The renal effects of PTH are**

    - It increases active calcium reabsorption at the level of the DCT
    - It decreases phosphate reabsorption in the PCT (and the distal tubule, to a lesser degree) through its action on the sodium phosphorus cotransporter
    - It stimulates calcitriol production by increasing 1α-hydoxylase levels

19. **Major stimuli for ADH release**

    - Hyperosmolality, hypovolemia, hypoglycemia, pregnancy, nausea.

Inhibitors for ADH release

- Hypo-osmolarity, hypervolemia, phenytoin and ethanol.

20. **Action of ADH**

- It facilitates the insertion of preformed water channels, known as AQP-2, into the luminal membrane of the principal cell (through V2 receptors)
- Increases systemic vascular resistance (through V1 receptor)
- Increased sodium reabsorption
- Increases potassium excretion
- Increases prostaglandin synthesis
- Increases ACTH secretion (through V3 receptors),
- Release of both factor VIII and von Willebrand factor from vascular endothelium.

21. **PCT**

Reabsorption of 60% of the glomerular filtrate:

- Reabsorbs 65% of the filtered **sodium, potassium and calcium.**
- Reabsorbs 80% of filtered **phosphate, water and bicarbonate.**
- Reabsorbs 100% of filtered **glucose and amino acids.**
- Reabsorbs 15% of filtered **magnesium.**

22. **Sodium is the most significant solute for the PCT because-**

- Only solute that is actively reabsorbed (through basolaterally located Na-K ATPase pump). (All other solutes are passively reabsorbed through Na+ coupled transport).
- Early reabsorption of Na+ creates an osmotic gradient that facilitate passive reabsorption of water.

23. **Thin descending LOH**

- High water permeability due to abundant expression of AQP-1

24. **Thin ascending LOH**

- Impermeable to water.
- High permeability for NaCl as well as urea

25. **Thick ascending LOH (TALH)**

- Reabsorbs 25% to 30% of the **sodium filtered across the glomerulus.**

- Reabsorbs 15% of the filtered **calcium.**
- Reabsorbs 60% to 70% of **magnesium.**
- Reabsorbs 10% to 20% of the **filtered bicarbonate.**
- Site of secretion of **Tamm-Horsfall mucoprotein or uromodulin.**

26. **Critical to the formation of the interstitial concentration gradient**–sodium reabsorption along the TAHL, in the absence of water reabsorption.

27. **DCT**
    - Reabsorbs 5% to 10% of the **sodium filtered through the glomerulus.**
    - Reabsorbs 10% to 15% of **calcium.**
    - Reabsorbs 5% to 10% of **filtered magnesium.**

28. **Cortical CD**
    - **Principal cells** (65%)–involved with NaCl reabsorption and K^+ regulation.
    - **Intercalated cells** (35%)–involved with acid secretion and K^+ regulation.

    Type A intercalated cells–involved with H^+ secretion.

    Type B intercalated cells–involved with bicarbonate secretion.

29. **Medullary CD**
    - **Impermeable to water in the basal state.**
    - Under the influence of ADH, permeability increases in both the inner MCT and outer MCT through the insertion of AQP-2 water channels.
    - **oMCT is relatively impermeable to urea,** both in the basal state and under ADH stimulation
    - **iMCT has a high basal permeability for urea and under the influence of ADH urea permeability** can further increase by 4 times.
        - o This allows a high concentration of urea to develop in the interstitium.
        - o This sustain the osmotic gradient that is responsible for water reabsorption and ultimately urinary concentration.

30. Total sodium deficit

- (Volume of distribution) × body weight (kg) × (125-plasma [Na^+]).
- Volume of distribution is 0.5 for men and 0.6 for women.
- The serum sodium concentration should be raised < 25 mEq/L in the first 48 hours, at a rate of <2 mEq/L/hr, and the target goal should be 125 mEq/L.
- If the hyponatremia is severe but chronic, the rate of correction should not exceed 8 to 12 mmol/L/day, or a cerebral demyelination syndrome may occur.

31. The water deficit

(Volume of distribution) × body weight (kg) × (plasma [Na]$^+$/140-1).

32. Urinary excretion of potassium can be increased in the kidney through:

- Increased aldosterone.
- High sodium load in the distal tubule.
- Acidosis.

Potassium is driven into the cells:

- Insulin.
- Bicarbonate.
- β-agonists.

33. Hypokalemia

- Increased losses through the gastrointestine or urine.
- Diuretics, laxatives, amphotericin, theophylline.
- Postobstructive diuresis.
- Adrenal adenoma, Cushing's syndrome and adrenal carcinoma.

34. Hyperkalemia

- Renal failure.
- Drugs (potassium-sparing diuretics, lithium, digoxin, ACE inhibitors).
- Chronic acidosis (e.g., renal tubular acidosis type 4).
- Hypoaldosteronism.

The classical ECG changes include a short QT interval, peaked T waves, and ultimately ventricular arrhythmias.

35. Treatment of hyperkalemia

Mild hyperkalemia without ECG changes- dietary restriction and reversal of underlying causes.

ECG changes require emergency therapy:

- Intravenous calcium gluconate and drugs to drive the potassium into the cell, including sodium bicarbonate, Insulin, and nebulized albuterol.

Therapy to remove potassium stores-

- potassium binding exchange resins (kayexalate, calcium resonium)

Hemodialysis can remove extracellular potassium the **most quickly and completely.**

36. **Anion gap**–difference between cations (Na^+) and anions (Cl and CO_2) in blood.

- Anion gap = $Na^+ - (Cl + HCO_3) = 140 - (105 - 24) = 11$.
- The normal range is 9 to 14 mEq/L.
- Predominant unmeasured anions include albumin and phosphate.
- Predominant unmeasured cations include Ca^{++}, Mg^{++} and gamma globulins.

37. **Hyperchloremic metabolic acidosis with normal anion gap**

- Hyperalimentation
- Ketoacidosis
- Diarrhea
- Ureterosigmoidostomy
- Enteric fistula
- Primary mineralocorticoid deficiency
- Hyper-aldosteronism

38.

	pH	**pCO2**
Metabolic acidosis	↓	↓
Metabolic alkalosis	↑	↑
Respiratory acidosis	↓	↑
Respiratory alkalosis	↑	↓

Broadly in metabolic disorders p H and p CO2 are in same directions

Broadly in respiratory disorders pH and pCO2 are in opposite directions

39. **RTA Type 1** (classical/distal).
    - **Most common form of RTA.**
    - Failure of H^+ secretion in the distal nephron (abnormalities in the H^+ ATPase).
    - Hypokalemic, hyperchloremic, non-anion gap metabolic acidosis.
    - Nephrolithiasis, nephrocalcinosis and elevated urine pH (>6.0).
    - Most common stone associated is **calcium phosphate** as a result of **hypercalciuria, hypocitraturia (most important) and increased urinary pH.**
    - **>70%** of adults with distal RTA have kidney stones.
40. **RTA Type 2** (proximal)
    - Failure of bicarbonate reabsorption in the proximal tubule.
    - **Stone formation does not occur.**
    - More common in children, and it can lead to growth retardation and metabolic bone disease.
41. **Type 4 RTA**
    - Impairment of cation exchange in the distal tubule with reduced secretion of both H^+ and K^+.
    - It is due to aldosterone deficiency or resistance.
    - **Hyperkalemia.**
    - Associated with CRF, seen in patients with interstitial renal disease and diabetic nephropathy.
42. **For operational purposes, hypertension in adults is defined as** a systolic pressure greater than 160 mm Hg or a diastolic pressure greater than 95 mm Hg or both (WHO)
43. **Definition of renovascular hypertension** is hypertension resulting from a renal arterial lesion that is relieved by correction of the offending lesion or removal of the kidney.
44. **Atherosclerosis**
    - Approximately 70% of all renovascular lesions are caused by atherosclerosis

- Predominantly in males.
- In older age groups.
- Progressive in 40%
- In the proximal 2 cm of the renal artery.

45. Intimal fibroplasia

- In children and young adults.
- Progressive
- Collagenous disease involving intima.

46. True fibromuscular hyperplasia

- In children and young adults.
- Progressive
- Diffusely involves media.

47. Medial fibroplasia

- **Most common of the fibrous lesions (70% to 80%)**
- In women between the ages of 25 and 50 years.
- Does not dissect, thrombose, or rupture, and seldom progresses after 40 year of age
- Involves both renal arteries.
- Angiographically, demonstrates a typical **"string of beads"** appearance.

48. Perimedial fibroplasia

- In young women between the ages of 15 and 30 years.
- Girlie disease.

49. Fibromuscular hyperplasia

- Extremely rare disease.
- In children and young adults.

50. Rate limiting step-Conversion of angiotensinogen to angiotensin I (AI) through the action of renin

Angiotensin I (AI) is converted to angiotensin II (A II) by angiotensin converting enzyme (ACE)

Angiotensinogen

- It functions as a serine protease inhibitor.
- The liver is the primary site of synthesis.

51. **Renin**

- Secreted from the juxtaglomerular cells of the afferent arteriole.
- The kidney is the major site of synthesis.

52. **The macula densa** is at the **thick ascending loop of henle** and comes in close proximity to the juxtaglomerular cells

    Signal for macula densa–controlled renin release is due to alteration of **tubular chloride concentration**

53. **Renin stimulation by:**

- Reduction of distal tubule salt delivery.
- Diminished cell stretch as a result of renal hypoperfusion.
- Stimulation of α-adrenergic nerves.
- Agents that increase adenylate cyclase activityβ-adrenergic agonists, prostaglandin E_2, prostaglandin I_2, dopamine, histamine and parathyroid hormone.

54. **Angiotensin II receptor subtypes:**

- **AT1 receptor**–located at glomeruli and tubulointerstitium.
- **AT2 receptor**–located at cortical blood vessels.

55. **Ischemic nephropathy (IN)**

- This occurs in bilateral severe stenosis or stenosis to a functionally or anatomically solitary kidney with deterioration of renal function
- It is the result of chronic hypoperfusion of the total functioning renal mass.

56. **Renal autoregulation fails to maintain the GFR when:**

- Renal perfusion < 70 mm Hg.
- Luminal diameter of the renal artery is stenosed by >70% of the original size.

57. **Risk factors strongly predictive of significant Atherosclerotic renal artery disease(ARAS)**

- Higher age
- Coronary artery disease
- History of congestive heart failure
- Female gender

- Peripheral vascular disease.
- An elevated serum creatinine level

58. Features s/o HTN associated with renovascular disease are:

- Onset of hypertension <30 years or >55 years.
- Sudden onset and shorter duration of hypertension.
- Hypertension that is difficult to control.
- Accelerated, malignant hypertension or hypertensive crises.

59. Diagnosis of RVHTN

- **Test that diagnose hyperactivity of the RAAS but provide no anatomic information of arterial lesion**–Plasma renin activity [PRA], captopril test, captopril renography, and RVR assays.
- Captopril renography and RVR assays can localize the ischemic kidney as well.
- **Anatomic delineation of the arterial lesion is obtained by** intra-arterial angiography.
- DUS, MRA, and spiral CTA can be used before angiography in cases in which clinical suspicion of RVH is not confirmed by functional tests.

60. Captopril test

- Measurement of peripheral PRA before and after an oral dose of captopril.
- Patients may continue to take β blockers, but all diuretics and ACE inhibitors need to be discontinued for at least 1 week before the test.
- The test is not reliable in patients who are azotemic, nor it is accurate for use in children.
- The low sensitivity of test makes it unsuitable for use as a general screening test for RVH.

61. Renal vein rennin–RVR assays are useful for localizing the ischemic kidney in unilateral RAS as well as the more ischemic kidney in bilateral cases.

62. Management of renovascular hypertension (RVH)

High suspicion

- Angiography (directly).

Low or moderate suspicion–captopril renography as a preliminary test.

- A positive test–angiography.
- Technically satisfactory negative study–no intervention.
- Technically unsatisfactory studies–DUS, MRA, or CTA (provide no functional information or prediction of cure after intervention).

63. **Revascularization for the preservation of renal function in patients with unilateral ARAS and an unobstructed contralateral renal artery**–no benefit.

    Revascularization to preserve renal function contraindicated with –serum creatinine level >4 mg/dL.

64. **Glomerular hyalinization indicates**–irreversible ischemic renal injury that obviates any benefit from revascularisation.

    Changes of **chronic reversible renal ischemia**–presence of tubular atrophy, interstitial fibrosis, and arteriolar sclerosis

65. **For surgical renal reconstruction**–aortorenal bypass with a free graft of autogenous hypogastric artery or saphenous vein.

66. **Percutaneous transluminal angioplasty (PTA)**
    - Performed in cases of FD.
    - Technical success > 90%.

67. **RAS in children is caused by**
    - Takayasu arteritis
    - Fibrous dysplasia
    - Middle aortic syndrome
    - Neurofibromatosis.

68. **Renal artery stents**
    - Adjunct to PTA
    - Oppose this recoil force and provide better results for angioplasty
    - Higher success of PTA with stenting in treating ostial ASO when compared with PTA alone.

69. **Renal artery aneurysm**
    - **Most common type–Saccular** aneurysms.

    Does not require operative intervention in
    - <2-cm, well-calcified renal arterial aneurysm, in an asymptomatic normotensive patient

Surgical removal is indicated for renal arterial aneurysms if:

- Aneurysm causing renal ischemia and hypertension.
- Dissecting aneurysm.
- Local symptoms such as flank pain or hematuria.
- Woman of childbearing age who is likely to conceive.
- Functionally significant renal arterial stenosis.
- Radiographic evidence of expansion on serial radiographs.
- Aneurysm containing a thrombus detectable on angiography with evidence of distal embolization.

70. **Renal arteriovenous fistulas**

- **Most common type**–Acquired fistulas.
- **Most common cause**–Iatrogenic trauma resulting from needle biopsy of the kidney.
- >70% of fistulas occurring after needle biopsy close spontaneously within 18 months.

71. **Renal arterial thrombosis** commonly involves the proximal or middle third of the main renal artery.

    Renal arterial embolization generally involves peripheral arterial branches.

72. **Page kidney**

- **Kidney compressed** by a subcapsular or perirenal process causing renal ischemia, inducing unilateral hypersecretion of renin and contralateral suppression.
- Causes of the perinephric process–blunt trauma, closed renal biopsy, anticoagulation and hemorrhage from a tumor.
- Some cases–resolves spontaneously.
- Medical antihypertensive therapy–control the BP until the hematoma resolves.
- If the hematoma does not resolve–drained percutaneously or surgically.

❑❑

Chapter 9

UPPER URINARY TRACT OBSTRUCTION AND TRAUMA

1. **Obstructive uropathy**–functional or anatomic obstruction of urinary flow at any level of the urinary tract
2. **Obstructive nephropathy**–obstructive uropathy + renal damage.
3.

	UUO	BUO
First phase (first 1 to 2 hours)	RBF ↑, P_T ↑, Vasodilation (PG and NO)	Lesser ↑ in RBF
Second phase (3 to 4 hours)	RBF ↓, P_T ↑ (angiotensin II)	
Third phase (>5 hours)	RBF ↓ P_T ↓	Greater ↓ in RBF
Triphasic pattern	Yes	No
Postobstruction diuresis	↑ urine flow ↑ FE_{Na} ↓ FE_K	↑↑ urine flow, ↑↑ FE_{Na} ↑ FE_K
Shift of blood flow	Outer to inner cortex	Inner to outer cortex

4. **Normal urine concentrating ability requires hypertonic medullary interstitial gradient because of**
   - Active salt reabsorption from the thick ascending LOH
   - Urea back flux from the inner medullary collecting duct
   - Water permeability of the collecting duct mediated by vasopressin and aquaporin water channels
5. **Dysregulation of aquaporin water channels contribute to the long-term polyuria and impaired concentrating capacity in the**
   - Proximal tubule
   - Thin descending loop
   - Collecting duct.
6. **Urinary enzymes (derived from the proximal tubule) elevated in patients with obstructed kidneys such as**
   - Alkaline phosphatase,

- γ-glutamyltransferase,
- *N*-acetyl-β-D-glucosaminidase
- Leucine aminopeptidase

7. **Obstruction leads to**
   - Elevated levels of angiotensin II, cytokines, and growth factors
   - Tubular cell apoptosis and cellular inflammation, increased net matrix formation, and tubulointerstitial fibrosis.

8. **Compensatory renal growth (CRG)**
   - Reduction in CRG occurs with increasing age
   - CRG is directly proportional to the duration of obstruction
   - CRG is less prominent with partial than with total UUO
   - Kidney enlarges, an increase in the number of nephrons or glomeruli does not occur

9. **Renal recovery after relief of obstruction is affected by:**
   - Duration of obstruction.
   - Degree of obstruction.
   - Patient's age.
   - Baseline renal function.
   - Renal cortical thickness
   - Compliance of collecting system
   - Presence of pyelolymphatic backflow

10. **DMSA**
    - Superior to tubular selective agents, such as DTPA or MAG3, **for the prediction of renal recovery.**
    - Better defines the functional cortex and is less affected by the dilated collecting system and dilution by undrained urine

11. **Resistive index** values > 0.7 reflects elevated resistance to blood flow and thus suggest obstructive uropathy

12. **Whitaker test:**
    - Measurement of renal pelvic pressure.
    - Infusion of either saline or contrast material at the rate of **10 mL/min.**

- Intrapelvic pressure of:
  - o <15 cm H_2O normal.
  - o **>22 cm H_2O–obstruction.**
  - o Between 15 and 22 cm H_2O–indeterminate.
- Sensitivity and specificity of 79% and 50%.

13. Nuclear renography

- Radiopharmaceutical tracers are **administered IV**, and their uptake and subsequent clearance can then be evaluated and quantitated scintigraphically.
- **Half-time**
  - o <10 minutes is normal,
  - o between 10 and 20 minutes is equivocal
  - o >20 minutes is considered obstructed
- Patients should be well **hydrated**
- **Bladder catheterization** should be performed to maintain low intravesical pressure (should be done in cases such as suspected LUT obstruction, VUR, neurogenic or noncompliant bladder, or low-lying, pelvic kidneys)
- Diuretic, typically furosemide (F), is administered 20 minutes after the tracer to induce a brisk diuresis **(F+20 study).**

14. Non contrast CT (NCCT)

- **Demonstrates calculi classically considered radiolucent when** evaluated by plain radiography, including uric acid, xanthine, dihydroxyadenine, and many drug-induced stones.
- **Exceptions**–calculi composed of protease inhibitors, which are not visualized by noncontrast CT

15. CT signs of obstruction

  - o ureteral dilatation
  - o nephromegaly
  - o decreased parenchymal density of the involved kidney as compared with the contralateral renal unit
  - o perinephric stranding, or fluid can facilitate the diagnosis of acute obstruction.
- NCCT is a **excellent technique for evaluating patients suspected of having chronic obstruction** who have renal insufficiency or other contrast risks

16. **Contrast CT**

- Significantly improved sensitivity for identification of the cause of obstruction compared with IVU.
- Excellent correlation between isotope and CT-estimated GFR.
- Useful in surgical planning for PUJO, with good sensitivity for detection of crossing vessel

17.

Accuracy	**MRI**	**IVU**
Obstruction due to stones	93%	96%
Obstruction related to strictures	100%	55%

The absence of ionizing radiation has allowed MRI use in the assessment of children, women of child-bearing age, and pregnant patients with flank pain and hydronephrosis

18. **Renal drainage**

Pregnant women

- <22 weeks–PCN better option.
- >22 weeks–DJ stenting better option.

Pyonephrosis–PCN should be strongly considered.

- For decompression of the renal collecting system, **ureteral stents and percutaneous nephrostomy catheters are equally effective (EAU Guidelines 2012).**

19. **Predictors of stent failure**

- Diagnosis of cancer.
- Metastatic disease requiring chemotherapy or radiation.
- Renal insufficiency.

20. **NSAIDs is first-line drugs for the management of renal colic** with narcotics being reserved as second-line drugs

21. **Postobstructive diuresis**

- Urine output of >200 mL/hr.
- Downregulation of sodium transporters with subsequent impaired sodium reabsorption in the TALH, prevents maintenance of the medullary interstitial solute gradient promoting a continued diuresis.
- The increased endogenous production and altered regulation of ANP induce a saline diuresis.

- Poor responsiveness of the collecting duct to ADH, due to a downregulation of aquaporin water channels in collecting duct and proximal tubule.

22. Retroperitoneal fibrosis (Ormond's disease) (RPF)

- 3:1 male-to-female ratio.
- Mean age at onset is 50 years.
- Centers around the distal aorta at L4-L5.
- In 70% of the cases, the disease is idiopathic.
- Malignancy in 8% to 10% of cases.
- If there is evidence of obstructive uropathy at presentation, therapy should be first directed at its correction by DJS or PCN
- Biopsy to exclude malignancy should be performed next.
- Medical treatment
  - o Prednisolone administered at an oral dose of 60 mg on alternate days for 2 months
  - o Tapered to 5 mg daily over the next 2 months.
  - o 5 mg is continued for a total of 2 years.
- Ureterolysis if medical therapy fails or if the patient is not a candidate for medical therapy.

23. Causes of RPF

- Hydralazine
- Haloperidol
- Methyldopa
- Methysergide
- β Blockers
- Ergotamine alkaloids
- Phenacetin
- Amphetamines

24. Pelvic lipomatosis

- 18:1 male-to-female ratio.
- On IVU, the bladder characteristically assumes a pear or gourd shape.

25. Endometriosis of the urinary tract

- Endometriosis is defined as presence of functional endometrial tissue in an ectopic site
- Affect 10% to 20% of women of reproductive age, with a peak incidence in the mid-20s
- Predominantly found in the bladder (80%).
- 80% of ureteral endometriosis is extrinsic and primarily involves the distal ureter.
- Left > Right.
- If renal function normal and minimal hydronephrosis **with no** functional obstruction–treatment is **gonadotropin-releasing** hormone agonists.
- If the patient does not desire future pregnancy- **treatment** is TAH +BSO
- If pregnancy is desired, lesser extirpative procedures, such as unilateral oophorectomy.

26. Circumcaval or retrocaval ureter

- Persistence of the posterior cardinal vein as the infrarenal cava.
- Failure of the supracardinal vein to develop into the infrarenal IVC (subcardinal vein persists as the infrarenal IVC)
- 2.8:1 male-to-female ratio.
- Present in the third or fourth decade of life.
- Majority involve right ureter, although **left-sided circumcaval ureter has been reported.**
- Type I crosses at the level of the L3 and type II crosses at the level of UPJ.
- Definitive diagnosis can be made noninvasively using three-dimensional CT imaging
- A spatulated ureteroureterostomy is performed **only if patient is symptomatic.**

27. Significant crossing vessels have been noted in 63% of cases of UPJ obstruction and 20% of cases of normal kidneys.

28. Differentiation between PUJO and MCKD by ^{99m}Tc-DTPA

29. In PUJO kidneys with <15% differential function–nonsalvageable in adults.

30. **Endopyelotomy**

- Termed by Badlani.
- **Full-thickness lateral incision** is given through the obstructing proximal ureter, from the ureteral lumen out to the peripelvic and periureteral fat.
- Site for percutaneous access- midposterior or superolateral calyx
- **Incision should be made–laterally** (Patient should be devoid of crossing vessels)
- **Indication**–UPJ obstruction + upper tract stone disease (because the stones can be managed concomitantly)
- **Contraindications include** a long segment (>2 cm) of obstruction, active infection, or untreated coagulopathy
- **Follow up**
  - o Stent is removed after 4 weeks,
  - o Further after 1 month diuretic scan is done.
  - o If the patient remains asymptomatic and the diuretic renography reveals normal drainage reevaluation is performed at 6 months and then at 12-month intervals

31. **Dismembered pyeloplasty**

Contraindication–UPJ obstruction associated with lengthy or multiple proximal ureteral strictures. UPJ obstruction is associated with a small, relatively inaccessible intrarenal pelvis

32. **The Foley Y-V-plasty**

Indication–repair of a UPJ obstruction secondary to a high ureteral insertion.

Contraindication–when transposition of lower pole vessels is necessary

Situations requiring concomitant reduction of redundant renal pelvis.

33. **The Culp-DeWeerd spiral flap**

Indication–for large, readily accessible extrarenal pelvis in which the ureteral insertion is already in a dependent, oblique position.

34. **Scardino-Prince vertical flap technique**–when a dependent UPJ is situated at the medial margin of a large, square ("box-shaped") extrarenal pelvis.

35. Ureterocalycostomy

Indication

- UPJobstruction associated with a relatively small intrarenal pelvis
- UPJ is associated with rotational anomalies such as horseshoe kidney
- Salvage technique for the failed pyeloplasty

36. Endourological management of ureteric stricture

- **Stent placement–**
  Adequate drainage is short lived in ureteral obstruction from extrinsic compression
- **Balloon dilatation–**not to be used in active infection or a stricture longer than 2 cm
  Best results of ballon dilation is obtained in patients with iatrogenic strictures compared with anastomotic stricture (85% vs 50%)
- **Endoureterotomy**
  - **Lower ureteral strictures are incised–**anteromedial direction.
  - **Upper ureteral strictures are incised–**laterally or posterolaterally.

37. Ureteric stricture with function <20%–nephrectomy.

- **<2 cm ureteric stricture with function >20%**–managed endourologically.
- **>2 cm ureteric stricture with function >20%**–lap/open repair.

38. Bridging various ureteral defect lengths.

Technique	**Ureteral Defect Length (cm)**
Ureteroureterostomy	2–3
Ureteroneocystostomy	4–5
Psoas hitch	6–10
Boari flap	12–15
Renal descensus	5–8

39. Psoas hitch

- The ipsilateral bladder dome is secured to the psoas minor tendon or the psoas major muscle.

- Avoid injury to the genitofemoral nerve and the femoral nerve in the vicinity when placing these sutures
- Additional mobility can be achieved by dividing the contralateral superior vesical artery

40. For boari flap

- Base of the flap–> 4 cm in width.
- Tip of the flap–> 3 cm in width.
- The flap length–estimated ureteral defect + 3 to 4 cm.
- Ratio of flap length to base width–3:1.

41. When treating left ureteroenteric strictures–the risk of hemorrhage is a consideration because the sigmoid mesentery can be in close proximity.

42. Transureteroureterostomy

- **Absolute contraindications**–presence of a diseased recipient ureter or a donor ureter of inadequate length.
- **Relative contraindications**–history of stones, RPF, urothelial malignancy, CPN and abdominopelvic radiation.

43. American association for the surgery of trauma organ injury severity scale for the Kidney:

- I–Microscopic or gross hematuria, urologic studies normal.
  - o Subcapsular hematoma, nonexpanding **without parenchymal laceration.**
- II–Nonexpanding perirenal hematoma confined to renal retroperitoneum.
  - o **Laceration <1 cm** parenchymal depth of renal cortex without urinary extravasation.
- III–**Laceration >1 cm** parenchymal depth of renal cortex without collecting system rupture or urinary extravasation.
- IV–Parenchymal laceration **extending through renal cortex, medulla, and collecting system.**
  - o Main renal artery or vein injury with contained hemorrhage.
- V–Completely shattered kidney.
  - o **Avulsion of renal hilum,** devascularizing the kidney.

44. CECT (EAU Recommendation 2012).

- All blunt trauma patients with gross hematuria and patients with microscopic hematuria and shock.

- All penetrating injuries with any degree of hematuria should be imaged.
- CT scan with enhancement of intravenous contrast material is the best imaging study for the diagnosis and staging of renal injuries in haemodynamically stable patients.
- CT is more sensitive and specific than IVP, ultrasonography or angiography.

45. **CT findings that suggest major injury** are:
    - Medial hematoma, suggesting vascular injury.
    - Medial urinary extravasation, suggesting renal pelvis or UPJ injury.
    - Lack of contrast enhancement of the parenchyma.
46. **Single shot IVU (EAU Recommendation 2012)**
    - Only a single film is taken 10 minutes after IV push of 2 mL/kg of contrast material.
    - Unstable patients who require emergency surgical exploration should undergo a one-shot IVP.
47. **Indications for surgical management (EAU Recommendation 2012):**
    - Haemodynamic instability.
    - Exploration for associated injuries.
    - Expanding or pulsatile peri-renal haematoma identified during laparotomy.
    - Grade 5 injury.
    - UPJ disruption

    Relative indications
    - Urinary extravasation.
    - Nonviable tissue.
    - Delayed diagnosis of arterial injury.
    - Segmental arterial injury.
    - Incomplete staging.
48. **Expectant management** (bed rest, prophylactic antibiotics, and continuous monitoring of vital signs)
    - In grade 1-4 blunt renal trauma, stable patients

- In grade 1-3 stab and low-velocity gunshot wounds, stable patients.

49. **Hysterectomy** was responsible for the majority (54%) of surgical ureteral injuries.

50. **American association for the surgery of trauma organ injury severity scale for the ureter**

Grade	Description
I	Contusion or hematoma without devascularization
II	<50% transaction
III	≥50% transaction
IV	Complete transection with <2 cm devascularization
V	Avulsion with >2 cm devascularization

51. **Principles of repair of complete ureteric injury.**
    - Debridement of ureteral ends to fresh tissue.
    - Spatulation of ureteral ends.
    - Placement of internal stent.
    - Watertight closure of reconstructed ureter with absorbable suture.
    - Placement of external, non-suction drain.
    - Isolation of injury with peritoneum or omentum.

52. **Options for damage control in ureteral injuries:**
    - Do nothing but plan a reoperation when the patient is more stable, usually within 24 hours
    - Place a ureteral stent and do nothing else
    - Exteriorize the ureter
    - Tie off the ureter and plan percutaneous nephrostomy

53. **Immediate recognition of ureteric injuries**

    Repair should be done immediately

54. **Delayed recognition of ureteric injuries**
    - Triad of fever, leukocytosis, and generalized peritoneal signs
    - Immediate attempt at placement of a double-J ureteral stent (but this is possible in only 20%)
    - In cases in which retrograde ureteral stent can not be placed, then place a PCN and make a gentle attempt at anterograde stenting of the injury.

- If this fails, wait 7 to 14 days to reattempt anterograde ureteral stenting.
- If the ureter ultimately cannot be stented, safest approach is to allow at least 6 weeks for complete healing of the wounds and then attempt open repair

55. **Ureteral perforation** can be treated by ureteral stenting, usually with no subsequent complications

56. **Options of reconstruction after ureteral injury (EAU Guildelines 2012)**

Upper third:

- Ureteroureterostomy.
- Transureteroureterostomy.
- Ureterocalycostomy.

Middle third:

- Ureteroureterostomy.
- Transureteroureterostomy.
- Boari flap and reimplantation.

Lower third:

- Direct reimplantation.
- Psoas hitch.
- Blandy cystoplasty.

Complete:

- Ileal interposition.
- Autotransplantation.

Chapter 10

RENAL FAILURE AND TRANSPLANTATION

1. **Acute kidney injury (AKI)**
   - Defined as a rapid reduction in renal function characterized by progressive azotemia, which may or may not be accompanied by oliguria.
   - The cardinal feature of AKI is a decline in glomerular filtration rate (GFR)
   - SCr is produced at a constant rate by muscle and accurately reflects GFR

2. **The causes of AKI are**
   - 45% - ATN
   - 21% - prerenal
   - 13% - acute or chronic renal failure
   - 10% - urinary tract obstruction,
   - 4% - glomerulonephritis/vasculitis
   - 2% - acute interstitial nephritis (AIN)
   - 1% - atheroembolic renal disease.

3. **The hallmark of prerenal azotemia** is its reversibility with treatment of the underlying cause and the lack of structural damage to the kidney.

   The "gold standard" is the response to appropriate fluid repletion, return of renal function to the previous baseline within 24 to 72 hours.

4. **AII** has selectively greater vasoconstrictor effects on the efferent than afferent arteriole

   Prostaglandins can cause afferent arteriolar vasodilation.

   AKI can be caused by- drugs that selectively block AII synthesis. (ACE inhibitors, and angiotensin II receptor blocker) or that inhibit prostaglandin synthesis (NSAIDs).

5. **Diagnosis of urinary extravasation**

   The drain creatinine is compared with the SCr.

   Ratios of 10 : 1 are virtually diagnostic for extravasation

6. **Urine Sediment in Acute Renal Failure**

Sediment Findings	Diagnosis
Normal	Prerenal/obstruction
Red blood cell casts, red blood cells	AGN
Eosinophils, WBC and sterile urine	AIN
Pigmented granular casts	ATN

7. **During prolonged ischemia**

   - Nephron structures located in the **outer medulla, are most sensitive to injury.**
   - **The S3 portion of the proximal tubule sustains the most severe injury.**

8. **The sentinel biochemical event in renal ischemia is** the depletion of ATP, which is the major energy currency for cellular work

9. **Low fractional excretion of sodium** (FE_{Na})

   - Hepatorenal syndrome.
   - Selected types of ATN, such as that due to IV contrast material.
   - Rhabdomyolysis.
   - Sepsis.
   - Multisystem organ failure.

   High fractional excretion of sodium (FE_{Na})

   - ATN.
   - Obstruction.

10. **Presence of marked oligoanuria suggests** urinary tract obstruction, renovascular occlusion, or cortical necrosis

11. Patterns of Urinary Indices in Acute Renal Failure

	Prerenal/Acute Glomerulonephritis	Acute Tubular Necrosis/ Obstruction
Urinary [Na^+] mEq/L	<20	>40
Urine: plasma creatinine	>30	<20
Renal failure index	<1	>1
FENa	<1	>1
Urinary osmolality	>500	<400

12. Complication of AKI

- Hyponatremia
- Hyperkalemia
- Hypermagnesemia
- Hyperphosphatemia
- Hypocalcemia
- Hypercalcemia (postrhabdomyolysis)
- Hyperuricemia
- Metabolic acidosis

13. Management of ATN

- **Isotonic fluid repletion.**
- Use of **diuretics** may increase urine output, but does not improve patient survival
    - o Both loop diuretics and mannitol wash out debris and casts
    - o Loop diuretics decrease active NaCl transport in the thick ascending limb of Henle and thereby limit energy requirements in the metabolically active segment
    - o Mannitol, an osmotic diuretic, ameliorates AKI by increasing RBF, increasing urine flow, reducing hypoxic cell swelling, protecting mitochondrial function, and scavenging free radicals
- If a trial of **dopamine** is considered, it should be limited to a 24- to 48-hour infusion.

- Role of **fenoldopam, ANP, dopamine, calcium channel blockers, and growth factors** is controversial

14. Dietary changes in AKI

Protein intake should not be severely restricted

Dietary phosphorus, potassium, and sodium chloride may be restricted.

In the critically ill patient, nutritional support via TPN or enteral feedings should be considered.

15. Hyperkalemia (If serum potassium exceeds 6 mEq/L)

Earliest ECG change–peaked T waves with subsequent broadening of the PR interval and eventual QRS broadening, which may mature into a sine wave form.

The stages of therapy for acute hyperkalemia include

(1) stabilizing the electrical membrane of the cardiac conduction system (IV Calcium)

(2) shifting potassium back intracellularly (IV Glucose and insulin or sodium bicarbonate)

(3) eventual elimination of potassium from the body. (Cationic binding resin–Kayexalate)

16. Dialysis treatment itself may have a detrimental impact on the course of AKI from ATN.

Three potential mechanisms is

- Fall in urine volume
- Dialysis-induced hypotension,
- Complement activation resulting from the blood-dialysis membrane interaction

17. The mortality rate for patients with ATN is consistently around 50%

18. Azotemic patients who require radiocontrast procedures

- IV hydration with isotonic fluids
- Use of nonionic contrast material in the lowest dose possible.
- Use of sodium bicarbonate as an isotonic fluid may be beneficial.
- *N*-acetylcysteine for 48 hours before the procedure

19. **Staging of CKD**

Stage	Description	GFR (mL/min/1.73 m^2)
1.	Kidney damage with normal or increased GFR	≥90
2.	Kidney damage with mild decrease in GFR	60 to 89
3.	Moderate decrease in GFR	30 to 59
4.	Severe decrease in GFR	15 to 29
5.	Kidney failure	<15 (or dialysis)

20. The National Institutes of Health Consensus Conference of 1993 recommended that patients with **CKD be referred to a nephrologist** when the SCr > 1.5 mg/dL in females and >2.0 mg/dL in males.

21. **Proposed criteria for initiation of renal replacement therapy (RRT):**

- Oliguria (urine output < 200 mL/12 hr) or anuria.
- Hyperkalemia ([K^+] > 6.5 mmol/L).
- Severe dysnatremia ([Na] > 160 or < 115 mmol/L).
- Severe acidemia (pH < 7.1).
- Azotemia ([urea] > 30 mmol/L).
- Pulmonary edema.
- Uremic encephalopathy, pericarditis, neuropathy.
- Drug overdose with dialyzable toxin.

22. **Renoprotective strategies (Goals 8 treatment)**

- Blood pressure control (130/80)- ACE inhibitor, salt restriction, diuresis
- Reduction in proteinuria (<0.5 g/day)- ACE inhibitor
- Glycemic–control (HbA1C <7%)- Oral hypoglycaemic agents
- Lipid lowering (LDL ≤70 mg/dL)- Statin
- Anemia management (Hb 11-12 g/dL)- Erythropoietin
- Lifestyle modifications- Ideal body weight, smoking cessation, exercise 3/week, depression modification

- Calcium × phosphorous product (<55)- Vitamin D supplementation, dietary phosphorous restriction

23. **Causes of anemia in CRF**
    - Decrease erythropoeitin production
    - Blood loss from hemodialysis
    - Low levels of iron and folic acid
    - Excessive destruction of red blood cells
24. **Drugs requiring no dose modification in renal failure**

    Antifungals
    - Ketoconazole
    - Miconazole

    Cephalosporins
    - Cefoperazone
    - Ceftrixone
    - Cefuroxime axetil

    Macrolides
    - Azithromycin
    - Erythromycin

    Pencillins
    - Dicloxacillin
    - Nafcillin
    - Moxifloxacin

    Tetracyclines
    - Doxycycline

    Chloramphenicol

    Clindamycin

    Linezolid
25. **Most common cause of ESRD**–(1) DM (2) hypertension (3) glomerulonephritis.
26. **Permanent renal failure**–irreversible GFR <10 mL/min or serum creatinine level >8 mg/dL.
27. **Predominant form of therapy for adults with ESRD**–in-center hemodialysis.

Predominant form of therapy for patients <20 years with ESRD–transplantation.

28. **Peritoneal dialysis:**

Indicated in

- Patients with desire for self-care.
- Long distance from a hemodialysis unit.
- Serious cardiac disease.
- Diabetes mellitus (DM).
- Small stature.

Not indicated in

- Obesity.
- Hernias.
- Poor hygiene.
- IBD.
- Obliterated peritoneal space.

29. **First long-term success with human renal allografting, was achieved by**–Murray in 1954.
30. **Probability of disease recurrence and the risk of secondary graft failure high in**–FSG, HUS and primary oxalosis.
31. **Indications for Pretransplant Nephrectomy**
    - Autosomal-dominant polycystic kidney disease (ADPKD).
    - Medically refractory hypertension.
    - Chronically infected kidneys.
    - Suspected renal or urothelial cancer.
    - Urolithiasis.
32. **The criteria for an ideal deceased kidney donor are**
    - Normal renal function
    - No hypertension requiring treatment or DM
    - No malignancy other than a primary brain tumor or treated superficial skin cancer
    - No generalized viral or bacterial infection, and negative assays for syphilis, hepatitis, HIV, and HTLV

- Acceptable urinalysis
- Age between 6 and 50 years,

33. **Advantages of LDN** (Laparoscopic donor nephrectomy)–decreased analgesic requirement, decreased length of hospital stay, and an earlier return to work.

    Disadvantages of LDN–increased operating time, donor surgeon preference for the left kidney, an increased need for special equipment, a longer warm ischemia time, and delayed graft function.

34. **First kidney graft is usually placed**–extraperitoneally in the contralateral iliac fossa by way of a rectus-preserving Gibson incision.

    (EAU Guidelines 2012)

    LDN offers equal urological complications, graft function and graft survival to ODN, with less post-operative morbidity, shorter convalescence and better cosmetic results.

    The use of **living donors has been associated with higher** success rates than seen with deceased donor donation.

    The **donor should always be left with the 'better' kidney.**

    Kidney removal through a transperitoneal approach has a higher number of splenic and intestinal complications compared with other surgical alternatives.

    UW–solution and HTK–solution are standard storage solutions and equally effective for both multiorgan-donors and kidney-only donors.

35. **Renal artery** is usually anastomosed to the end of the internal iliac artery or to the side of the external iliac artery.
    - The **renal vein,** is usually anastomosed end to side to the external iliac vein.
    - **Urinary tract reconstruction** is by anti-reflux ureteroneo-cystostomy.

36. **MHC genes**–short arm of chromosome 6.

37. **Rejection**
    - **Hyperacute rejection (HAR)**
      - o Occurs immediately after renal revascularization.
      - o Irreversible process mediated by preformed circulating

cytotoxic antibodies that develop after pregnancy, blood transfusions, or an earlier failed transplantation.

- **Accelerated rejection**
  - o Occurs within days to weeks.
  - o Does not respond to antirejection therapy.
  - o It is mediated by humoral and cellular components of the immune response.
- **Acute cellular rejection (ACR)**
  - o Much more common than HAR, occurring in 10-40% of transplants.
  - o Usually occurs from 5 days post transplant.
  - o Most likely within the first 3 months, though may occur after this time.
  - o Usually responds well to steroid bolus treatment.
- **Acute humoral rejection (AHR)**
  - o Much less frequent than ACR, occurring in 5-20% of transplants.
  - o Most likely within the first 3 months post-transplant.
  - o Presence of certain histological features and/or positive C4d immunostaining and/or anti-HLA antibodies.
  - o Worse prognosis than ACR because more difficult to treat.
- **Chronic rejection**
  - o Gradual decline in renal function associated with interstitial fibrosis, vascular changes, and minimal mononuclear cell infiltration.

38. **Banff classification** is now accepted as the standard schema for diagnosing rejection.

39. **Triple maintenance immunosuppression**
    - Prednisone + cyclosporine or tacrolimus + azathioprine or mycophenolate mofetil.

40. **Action of immunosuppresants**
    - Cyclosporine or tacrolimus- calcineurin and IL2 inhibitors
    - Azathioprine or mycophenolate mofetil- purine antagonists
    - Sirolimus- inhibits cell cycle progression
    - Antithymocyte globulin- depletes T lymphocyte
    - Basililiximab and Daclizumab- blocks IL2 receptor

41. To differentiate between lymph/urine or blood in drain

- Creatinine concentration →Lymph=serum.
- Creatinine concentration→Urine > serum.
- Hematocrit level→Blood > Lymph and urine.

42.

	Tacrolimus/ cyclosporine toxicity	**Acute rejection**
Fever	No	Yes
Urine output	Normal	↓
Graft size	Stable	↑
Serum creatinine level rise	Slow	Rapid

43. New onset DM

- This is due to the diabetogenic effects of glucocorticoids and calcineurin inhibitors.
- The incidence is higher with tacrolimus than in those treated with cyclosporine.

44. Exclusion criteria for living donors (EAU Guidelines 2012)

Absolute contraindications

- Age < 18 years.
- Uncontrolled hypertension.
- Diabetes mellitus.
- Proteinuria (> 300 mg/24 h).
- Abnormal GFR for age.
- Microscopic haematuria.
- High risk of thromboembolism.
- Medically significant illness (chronic lung disease, recent malignant tumor, heart disease).
- History of bilateral kidney stones.
- HIV positive.

Relative contraindications

- Active chronic infection (e.g., tuberculosis, hepatitis B/C, parasites).
- Obesity.
- Psychiatric disorders.

❑❑

Chapter 11

URINARY LITHIASIS AND ENDOUROLOGY

1. **Demography of stone disease**

   - Incidence has increased in all age groups and in both men and women
   - Peak incidence in men from 30 to 69 years
   - Adult men more commonly affected than adult women (struvite stones are more common in women)
   - Highest prevalence of stone disease in whites, followed by Hispanics, Asians, and African-Americans
   - Higher prevalence of stone disease is in southeast
   - Highest incidence of stone disease in the summer months. (July through September)
   - Heat exposure and dehydration constitute occupational risk factors for stone disease
   - Obesity and weight gain are risk factors

2. **Stage of saturation**

   Undersaturation-

   - Crystals will not form
   - Existing stones will dissolve

   Metastable

   - Crystal growth and aggregation will occur but de-novo nucleation is very slow
   - Hetrogenous nucleation (epitaxy) may occur
   - Matrix may be involved
   - Inhibitors will prevent crystallization

   Unstable

   - Inhibitors will not be effective
   - Nucleation will occur

3. **Transit of urine through the nephron,** takes 5 to 7 minutes

4. **Inhibitors of Stone Formation**

	Nucleation	Growth	Aggregation
Magnesium			–
Citrate			–
Nephrocalcin	–	–	–
Tamm-Horsfall mucoprotein		–	–
Uropontin	–	–	–
Bikunin	–		–

– → inhibits

5. **Randall plaques**–calcium apatite constitute the main component of the plaque

6. **Matrix**
   - Noncrystalline component of renal calculi
   - Constitute 2.5% of the weight of the stone
   - Radiolucent
   - Heterogeneous mixture consisting of 65% protein, 9% nonamino sugars, 5% glucosamine, 10% bound water, and 12% organic ash

7. **Most potent stimulator of intestinal calcium absorption**–1, 25-Dihydroxyvitamin D3

   Most potent stimulus for PTH secretion–decrease in serum calcium

8. **Oxalobacter formigenes**
   - Oxalate-degrading bacteria.
   - Utilize oxalate as an energy source and reduce intestinal oxalate absorption.
   - Stone formers have reduced levels of oxalobacter compared with non-stone-formers.

9. **The most common component of urinary calculi is calcium (75%)**

10. **Incidence on the basis of stone composition**
    - Calcium oxalate - 60%
    - Mixed calcium oxalate and hydroxyapatite, 20%
    - Brushite stones- 2%.

- Uric acid and struvite (magnesium ammonium phosphate)- 10%
- Cystine- 1%

11. **Hypercalciuria**–urinary calcium> 200 mg /day.

    Hyperoxaluria–urinary oxalate >40 mg/day.

    Hyperuricosuria–urinary uric acid >600 mg/day.

12. **Absorptive hypercalciuria**
    - Type I when urinary calcium remains high despite a low calcium diet.
    - Type II when urinary calcium normalizes with a restricted calcium intake.
13. **In renal hypercalciuria**
    - Impaired renal tubular reabsorption of calcium results in ↑ urinary calcium levels leading to secondary hyperparathyroidism.
14. **Resorptive hypercalciuria**
    - Associated with primary hyperparathyroidism.
15.

	Absorptive	**Renal**	**Resorptive**
Serum calcium	Normal	Normal	Elevated
Parathyroid function	Suppressed	Stimulated	Stimulated
Fasting urinary calcium	Normal	Elevated	Elevated
Intestinal calcium absorption	Elevated	Elevated	Elevated

16. **Most common cause of hypercalcemia in an outpatient setting**– primary hyperthyroidism

    Most common cause of hypercalcemia in hospitalized patients– malignancy

17. **Primary hyperparathyroidism** is the cause of nephrolithiasis in about 5% of cases.
18. **Primary hyperoxaluria type 1**–mutations in aminotransferase (AGT), gene.

    Primary hyperoxaluria type 2–mutation in glyoxylate reductase/ hydroxy pyruvate reductase (GRHPR) gene.

19. **At pH < 5.5**, the undissociated form of uric acid predominates, leading to uric acid and/or calcium oxalate stone formation.

    At pH >5.5, sodium urate formation promotes calcium oxalate stone formation through heterologous nucleation.

20. **Hypocitraturia as an isolated abnormality in**–10% of calcium stone formers.

21. **Role of citrate in prevention of stone formation**
    - Reduces urinary saturation of calcium salts by complexing with calcium
    - Directly prevents spontaneous nucleation of calcium oxalate
    - Inhibits agglomeration and sedimentation of calcium oxalate crystals as well as the growth of calcium oxalate and calcium phosphate crystals
    - Normal urinary citrate levels can enhance the inhibitory effect of Tamm-Horsfall glycoprotein

22. **Main determinants of uric acid stone formation**–↓ pH, ↓ urine volume, and hyperuricosuria.

    The most important pathogenetic factor is low urine pH

23. **Cystinuria**
    - **AR** disorder characterized by a defect in intestinal and renal tubular transport of dibasic amino acids.
    - Results in excessive urinary excretion of cystine, lysine, ornithine, and arginine (COAL).
    - Present at a young age and may have affected first-degree relatives.
    - Stones are yellow and waxy in appearance and are relatively faint on plain radiography

24. **Prerequisite for formation of infection stones**–infection with urease-producing bacteria.
    - The most common urease producing pathogens are **Proteus,** Klebsiella, Pseudomonas and Staphylococcus species.
    - E Coli does not produce urease
    - The urine pH is usually greater than 6.5 and 7.0.

25. **Xanthine stones**
    - Radiolucent
    - Inherited disorder in the catabolic enzyme xanthine dehydrogenase or xanthine oxidase, which catalyzes the conversion of xanthine to uric acid.
    - Xanthine that accumulate in XDH deficiency lead to xanthine stones

26. **In developing countries, bladder calculi in children**–ammonium acid urate

27. **Medication that directly promote stone formation.**
    - Indinavir
    - Triamterine
    - Guaifenecin
    - Ephedrine
    - Silica

    Medication that indirectly promote stone formation.
    - Thiazides
    - Loop diuretics
    - Carbonic anhydrase inhibitors
    - Antiepileptics- topiramate, zonisamide
    - Laxatives
    - Cytotoxic agents

28. **Anatomic predisposition to stones**
    - PUJ obstruction (20%)
    - Horseshoe kidney (20%)
    - Caliceal diverticula (40%)
    - Medullary sponge kidneys

29. **Overall risk of stone formation in gravid and nongravid women** is–similar.

30. **(EAU Guidelines 2012)**
    - **To confirm stone diagnosis** in patients with acute flank pain–**NCCT should be used,** because it is superior to IVU.
    - **Planning treatment for renal stones**–contrast study (CECT or IVU) is indicated.

31. **Risk of recurrence within the subsequent 10 years for first-time stone formers**–50%.

32. **Indications for a Metabolic Stone Evaluation**
    - Recurrent stone formers.
    - Strong family history of stones.

- Pathologic skeletal fractures, osteoporosis.
- History of UTI or gout.
- Solitary kidney.
- Anatomic abnormalities.
- Renal insufficiency.
- Stones composed of cystine, uric acid or struvite.

33. Microscopic Appearance of Common Urinary Calculi

Chemical type	**Appearance**
Calcium oxalate monohydrate	Hourglass
Calcium oxalate dihydrate	Envelope, tetrahedral
Calcium phosphate–apatite	Amorphous
Brushite	Needle shaped
Magnesium ammonium phosphate (struvite)	Rectangular, coffin–lid
Cystine	Hexagonal
Uric acid	Amorphous shards, plates

34. Mineralogic Names of Renal Calculi

Calcium oxalate monohydrate	–	**Whewellite**
Calcium oxalate dihydrate	–	**Weddellite**
Calcium hydrogen phosphate dihydrate	–	**Brushite**
Tricalcium phosphate	–	**Whitlockite**
Carbonite-apatite	–	**Carbonite-apatite**
Magnesium ammonium phosphate	–	**Struvite**

35. Up to 70% of adults with distal RTA have kidney stones

36. Hyperuricosuric calcium nephrolithiasis patients present with normal urinary pH and hyperuricosuria, accompanied sometimes by hypercalciuria.

Gouty diathesis patients have a low fractional excretion of urate (that contributes to hyperuricemia) and low urinary pH (that leads to increased amount of undissociated uric acid)

37. Causes of acquired RTA

- Recurrent pyelonephritis
- Renal transplantation
- Acute tubular necrosis

- Analgesic nephropathy
- Sarcoidosis
- Idiopathic hypercalciuria
- Primary hyperparathyroidism
- Obstructive uropathy

38. **Conservative medical management**

- Forced increase in **fluid intake** to achieve a daily urine output of 2 liters.
- **Caffeine intake** may increase the risk of stone recurrence in calcium stone formers.
- **Lemonade and orange juice** increases urine volume as well as increased urinary citrate excretion.
- **Animal protein restriction, moderate calcium ingestion and reduced sodium diet** will decrease stone episodes.
- **Increased BMI, larger waist size and weight gain** correlated with an increased risk of stone episodes.
- **Low-carbohydrate, high-protien diet,** increases the risk for stone formation
- **Vitamin C** in large doses may increase the risk of stone recurrence

39. **Recommendations for pharmacological** treatment of patients with specific abnormalities in urine composition.

Urinary risk factor	**Suggested treatment**
Hypercalciuria	– Thiazide + potassium citrate
Hyperoxaluria	– Oxalate restriction
Hypocitraturia	– Potassium citrate
Enteric hyperoxaluria	– Potassium citrate, calcium supplement, oxalate absorption
Distal renal tubular acidosis	– Potassium citrate
Primary hyperoxaluria	– Pyridoxine
Cystinuria	– α-Mercaptopropionylglycine (Thiola)

40. **Major goal in the management of gouty diathesis** is to increase the urinary pH above pH 5.5., preferably between 6.0 and 6.5

41. **Acetohydroxamic acid**

- **Urease inhibitor.**
- **Reduce the urine saturation of struvite** and therefore retard stone formation.
- Most common side effect–**deep venous thrombosis (15%).**

42. **Bladder stones**–uric acid (in non-infected urine) or struvite (in infected urine).

43. **Neonatal nephrocalcinosis**

- Caused by loop diuretics.
- Cessation of loop diuretics is essential.
- It may be reversed by the use of thiazides

44. **Urolithiasis in pregnancy**

- No net increase or decrease in the risk of calculi formation during pregnancy
- USG is first-line imaging study to search for calculi during pregnancy
- A limited IVP consisting of one scout image followed by one plate taken 30 minutes after the injection of contrast may be sufficient.
- Ureteroscopy, with holmium laser lithotripy, performed later during pregnancy is safe and free of increased risk to the fetus or mother
- Conservative management should be the first-line treatment for all non-complicated cases **(65%-85% passes stone spontaneously). EAU Guidelines 2012**

45. **Location of kidneys**

- The longitudinal axis of the kidneys parallels the lateral edges of the psoas muscles
- Kidneys are 30^0 from vertical with the lower poles lateral to the upper poles.
- Kidneys are 30^0 off the frontal plane, with the lower poles anterior to the upper poles.
- Lateral aspect of kidney posterior to the medial aspect, by 30^0.

46. Renal anatomy

- The renal papillae drain into the minor calyces
- Minor calyces are the most peripheral portions of the intrarenal collecting system
- The outermost wall of the calyx, into which the papilla is set, is the calyceal fornix.
- There are 5 to 14 minor calyces in each kidney (mean of 8 minor calyces)
- There are three drainage zones: the upper pole, the middle region, and the lower pole.
- The minor calyces, drain into major calyces, which further drain by infundibula into the renal pelvis

47. The lumbar notch

- Also known as the superior lumbar triangle or Grynfelt lumbar triangle
- Reliable landmark for blind percutaneous renal access
- Boundaries
  - o Superior border is the 12th rib and latissimus dorsi muscle
  - o Lateral border is the transversus abdominis and external oblique muscles
  - o Medial border is the quadratus lumborum and sacrospinalis muscles
  - o Inferior border is the internal oblique muscle.

48. History

- **Inferior pyelonephrolithotomy**–Zuckerkandl.
- **Extended pyelolithotomy**–Gil-Vernet.
- **Anatrophic nephrolithotomy**–Smith and Boyce.
- **Extended pyelolithotomy combined with multiple radial nephrotomies**–Wickham.
- **Term endourology**–Arthur Smith.
- **First urologic use of flexible endoscope**–Marshall.
- **First used rigid ureteroscope**–Goodman.
- **First percutaneous access** to remove a renal stone–Fernstrom and Johannson.

49. **Best predictor of post-PNL urosepsis**–stone culture or renal pelvic urine culture.

50. **Calyceal stones**

- Most calyceal stones, in the absence of intervention, are likely to increase in size and cause symptoms of pain or infection
- Small (<5 mm), nonobstructive, asymptomatic stones can be observed

51. **Most staghorn stones are composed of struvite**

52. **Staghorn calculi**

- Partial- renal pelvic calculi extending into two calyceal groups
- Complete- renal pelvic calculi extending into all major calyceal groups, filling at least 80% of the collecting system
- Most accurate method to estimate the volume of a staghorn calculus is 3D CT

53. **Indication for active removal of kidney stones (EAU Guidelines 2012)**

- Obstruction caused by stones.
- Infection.
- Symptomatic stones (e.g., pain, haematuria).
- Stones > 15 mm.
- Stones < 15 mm if observation is not the option of choice.
- > 2-3 years stone persistence.

54. **Single most important factor in determining the appropriate treatment modality for a patient with renal calculi**–Stone burden (size and number).

55. **Most resistant to SWL–Cystine and brushite calculi**

Following in descending order of resistance calcium oxalate monohydrate, struvite, calcium oxalate dihydrate, and uric acid stones.

- Patients with brushite, cystine, calcium oxalate monohydrate should be treated by SWL only when the stone burden is small (i.e., <1.5 cm).
- Those patients with larger stones should preferentially be treated with PNL or ureteroscopy

56. Recommendations for kidney stones (EAU Guidelines 2012)

- SWL< 2 cm within the renal pelvis and upper or middle calices.
- PNL> 2 cm stones within the renal pelvis and upper or middle calices.
- SWL for the lower pole <1.5 cm.
- PNL / flexible URS for the lower pole >1.5 cm.

57. Management of symptomatic lower pole renal calculus

- **<1 cm-**
  - HU <1000, Skin Surfact Distance (SSD) <10 cm, favorable anatomy–**ESWL**
  - HU>1000, SSD>10 cm, unfavorable anatomy–**URS (Flexible)**
- **>2 cm- PNL**
- **1-2 cm- PNL/URS**

58. Antibiotic prophylaxis in indicated for all URS, PNL and ESWL

59. Matrix calculi

- Soft stones.
- Composed of 65% organic matter (2% to 3% in non-infected urinary calculi).
- Matrix stones are radiolucent.
- Often associated with urea–splitting bacteriuria.
- SWL is not an effective treatment modality for patients with these stones.
- Best treated with PNL.

60. Indinavir stones

- The mean time from the initiation of indinavir therapy until the acute stone episode was 21.5 weeks
- >75% stones pass spontaneously
- Hydration and analgesic therapy are recommended.
- Indinavir therapy may need to be temporarily or permanently discontinued.

61. In ureteropelvic obstruction with stone options are

- Open pyeloplasty and stone extraction
- PNL with concomitant endopyelotomy
- Laparoscopic pyeloplasty with concomitant pyelolithotomy

62. In calyceal diverticulum stone

- Direct percutaneous approach.
- Dilation and incision of the diverticular neck.
- Fulguration of the diverticular epithelium.

63. Horse shoe kidney

- <1.5 cm and nonobstructed urine drainage- SWL
- >1.5 cm→PNL.

Upper pole access is useful in horseshoe kidneys because

- easiest calyx to enter
- puncture rarely needs to be supra-co ,tal
- provides excellent access to most of the kidney and the ureter owing to the alignment of long axis of the moiety

The initial entry into a horseshoe kidney is more medial than in normal kidneys

64. In morbidly obese patients

- For SWL the skin surface distance was a stronger predictor of treatment failure than the BMI.
- Outcome of PNL is independent of the patient's BMI.
- For morbidly obese patients who do not harbor an excessively large stone burden the ureteroscopic approach may be preferable

65. Coagulopathy due to pharmacologic therapy that cannot be safely discontinued, ureteroscopy with holmium:YAG laser lithotripsy is the preferable approach.

66. After SWL follow up by–abdominal radiography and ultrasonography.

After PNL follow up by–flexible nephroscopy considered the "gold standard".

- Routine use of flexible nephroscopy has been challenged by studies showing the **high sensitivity of CT** in detecting residual stones after PNL.

67. For ureteric stone most significant measurement affecting the likelihood of stone passage–width of the stone.

For patients with stones of <5 mm , conservative management should be considered

68. Rates of spontaneous passage

- Stones <4 mm, 4 to 6 mm, and >6 mm were 80%, 60% and 20%, respectively.
- Proximal, middle and distal ureter were 20%, 45% and 70%, respectively.

69. Indication for active removal of ureteral stones (EAU Guidelines 2012)

- Stones with low likelihood of spontaneous passage.
- Persistent pain despite adequate pain medication.
- Persistent obstruction.
- Renal insufficiency (renal failure, bilateral obstruction, single kidney).

70. Recommended treatment options (EAU Guidelines 2012)

	First choice	Second choice
Proximal ureter <10 mm	SWL	URS
Proximal ureter >10 mm	URS or SWL	PNL
Distal ureter <10 mm	URS or SWL	
Distal ureter >10 mm	URS	SWL

71. Medical expulsive therapy (MET) (EAU Guidelines 2012)

- 1995% of ureteric **stones up to 4 mm pass** within 40 days.
- In patients with newly diagnosed **ureteral stones < 10 mm**, and if active removal is not indicated–observation with periodic evaluation is optional initial treatment.
- **Tamsulosin is significantly better than nifedipine** in relieving renal colic and facilitating and accelerating ureteral stone expulsion.
- Insufficient data exist to support the use of corticosteroids in combination with alpha-blockers as an accelerating adjunct.
- MET has an expulsive effect also on **proximal ureteral stones.**

72. Intracorporeal lithotripter

	Advantages	Disadvantages
EHL	• Least costly. • Smaller probes	• Damage mucosa • Ureteral perforation

	• Probe flexibility	• Retrograde propulsion of fragments • Larger size of fragments
Holmium laser	• Fragment all stones regardless of composition • Safest, most effective, versatile intracorporeal lithotripters • Reduces the likelihood of retropulsion of the stone	• High cost of the device
Ballistic	• Low cost and low maintenance • Least risk of ureteral perforation	• High rate of stone retropulsion
Ultrasonic	• Combination of stone fragmentation and simultaneous fragment removal	• Rigid nature of ultrasonic probes and there small diameter

73. The holmium laser

- Solid-state laser system
- Operates at a wavelength of 2140 nm in the pulsed mode.
- Highly absorbed by water
- The zone of thermal injury associated with laser ablation ranges from 0.5 to 1.0 mm
- Holmium laser lithotripsy occurs primarily through a **photothermal mechanism** that causes stone vaporization
- No significant cyanide toxicity from holmium laser lithotripsy

74. Laser fiber

- Only the 200-µm and 365-µm fibers are used for flexible intracorporeal lithotripsy.
- In treatment of ureteral stones, the end-firing fiber is more effective
- 550-µm side-firing fiber is more effective than the end-firing fiber during PNL

75. Holmium laser lithotripsy technique

- Keep the fiber tip in view at all times.

- Start at low settings and increase only as necessary.
- Work from the inside of the stone outward.
- Keep the fiber tip at least 2 mm from the urothelium.
- One person should control the fiber and the foot pedal.
- Do not discharge the laser fiber inside the working channel
- Laser fiber should extend at least 2 mm beyond the tip of the endoscope to avoid destroying the lens system

76. ESWL

	Advantages	**Disadvantages**
Electrohydraulic (spherically expanding SW)	• Effectiveness in breaking kidney stones	• Substantial pressure fluctuations from shock to shock • Short electrode life.
Electromagnetic (Plane or cylindrical SW)	• More controllable and reproducible • Less pain. • Small focal point can be achieved with high-energy densities, which increase its effectiveness in breaking stones.	• Increased rate of subcapsular hematoma formation
Piezoelectric	• Focusing accuracy • Long service life • Possibility of an anesthetic-free treatment	• Insufficient power to break stone effectively

77. For the shockwave

- Electrode is placed at one focus (termed F1) of an ellipsoid
- Target (the kidney stone) is placed at the other focus (termed F2)

78. A typical pressure pulse generated by an EHL is

- Initial short and steep compressive front with pressures of about 40 MPa that is followed by a longer, lower amplitude negative (tensile) pressure of 10 MPa
- Entire pulse duration is 4 μsec.

79. Mechanism by which stone fragmentation occurs-

- Spall fracture
- Squeezing-splitting or circumferential compression
- Shear stress
- Superfocusing
- Cavitation
- Dynamic fracture

80. Contraindications of ESWL (EAU Guidelines 2012)

- Pregnancy.
- Bleeding diatheses
- Uncontrolled UTIs.
- Severe skeletal malformations and severe obesity.
- Arterial aneurysm in the vicinity of the stone.
- Anatomical obstruction distal to the stone.

81. Risk factors for SWL

- Age
- Obesity
- Coagulopathies
- Thrombocytopenia
- Diabetes mellitus
- Coronary heart disease
- Preexisting hypertension

82. PCNL

Open system	**Closed system**
With amplatz working sheath	Nephroscope serving as its own sheath
High flow and low pressure	Low flow, high pressure
Tract is larger and bleeding may be more	Nephrostomy track is smaller and bleeding may be reduced

83. First line of treatment of steinstrasse (EAU Guidelines 2012)

Asymptomatic	**Symptomatic**	**Symptomatic + fever**
MET	URS	PCN

84. Safest approach to pelvicalyceal system in PNL

- Through **posterior calyx** (transparenchymal route stabilizes nephrostomy catheter).
- Puncture through **fornix** is safe.
- Preferred point of entry is along the axis of calyx **through papilla.**

85. Approach to be avoided in PNL

- **Anterior calyceal puncture** avoided as access to renal pedicle is difficult because it requires directing the guidewire backwards.
- **Direct renal pelvis puncture** is avoided as it causes increase risk of injury to posterior branch of renal artery.
- **Medial puncture** is avoided as risk of injuring large vessels increases.
- Percutaneous access should not be **directly into an infundibulum or the renal pelvis,** as it increases the risk of vascular injury

86. During PNL hemorrhage requiring transfusion is 0.5% to 4%

Factors associated with hemorrhage during percutaneous surgery include

- Multiple access sites
- Supracostal access
- Increase tract size
- Tract dilation with methods other than balloon dilation,
- Prolonged operative time
- Renal pelvic perforation

87. If there is bleeding from the PCN tract

Best management is to occlude a nephrostomy tube, apply pressure to the incision, and let the collecting system clot of hemorrhage

If refractory to this hemostatic measures, then use of a Kaye nephrostomy tamponade balloon

88. Delayed hemorrhage is usually due to arteriovenous fistulas or arterial pseudoaneurysms, with the latter being more common

- Angiography, is diagnostic in more than 90% of cases.
- Treatment is selective angio-embolization, which is highly effective

89. In renal pelvic perforation–insert nephrostomy tube plus an internal ureteral stent to optimize drainage

After 2 to 7 days perform nephrostogram and then tube removal

90. **Colon injuries** from percutaneous renal surgery are mostly extraperitoneal and can be managed conservatively by draining the colon and urinary collecting system separately.

91. **Chest complications**

Chest radiography is recommended following all cases of supracostal percutaneous renal access.

If a hydrothorax is noted on the postoperative CXR then place a small-caliber tube only if-

- Effusion is large
- Evidence of respiratory compromise
- Hemodynamic instability.

92. **Normal saline should be the irrigant for percutaneous renal surgery**

Irrigation with water during percutaneous renal surgery risks intravascular hemolysis

93. **If pus is aspirated on initial percutaneous to the upper urinary tract**, the safest measure is to abort the procedure and leave a nephrostomy tube for drainage.

94. **Complications of URS:**

Intraoperative complications 3.6%

- Mucosal injury 1.5%.
- Ureteral perforation 1.7%.
- Significant bleeding 0.1%.
- Ureteral avulsion 0.1%.

Early complications 6.0%

- Fever or urosepsis 1.1%.
- Persistent haematuria 2.0%.
- Renal colic 2.2%.

Late complications 0.2%

- Ureteral stricture 0.1%.
- Persistent vesicoureteral reflux 0.1%.

95. **Steinstrasse**

- Complication of SWL
- Most cases resolve spontaneously.
- Percutaneous nephrostomy alone has a success rate of more than 70%.

- Ureteroscopic intervention–success rate approaching 100%.
- Additional SWL may be successful, but the results are less predictable

96. Indications for ureteroscopy rather than SWL in ureteral stone disease:

- Salvage for failed shockwave lithotripsy (SWL).
- Hard stone (calcium oxalate monohydrate, cystine, brushite).
- Morbidly obese (>300 lb or above the focusing limit of the lithotriptor).
- Uncorrectable bleeding diathesis
- Multiple proximal ureteral stones.
- Stones >1 cm.
- Radiolucent stones.

97. Most common injured vessel in endourologic procedures– posterior segmental artery.

98. ALARA: as low as reasonably achievable.

- The maximum yearly whole-body exposure recommended by the National Council on Radiation Protection **is 5000 mrem, or 5 rem.**

99. Choosing Appropriate Nephrostomy Tube Drainage

Clinical indication management	Suggested nephrostomy tube and tract
Acute obstruction, simple temporary drainage	Pigtail, cope loop catheter
Uncomplicated percutaneous renal surgery	Tubeless
Complicated percutaneous renal surgery	Councill tip catheter, Kaye tamponade catheter
Minor mucosal damage or post-endopyelotomy care	Malecot re-entry tube, Endopyelotomy stent (14 Fr/7 Fr)
Long-term drainage, administration of topical chemotherapy, pyelopyelostomy	Circle loop nephrostomy tube

❑❑

Chapter 12

NEOPLASM OF UPPER URINARY TRACT

1. **Features suggestive of malignancy on intravenous pyelography include**
   - calcification within the mass
   - increased tissue density
   - irregularity of the margin
   - distortion of the collecting system
2. **Sonographic criteria for simple cysts**
   - Smooth cyst wall.
   - Round or oval shape without internal echoes.
   - Through-transmission with strong acoustic shadows posteriorly.
3. **Single most important radiographic test** for delineating the nature of a renal mass (thin-slice) renal CT scan.
4. **Any renal mass that enhances with IV administration of contrast material on CT scanning by >15 HU**–RCC until proved otherwise.
5. **Solid masses with <20 HU**–indicative of fat are diagnostic of AMLs.
6. **Renal pseudotumors**–hypertrophied column of Bertin.

   Diagnosis of a pseudotumor–confirmed by isotope renography with DMSA.
7. **Category I Bosniak lesions**
   - Uncomplicated, simple, benign cysts of the kidney.
   - Most common renal cystic lesions.
   - In absence of associated symptoms, no treatment is necessary.
8. **Category II Bosniak lesions**
   - Minimally complicated cysts that are benign.
   - Septated cysts, cysts with minimal calcium in the wall or septum, infected cysts and hyperdense (high-density) cysts.
   - Risk of malignancy is 0% to 5% and lesions should be observed with periodic imaging.

9. **Category III Bosniak lesions**
   - More complicated renal cysts that are indeterminate and cannot be confidently distinguished from malignant neoplasms.
   - Irregular margin, thickened septa and thick irregular calcification.
   - Risk of malignancy–50%.
   - Surgically treated. When possible, a nephron-sparing procedure should be performed **(EAU Guidelines 2012).**
10. **Category IV Bosniak lesions**
    - Large cystic components; irregular, shaggy margins; and, most important, some solid enhancing portions that provide a definitive diagnosis of malignancy.
    - Risk of malignancy–75% to 90%.
    - Require surgical treatment.
11. **Most lethal of the urologic cancers**–RCC (2% to 3% of all adult malignant neoplasms).

    2% to 3% RCC is familial.
12. **RCC in children**
    - RCC is as common as Wilms' tumor during the second decade of life.
    - Stage for stage, children and young adults with RCC may respond better to surgical therapy
    - Formal lymphadenectomy has thus been recommended at the time of radical nephrectomy when RCC is suspected in children or young adults
13. **Risk factor for RCC**
    - Tobacco exposure
    - Hypertension
    - Obesity
14. **Familial RCC syndromes**

Syndrome	**Gene**	**Manifestation**
VHL	VHL Gene (3p)	Clear RCC
Hereditary papillary RCC	c MET (7q)	Type 1 papillary RCC
Familial leiomyomatosis and RCC	Fumarate hydratase	Type 2 papillary RCC

Birt-Hogg-Dubé	BHD1 gene	Chromophobe RCC, Oncocytoma, Clear cell RCC

15. VHL

Major manifestations include the development of

- Clear cell RCC
- Pheochromocytoma
- Retinal angiomas
- Hemangioblastomas of the brainstem, cerebellum, or spinal cord
- Islet cell tumors
- Endolymphatic sac tumor

16. RCC develops in about 50% of patients with VHL disease.

Early age at onset, bilateral and multifocal involvement.

17. Most common cause of mortality in patients with VHL–RCC.

18. VHL gene

- Located at chromosome 3p25-26.
- Role as a tumor suppressor gene for both sporadic and familial forms of clear cell RCC.
- Both alleles of the VHL gene must be mutated or inactivated for development of the disease

19. Inactivation or mutation of the VHL gene →dysregulated expression of the Hypoxia inducible factors → upregulation of the expression of VEGF → pronounced neovascularity associated with clear cell RCC

20. Type I papillary RCC

- Consists of Basophilic cells with scant cytoplasm.
- More common than type II.
- Associated with hereditary papillary RCC (HPRCC).

Type II papillary RCC

- Patients commonly develop cutaneous and uterine leiomyonas.
- Renal tumors are solitary and unilateral (unusual for familial RCC)
- More aggressive

- Consist of eosinophilic cells and abundant granular cytoplasm.

21. **Birt-Hogg-Dubé syndrome**

- Patients develop cutaneous fibrofolliculomas, lung cysts, spontaneous pneumothoraces, and a variety of renal tumors.
- Renal tumors include chromophobe RCC, oncocytomas, and hybrid or transitional tumors.
- AD pattern of inheritance
- Renal tumors are often bilateral and multiple

22. **RCC expresses a variety of tumor associated antigen**

- PRAME, RAGE-1, MUC-1and gp47.
- **Most specific-** CA-9 (also known as MN-9)

23. **Prognostic factors**

- **VEGF** is suppressed by the wild-type VHL protein under normal conditions and is upregulated during tumor development.
- Decreased proliferative index **(Ki-67)** has correlated with improved survival in clear cell RCC.
- Increased expression of **TGF-α** and its receptor tyrosine kinase, EGFR contribute to tumorigenesis.
- **The hepatocyte growth factor** and its receptor, the c-*MET* proto-oncogene, contribute to the pathogenesis of RCC
- Upregulation of **E-cadherin**, mediate adhesion between cancer cells and has correlated with improved outcomes.
- **High CA-9** expressions has correlated with improved survival.
- **G250 monoclonal antibody,** is expressed almost ubiquitously by clear cell RCC and only rarely by other RCC subtypes
- Increased expression of proteases, such as **plasmin and the matrix metalloproteinases**, has correlated with reduced survival in RCC
- The most important **primary prevention for RCC** is to eliminate cigarette smoking and to avoid obesity.

24. **Spontaneous regression of RCC**

- 0.3% to as high as 7%,
- Most spontaneous regressions have been noted in patients with pulmonary metastases and have occurred after cytoreductive nephrectomy, with a median duration of 6 months

25. **RCCs are not grossly infiltrative**, with the notable exception of collecting duct RCC and sarcomatoid variants.

26. RCC

- **Cystic degeneration** in 10% to 20%.
- **Calcification** can be stippled or plaque-like in 10% to 20%.
- **Frank invasion and perforation** of the collecting system in 20%.
- **Involvement of the venous system** in 10%.
- **Bilateral involvement** can be synchronous or asynchronous in 2% to 4% (more common in familial RCC such as VHL)
- **Multicentricity,** is found in 10% to 20% of cases, (common in papillary histology and familial RCC)
- **Paraneoplastic syndromes** in 20% of patients with RCC.

27. **Fuhrman's Classification:** System for nuclear grade in RCC is based on nuclear size, nuclear outline and nucleoli.

28. **In RCC tumor in the contralateral kidney** is likely to be an independent growth if it is synchronous or a metastasis if it is asynchronous.

29.

RCC variant	Characterstics	Gene abnormalities
Conventional (clear)	• 70% to 80% of all RCCs • Garden variety • Most responders in immunotherapy • Hypervascular • Worst prognosis • Originate from proximal tubule	VHL gene (3p25-26) mutation or hypermethylation
Chromophilic (papillary)	• In ESRD and ARCD • Hypovascular • Derived from medulla • Originate from proximal tubule • Multicentric	Trisomy of chromosomes 7 and 17

Chromophobe cell carcinoma	• Plant cells" with pale Cytoplasm and perinuclear clearing or "halo." • Electron microscopic-numerous microvesicles • Hypovascular • Arising from collecting duct	Loss of multiple chromosomes (1, 2, 6, 10, 13, 17, 21)
Collecting duct (Bellini's duct carcinoma)	• Affinity for the Ulex europaeus lectin • Expression of HMW keratins (34βE12)support a collecting duct origin • Infiltrative • Originate from collecting duct • Poor prognosis	Loss of chromosomes 1, 6, 8, 11, 21 and γ
Renal medullary Carcinoma	• Associated with sickle cell trait • Originate from collecting duct	

30. **Sarcomatoid differentiation** is found in 1% to 5% of RCCs

    Sarcomatoid differentiation is characterized by

    - spindle cell histology
    - positive staining for vimentin
    - infiltrative growth pattern
    - aggressive local and metastatic behaviour
    - poor prognosis
    - common in clear cell RCC or chromophobe RCC

31. **RCCs detected incidentally**–>50%.

    Approximately one third of all newly diagnosed RCC patients present with synchronous metastatic disease

32. **RCC triad**–flank pain, gross hematuria and palpable abdominal mass.
33. RCC–**internist's tumor and radiologist's tumor.**

34. Bisphosphonate therapy

- Standard of care for patients with hypercalcemia of malignancy.
- Zoledronic acid, 4 mg intravenously every 4 weeks (must be withheld in the presence of renal insufficiency).

35. Hypertension associated with RCC can be due to

- Secondary to increased production of renin directly by the tumor
- Compression or encasement of the renal artery or its branches, effectively leading to renal artery stenosis
- Arteriovenous fistula within the tumor
- Polycythemia
- Hypercalcemia
- Ureteral obstruction
- Increased intracranial pressure associated with cerebral metastases

36. Stauffer's syndrome

- 3% to 20% of cases.
- Elevated serum alkaline phosphatase, PT, bilirubin and transaminases
- Hypoalbuminemia
- Thrombocytopenia and neutropenia.
- Fever and weight loss.
- Hepatic metastases must be excluded.
- Biopsy, when it is indicated, often demonstrates nonspecific hepatitis associated with a prominent lymphocytic infiltrate.
- Elevated serum levels of IL-6.
- Hepatic function normalizes after nephrectomy in 60% to 70% of cases

37. Screening for Renal Cell Carcinoma: Target Populations

- Patients with end-stage renal failure.
- Patients with known von Hippel-Lindau syndrome.
- Relatives of patients with von Hippel-Lindau syndrome.
- Relatives of patients with other familial forms of RCC.
- Patients with tuberous sclerosis.

(Patients with ADPKD–Routine screening not justified)

38. **Tuberous sclerosis**
    - Autosomal dominant disorder
    - Adenoma sebaceum
    - Epilepsy
    - Mental retardation
    - Renal cysts
    - AMLs
    - Increase incidence of RCC

39. **International TNM Staging System (2009) for Renal Cell Carcinoma**

    T1a: Tumor $\leq$ 4.0 cm and confined to the kidney

    T1b: Tumor > 4.0 cm and $\leq$ 7.0 cm and confined to the kidney

    T2a: Tumor > 7.0 cm and $\leq$ 10.0 cm and confined to the kidney

    T2b: Tumor > 10.0 cm and confined to the kidney

    T3a: Tumor grossly extends into the renal vein or tumor invades sinus fat but not beyond Gerota's fascia

    T3b: Tumor grossly extends into vena cava below diaphragm

    T3c: Tumor extends into the vena cava above the diaphragm or invades the wall of the vena cava

    T4: Tumor invades beyond Gerota's fascia (including extension into ipsilateral adrenal gland)

    N1: Metastasis in a regional lymph node

    M1: Distant metastasis present

40. **Risk for ipsilateral adrenal involvement**
    - Patients with an enlarged adrenal gland on CT.
    - Upper pole tumor location.
    - Extensive malignant replacement of the kidney.
    - Palpably abnormal adrenal gland.

41. **Enlarged hilar or retroperitoneal lymph nodes >2 cm** in diameter on CT–harbor malignant change, but should be confirmed by percutaneous aspiration or surgical exploration.

42. **CT for detection of renal venous tumor thrombus and inferior vena caval involvement**–78% and 96%, respectively.

43. MRI

- Investigation of choice for staging of inferior vena caval tumor thrombus.
- Provides reliable information about both the cephalad and caudad extent of the thrombus and can often distinguish bland from tumor thrombus.
- **Venacavography** is best reserved for patients with equivocal MRI findings and for patients who cannot tolerate MRI or have other contraindications to MRI.

44. Limitations for percutaneous renal biopsy or aspiration

- Difficulty in interpreting due to inherent similarities between the eosinophilic variants of RCC and oncocytoma.

45. Indications for percutaneous renal biopsy

Patients suspected of having metastatic disease, renal abscess, or lymphoma(all of these are primarily managed).

46. Kattan staging system includes

- Manner of presentation (incidental, or local versus systemic symptoms).
- Tumor histology.
- Tumor size.
- Pathologic stage to develop a nomogram that predicts cancer-free survival after nephrectomy (no tumor grade).

47. **UCLA Integrated Staging System**–This classification system incorporates stage, grade, and performance status and provides estimates of 2-year and 5-year survival rates.

48. SSIGN score for clear cell RCC incorporates

1997 TNM stage, tumor size, nuclear grade, and presence of tumor necrosis to predict recurrence and survival after radical nephrectomy

49. **Twenty percent of solid, enhancing, clinical T1 renal masses are benign,** most often oncocytomas or atypical AML

50. **For T1 tumors**–Surgical therapy **(EAU Guidelines 2012)**

- Nephron-sparing surgery should be performed whenever possible.
- Laproscopic radical nephrectomy (LRN) should not be performed in patients with T1 tumors for whom partial resection is indicated.

- Extended lymphadenectomy does not improve survival and can be restricted to staging purposes.
- Adrenalectomy (together with nephrectomy) is not needed in most patients

For T2 tumors–Laparoscopic radical nephrectomy (LRN) **(EAU Guidelines 2012)**

51. Postoperative Surveillance after Radical Nephrectomy for Localized RCC

Pathologic Tumor Stage	History, Examination and Blood Tests	Chest Radiograph Scan	Abdominal CT
T1 N0 M0	Yearly	—	—
T2 N0 M0	Yearly	Yearly	Every 2 years
T3 N0 M0	Every 6 months for 3 years, then yearly	Every 6 months for 3 years, then yearly	At 1 year, then every 2 years

Postoperative Surveillance after Partial Nephrectomy for Localized RCC

Pathologic Tumor Stage	History, Examination and Blood Tests	Chest Radiograph Scan	Abdominal CT
T1 N0 M0	Yearly	—	—
T2 N0 M0	Yearly	Yearly	Every 2 years
T3 N0 M0	Every 6 months for 3 years, then yearly	Every 6 months for 3 years, then yearly	**Every 6 months for 3 years, then every 2 years**

52. Partial nephrectomy (PN)

- 3D volume rendered CT (or MRI) is a noninvasive imaging modality that can accurately depict the renal parenchymal and vascular anatomy
- A functioning renal remnant of at least 20% of one kidney is necessary to avoid ESRD.
- PN is now standard of care for the management of clinical T1 renal masses in the presence of a normal contralateral kidney
- PN provide effective initial treatment of patients with RCC and VHL disease but tumor size should be > 3.0 cm
- Laparoscopic approach (LPN) can provide more rapid convalescence but has been associated with an increased risk of

major urologic complications and longer warm ischemia times when compared with traditional OPN.

- OPN is preferred for complex cases such as tumor in the renal hilum, tumor in a solitary kidney, or multiple tumors.

53. **For screening of hyperfiltration nephropathy**–24 hour urinary protein measurement should be obtained yearly in patients with a solitary remnant kidney

    ACEI therapy and a low-protein diet may improve the long-term renal functional outcome for patients with remnant kidney after PN

54. **Thermal ablative therapies(TA)**

    Renal cryosurgery and radiofrequency ablation (RFA), are alternative to nephron-sparing treatments for patients with localized RCC

    The ideal candidates for TA procedures

    - Patients with advanced age or significant comorbidities who prefer a proactive approach but are not optimal candidates for conventional surgery
    - Patients with local recurrence after previous nephron-sparing surgery
    - Patients with hereditary renal cancer who present with multifocal lesions for which multiple PNs might be cumbersome if not impossible
    - Kidney may be an anatomically favored organ for cryosurgery because
        - Can be laparoscopically mobilized, thereby minimizing the risk of injury to adjacent vital structures
        - Usually presents with unifocal, well-circumscribe malignancy

55. **Established prerequisites for successful cryosurgery include**

    - Rapid freezing
    - Gradual thawing
    - Repetition of the freeze-thaw cycle.

56. **The mechanism underlying tissue cryodestruction is**-immediate cellular damage and delayed microcirculatory failure

    Target lethal temperature of −20° C should be achieved at a distance of 3.1 mm inside the leading edge of the ice ball

57. Patients managed with observation and serial renal imaging

- **Indication**–small, solid, enhancing, well-marginated, homogeneous renal lesions, who are elderly or poor surgical risks.
- **Contraindication**–>3 cm, poorly marginated, or non-homogeneous solid renal lesions. Observation is also not advisable in younger, otherwise healthy patients with small, solid tumors that have radiographic characteristics consistent with RCC.

58. 3-cm rule for intervention is applied in patients

- To reduce the number of surgical interventions, to optimize renal function, and to minimize the risk of metastatic disease.
- This recommendation applies to patients with
  - VHL
  - Hereditary papillary RCC
  - Birt-Hogg-Dubé syndromes
  - (Hereditary leiomyomatosis is an exception in that tumors in this syndrome are more aggressive and should be managed accordingly, even when <3 cm)

59. Staging of the level of IVC thrombus :

I- adjacent to the ostium of renal vein

II- extending up to the lower aspect of the liver

III- involving the intrahepatic portion of the IVC but below the diaphragm

IV- extending above the diaphragm.

60. Level I thrombi

- Isolated by a Satinsky clamp and are thus readily removed.

Level II thrombi

- Sequential clamping of the caudal IVC, contralateral renal vein, and cephalad IVC along with mobilization of the relevant segment of the IVC and occlusion of lumbar veins.

61. Level III thrombi

- Mobilization of the liver and exposure of the intrahepatic IVC will allow the thrombus to be mobilized proximal to the hepatic veins, and dissection can then proceed as for a level II thrombus.

- If this is not possible, the IVC can be clamped above the liver and a Pringle maneuver can be performed (portal triad is temporarily occluded)
- Venovenous bypass.

62. Level IV IVC thrombi

- Managed with cardiopulmonary bypass and hypothermic circulatory arrest

63. Local recurrence after nephrectomy

- Only about 40% of local recurrences are isolated
- Majority of patients with local recurrence also have systemic disease, and a thorough metastatic evaluation should be pursued
- Surgical resection of isolated local recurrence of RCC after RN should be considered, because it can provide long-term cancer-free status for 30% to 40% of patients

64. Renal sarcoma

- Less common but more lethal than sarcoma of any other genitourinary site, including the prostate, bladder and paratesticular region.
- Most important prognostic factors for sarcomas are margin status and tumor grade
- Leiomyosarcoma has been the **most common histologic subtype.**

65. Hypovascular renal tumors

- Sarcoma
- Lymphoma and leukemia
- Metastatic tumors
- Carcinoid
- Small cell carcinoma of kidney
- Primitive neuroectodermal tumor

66. Lymphoma or leukemia

- Suspected in patients with massive retroperitoneal lymphadenopathy, splenomegaly, or lymphadenopathy in other regions of the body or atypical regions within the retroperitoneum.

- If renal involvement is suspected, confirm with percutaneous biopsy.
- If lymphoma or leukemia is confirmed, the kidney should be spared, and complete staging of the neoplasm should be performed.
- The classic chemotherapy regimen for non-Hodgkin's lymphoma is the CHOP- cyclophosphamide, doxorubicin, vincristine, and prednisolone
- Nephrectomy is seldom indicated except in patients with uncontrollable hemorrhage.
- Patient with primary renal lymphoma–nephrectomy + systemic chemotherapy.

67. Carcinoid tumors:

- Arise from neuroendocrine cells.
- Increase in urinary and plasma serotonin.
- Majorty asymptomatic.
- NSS if diagnosis suspected preoperatively.
- Good prognosis.

68. Primary neuroectodermal tumor (PNET)

- On microscopic examination, reveal Homer-Wright rosettes
- A characteristic t(11;22)(q24;q12) translocation is highly specific for PNET

69. Adult Wilms' tumor

- Wilms tumor is the most common abdominal malignant neoplasm in children
- 3% of Wilms tumors are seen in adults
- Present with advance disease and prognosis is worst than in children.

70. Metastatic tumors.

- Multifocal
- Most common malignant neoplasms in the kidney, outnumbering primary renal tumors
- Increase incidence because of high blood flow and profuse vascularity of the kidney

71. Predictors of a poor outcome in metastatic RCC

- Poor performance status (Karnofsky score <80)
- Elevated serum lactate dehydrogenase (LDH) level (>1.5 times upper limit of normal)
- Low hemoglobin (less than the lower limit of normal)
- Elevated corrected calcium concentration (>10 g/dL)
- Lack of prior nephrectomy

Adverse factors	Overall survival (months)
Nil	20
1-2	10
>3	4

72. Cytoreductive nephrectomy

Indication

- In patients with metastatic RCC who are likely candidates for subsequent cytokine therapy
- Palliative intention

73. Cytoreductive nephrectomy can be performed with palliative intent in patients with

- Intractable pain
- Hematuria
- Constitutional symptoms
- Paraneoplastic manifestations such as hypercalcemia, erythrocytosis, secondary thrombocytosis, or hypertension

74. Factors that are associated with an improved outcome after metastasectomy, includes

- Complete resection
- Presence of solitary metastatic lesions
- Age <60 years
- Smaller tumor size
- Presence of pulmonary metastases
- Development of metachronous metastatic disease

75. Metastatic RCC (EAU Guidelines 2012)

- In patients with synchronous metastatic spread, metastasectomy should be performed where disease is resectable and the patient has a good performance status.
- Prognosis is worse in patients who have surgery for metachronous metastases.
- Metastasectomy should be performed in patients with residual and resectable metastatic lesions previously responding to immuno-therapy.

76. First-line treatment for mRCC in selected cases with clear-cell histology and good prognostic factors:

- Monotherapy with IFN-alpha or high-dose bolus IL-2.
- Cytokine combinations, with or without additional chemotherapy, do not improve overall survival compared with monotherapy.

77. Cytokine therapy

Interferon

- Overall response rates of 16% to 26% in patients treated with interferon-α
- Durable complete responses with this agent are relatively rare (<2%).

IL-2

- Response rates in the range of 15% to 20%
- 7% to 9% of patients receiving high-dose IL-2 achieve complete regression

Combination of IL-2 and interferon

- Higher response rate (18.6%) however no difference in1-year event-free survival

78. Target therapy

Bevacizumab

- Humanized monoclonal antibody against VEGF-A, was the first VEGF pathway antagonist

Sorafenib

- Oral receptor kinase inhibitor with activity against VEGFR2, PDGF receptor-β, and raf-1.

Sunitinib

- It is a potent inhibitor of VEGFR2, PDGFR- β, c-*KIT*, and fms-like tyrosine kinase-3.
- Diarrhea, dermatologic manifestations such as rash and hand-foot syndrome, fatigue, asthenia, and hypertension are side effects.
- Bone marrow suppression, decline in left ventricular ejection fraction, and hypothyroidism occur.
- Most widely used agent in the initial management of metastatic clear cell RCC patients

Temsirolimus and everolimus

- Inhibitors of mammalian target of rapamycin
- Temsirolimus is a reasonable front-line choice in patients presenting with high-risk features

79. Recommendations for systemic therapy for metastatic RCC (EAU recommendation 2012)

Treatment risk		Recommended agent
Low or intermediate	1st–line therapy	Sunitinib
		Bevacizumab + IFN-α
High risk	1st–line therapy	Temsirolimus
Prior cytokine failure	1st–line therapy	Pazopanib
	2nd–line therapy	Sorafenib

80. Simple cysts

- Most common benign renal lesions.
- >70% of all asymptomatic renal masses.
- Prevalence increases with age, and renal cysts can be found in more than 50% of patients older than 50 years.

81. Renal cortical adenoma

- Incidence increases with age and male sex,
- Associated with acquired renal cystic disease that results in end-stage renal failure

82. In metanephric adenoma

- Rare benign tumor with female predominance
- Polycythemia seen in 10% of patients
- Frequently expressed-WT1, S100
- Poorly expressed- α-Methylacyl- CoA racemase (AMACR)

83. Oncocytoma

- 3% to 7% of all solid renal masses.
- Prominent necrosis or hypervascularity is lacking.
- Uniform round or polygonal eosinophilic cells predominate.
- Packed with numerous large mitochondria **(megamitochondria).**
- The **central stellate scar** observed on CT scan.
- **Spoke-wheel pattern** of feeding arteries observed on angiography.
- Except for AML, most of these less common renal tumors cannot be differentiated from RCC on the basis of radiology and should therefore be treated in the same way as RCC **(EAU Guidelines 2012).**

84. Angiomyolipoma (AML)

- AML is most common renal tumor associated with spontaneous hemorrhage, followed by RCC.
- **20% to 30% of AMLs are found in patients with Tuberous sclerosis (TS)**
- **50% of patients with TS develop AMLs.**
- **AML in TS**
  - o More likely to be bilateral and multicentric.
  - o Mean age at presentation is 30 years.
  - o F: M predominance is 2:1.
- **AML with no TS**
  - o More pronounced female predominance.
  - o Present, during the fifth or sixth decade.
- Massive retroperitoneal hemorrhage from AML, known as **Wunderlich's syndrome.**
- The presence of fat (confirmed on nonenhanced thin-cut CT by a value of −20 HU or less) within a renal lesion is considered the diagnostic hallmark
- In 14% of AMLs, fat cannot be identified with CT.
- On USG is a well circumscribed, **highly echogenic lesion**, often associated with shadowing.
- **Aneurysmal dilation** is found in 50% of AMLs when they are visualized by angiography.

- **HMB-45**, a monoclonal antibody raised against a melanoma-associated antigen, is characteristic for AML.
- **Management**
  - The treatment of choice in cases of **acute hemorrhage** is selective renal angioembolization
  - **Asymptomatic, <4 cm AMLs**–observed expectantly, with repeated evaluation and imaging at 6- to 12-month intervals.
  - **Symptomatic and/or >4 cm**–surgery, thermal ablation, and selective arterial embolisation. When possible, a nephron-sparing procedure should be performed **(EAU Guidelines 2012).**

85. Cystic nephroma

- Bimodal age distribution and a benign clinical course.
- Male predominance is observed in children. Children present with an asymptomatic abdominal mass.
- Female predominance is observed in adults.

86. Reninoma

- Benign renal tumor is the renin-secreting juxtaglomerular tumor, or reninoma.
- Specialized form of a hemangiopericytoma, derived from the juxtaglomerular cell.
- Most are small (<3 cm), solitary and hypovascular.
- Hypersecretion of renin and includes hypertension and hypokalemia and associated symptoms such as polydipsia, polyuria, myalgia and headaches.
- Almost all patients may be cured with surgical excision.

87. Summary of Other Renal Tumors

Entity	Malignant potential	Treatment
Sarcomatoid variants of RCC	High	Surgery
Multilocular clear cell RCC	Low, no metastasis	Surgery, NSS
Papillary adenoma	Benign	Observation
Ca collecting duct of Bellini	High, very aggressive	Surgery
Renal medullary carcinoma	High, very aggressive	Surgery
Translocation carcinoma	Intermediate	Surgery, NSS
Spindle cell carcinoma	Intermediate	Surgery, NSS

Metanephric adenoma	Benign	Surgery, NSS
Oncocytoma	Benign	Observation /Surgery
Angiomyolipoma	Benign	Treatment when >4 cm

88. Retroperitoneal tumor

- 50% of all retroperitoneal tumors are sarcomas.
- 15% to 20 % are benign lesions such as lipomas
- Liposarcomas are among the most common of primary retroperitoneal tumors
- Leiomyosarcomas account for less than 10% of all soft tissue sarcomas yet a significant percentage of retroperitoneal sarcomas because almost half of them appear in this region
- The most common lesion associated with radiation is malignant fibrous histiocytoma

Lipomas

- Consist almost entirely of mature fat and are uncommonly found in the retroperitoneum.
- Most common soft tissue tumor in humans.

89. Myelolipoma

- Usually occurs in the adrenal gland
- In patients > 40 years and are mostly <5 cm
- The adrenal gland can create inferior renal displacement due to a radiolucent mass.

90. Upper urinary tract urothelial tumors involving the renal pelvis or ureter, accounts for 5% to 7% of all renal tumors and about 5% of all urothelial tumors

91. The incidence of upper tract recurrence has been shown to be higher in

- Patients with CIS than in patients with noninvasive papillary TCCs
- Patients treated with cystectomy for CIS rather than for invasive cancer

92. Risk factors for upper urinary tract tumors

- Balkan nephropathy
- Smoking

- Coffee intake
- Analgesics
- Aniline dyes
- βnaphthylamine
- Benzidine
- Chronic bacterial infection associated with urinary stones and obstruction
- Lynch syndrome II.

Balkan nephropathy and those seen in association with analgesic abuse and arsenic endemic areas, have an even higher tendency to multiple and bilateral recurrences than do sporadic tumors.

93. **Tumors of renal pelvis are more common** than ureteral tumors.
    - **Ureteral tumors more common in the lower** than in the upper ureter.
    - 70%–distal ureter, 25%–midureter and 5%–proximal ureter.
94. **Bilateral involvement (either synchronous or metachronous)** occurs in–1.6% to 6% of sporadic upper tract transitional cell cancers.
95. **Patients with upper tract tumors are at risk for development of bladder cancer**–(15% to 75%) within 5 years of the development of the upper tract cancer.

    Upper tract cancers have been reported to develop in 2% to 4% of patients with bladder cancer, with a mean interval to recurrence of 17 to 170 months.
96. **Stage**–most important predictor of survival in patients with upper tract urothelial tumors.

    High grade–more likely to invade the connective tissue, muscle and surrounding tissues.
97. **Transitional cell carcinoma**
    - TCC makes up more than 90% of upper urinary tract tumors
    - Relative thinness of the muscle layer of the renal pelvis and ureter makes invasion through the muscle coat an earlier event.

    Squamous cell carcinoma
    - Frequently associated with chronic inflammation or infection or with analgesic abuse
    - Six times more frequently in the renal pelvis than in the ureter

- Generally moderately to poorly differentiated and more likely to be invasive at the time of presentation.

Adenocarcinoma

- Associated with long term obstruction, inflammation, or urinary calculi
- These tumors typically present at advanced stage and display a poor prognosis.

98. **Most common presenting symptom** of upper tract urothelial tumors is hematuria.

    Most common finding on imaging studies–filling defect.

99. **Imaging for upper tract malignancies**
    - With CT urography, the sensitivity of 100%, with a specificity of 60% and a negative predictive value of 100%
    - Diagnostic accuracy can be improved from 75% with IVU/ RGU alone to 90% when it is combined with ureteroscopy

100. **TCC has an average density**–46 HU (range of 10 to 70 HU).

     Radiolucent uric acid stones has an average density–100 HU (range, 80 to 250 HU).

101. **Ureteral tumors are low grade and low stage in**–55% to 75%.

     Renal pelvic tumors are papillary in–85%.

102. **Staging of upper urinary tract tumor**

Ta	Papillary noninvasive carcinoma
Tis	Carcinoma in situ
T1	Tumor invades subepithelial connective tissue
T2	Tumor invades the muscularis
T3	Tumor invades periureteral fat [for renal pelvis only] Tumor invades beyond muscularis into perinephric fat or the renal parenchyma
T4	Tumor invades adjacent organ, or through the kidney into the perinephric fat
N1	Metastasis to a single lymph node, <2 cm
N2	Metastasis in a single lymph node, 2 cm - 5 cm or multiple lymph nodes, none more than 5 cm
N3	Metastasis in a lymph node, >5 cm
M1	Distant metastasis

103. (EAU Guidelines 2012) for the diagnosis of Upper Urinary Tract-Urothelial Cell Carcinoma (UUT-UCC)

Recommendations

- Urinary cytology.
- Cystoscopy to rule out a concomitant bladder tumor.
- CT urography.

104. (EAU Guidelines 2012) Indications for radical nephroureterectomy (RNU) for UUT-UCC

- Suspicion of infiltrating UUT-UCC on imaging.
- High-grade tumor (urinary cytology).
- Multifocality (with two functional kidneys).

Techniques for RNU in UUT-UCC

- Open and laparoscopic access are equivalent in terms of efficacy.
- Bladder cuff removal is must.
- Lymphadenectomy is recommended in case of invasive UUT-UCC.

Indications for conservative management of UUT-UCC

- Unifocal tumor.
- Small tumor.
- Low-grade tumor (cytology or biopsies).
- No evidence of an infiltrative lesion on CT urography.
- Understanding of close follow-up.

Techniques used in conservative management of UUT-UCC

- Laser should be used in case of endoscopic treatment.
- Flexible ureteroscopy is preferable over rigid ureteroscopy.
- Open partial resection is an option for pelvic ureteral tumors.
- A percutaneous approach remains an option in small low-grade caliceal tumors unsuitable for ureteroscopic treatment.

105. Radical nephroureterectomy with resection of a bladder cuff is gold standard for

- Large, high grade and invasive
- Large, multifocal or rapidly recurring

- Medium-grade, noninvasive tumors of the renal pelvis or proximal ureter.

Radical nephroureterectomy and dialysis

Offer the best chance of cure and survival in patients with a large, invasive, high-grade, organ-confined renal pelvis tumor (T2, N0, M0) in a solitary kidney.

106. The entire ureter, including the intramural portion and ureteral orifice, should be removed or the risk of tumor recurrence in a remaining **ureteral stump is 33% to 75%.**

107. Pluck technique, should be reserved for proximal, low-grade tumors urothelial tumors.

108. The rationale for regional lymphadenectomy

- Adds little time or morbidity to the surgery.
- Important for prognosis, and may occasionally have therapeutic value.

109. Segmental ureterectomy for:

- Grade 1 to grade 2, stage Ta to stage T1 tumors of the proximal ureter or midureter that are not amenable to complete ablation by endoscopic means because of size or multiplicity.
- Segmental excision also is offered for grade 1 to grade 2, stage T2 tumors of the proximal ureter or midureter.

Distal ureterectomy and neocystostomy for:

- Low-grade, low-stage tumors that are not controlled by endoscopic means.
- Ureteral excision may also be suitable for some high-grade, locally invasive tumors of the distal ureter.

110. Isolated urine cytology positive

- By definition, the patient should have normal IVU and RGP, normal cystoscopy, and normal biopsy findings from the bladder and urethra.
- Ureteropyeloscopy is indicated in such cases.

111. Crossing vessel responsible for UPJ obstruction is–aberrant posterior segmental artery passing anterior to the PUJ

112. **The kidney has four constant vascular segments**, which are termed apical, anterior, posterior and basilar. The anterior segment is the largest.

113. Unlike the arterial structure of the kidney, the **renal venous system is characterized by a rich anastomotic network** between the various renal segments.

Ligation and division of segmental veins can be done without compromising drainage

114. **Renal artery embolization (RAE)**

Indication

- For palliation of inoperable renal tumors, to control bleeding
- For multimodal treatment of hypervascular metastatic disease

Benefits of preoperative RAE-

- Shrinkage of an arterialized tumor thrombus to ease surgical removal, and reduce blood loss
- Ability to ligate the renal vein before the renal artery at time of nephrectomy
- Modulation of the immune response

Complication

- The postinfarction syndrome, characterized by flank pain, nausea, and fever. Occurs in 75% of patients (most common complication)

115.

Approach	**Advantages**	**Disadvantages**
Flank	• For surgery on lower renal pole, UPJ, and upper ureter • For simple nephrectomy, PCN insertion, and drainage of perinephric abscess • Prevents peritoneal contamination	• Provides poor access to renal hilum and renal vasculature • Poor option for radical or partial nephrectomy

Thoracoabdominal	• For radical nephrectomy and partial nephrectomy of large renal masses, especially those of the upper pole and those with venous extension	• Longer operative time • Greater potential pulmonary morbidity
Dorsal lumbotomy	• Useful for simple nephrectomy for small atrophic kidney • Simultaneous bilateral simple nephrectomies in ESRD • Fresh tissue planes in patients with numerous prior abdominal or flank procedures • No muscles are transacted	• Poor control of the renal vessels
Abdominal	• Exposure in the area of the renal pedicle is excellent	• Ileus, adhesions, and possible bowel obstruction

116. The chevron incision

- Bilateral anterior subcostal approach
- Advantageous for renovascular surgery and radical nephrectomy with IVC tumor thrombectomy.
- Exposure of the renal pedicles and great vessels is good

117. Key step of a simple nephrectomy

Division of the artery followed by the vein and than division of the ureter

118. Indications for surgical or percutaneous (angioplasty or stenting) renal revascularisation

- Hypertension not responsive to multimodal medical therapy
- ACE-I induced GFR reduction or elevation of creatinine concentration
- Congestive heart failure (recurrent and difficult to manage)

- Favorable renal biopsy (salvageable glomeruli)
- Creatinine concentration <4.0 mg/dL
- Evidence of collateral circulation and renal size >7 cm
- Positive nuclear function study
- Doppler resistive index <0.80
- Lateralization of renin on renal vein sampling
- Progressive occlusion

119. Almost all disease processes affecting renal artery patency, can be bypassed with an aortorenal graft

The preferred graft in adults and also the most common graft material used for restoration of renal blood flow–autogenous saphenous veins

120. The kidney with a totally occluded renal artery may be revascularized when the following criteria are fulfilled:

- Angiographic demonstration of a nephrogram
- Proximal occlusion with retrograde filling of distal circulation
- Intraoperative back-bleeding from a renal arteriotomy distal to the occlusion
- Intraoperative frozen section or preoperative biopsy of an intact glomerular architecture.

121. Periods of warm ischemia beyond 30 minutes–significant, immediate functional loss.

122. Hypothermia (temperature of 20°C to 25°C) provides complete renal protection from arterial **occlusion of up to 3 hours.**

123. Renal functional impairment is less

- **Renal artery (RA) alone** is continuously occluded (as compare to RA and RV occlusion).
- **Continuous arterial occlusion** rather than intermittent clamping of the renal artery with short periods of recirculation.
- **Simple arterial occlusion** rather than manual renal compression.

124. Patients with > 50% reduction in overall renal mass are at the greatest risk for proteinuria, glomerulopathy and progressive renal failure.

125. Multiple cyst punctures and unroofing of cysts **(Rovsing's operation)** do not appear to improve renal function or to prevent further deterioration.

126. **Open biopsy is usually preferred to the percutaneous technique in:**

- Solitary kidney, coagulopathy, atypical anatomy, or other factors that may increase the risk of a closed biopsy.
- An open biopsy also provides more tissue for study and minimizes the potential for complications such as arteriovenous fistula, perirenal hematoma and gross hematuria.

127. **Nephroptosis**

- Diagnosis by color doppler imaging in the supine and upright positions.
- Descent of the symptomatic kidney by two vertebral bodies and obstruction or diminished flow to the symptomatic side

128. **Access options for laparoendoscopic single site surgery (LESS) are**–Keyhole, Triport, Uni-x and Gelport

129. **Most common cause of conversion to open surgery with laparoscopic renal surgery**–vascular injuries.

- This is more commonly seen in patients undergoing nephrectomies for chronic inflammatory processes.

130. **Complete destruction of normal renal parenchyma occurs at temperatures <19.4° C.** Cancer cells may need even lower temperatures for reliable cell death.

131. **The adequacy and reproducibility of tissue destruction during cryoablation is dependent upon several parameters:**

- Minimum preferred target temperature is < −40° C.
- Double freeze-thaw cycle is the standard of care
- Performed under real-time imaging with the treatment area 1 cm beyond tumor margin
- Initial freeze cycle of 8 to 10 minutes and a second freeze cycle of 6 to 8 minutes.
- Passive thaw is preferred for initial freeze cycle
- Active thaw is preferred following the second freeze cycle

132. **Heating >60° C** results in instantaneous and irreversible coagulation necrosis of all biologic tissues, with denaturation of cellular proteins, melting of lipids, and disintegration of cell membranes.

133. **Adequacy and reproducibility of tissue destruction during RFA is dependent upon several parameters:**

- Mean treatment temperature of 105° C is preferred
- Number of cycles
  - o Tumors <2 cm are treated with two cycles of 5 minutes
  - o Tumors 2 to 3 cm are treated with two cycles of 7 minutes
  - o Tumors >3 cm are treated with two cycles of 8 minutes
- Application of energy
  - o Needles placed directly into tissue (dry RFA)
  - o Ionic solutions perfuse into tissues to decrease carbonization and act as energy conductor (wet RFA).
- More complete necrosis and superior treatment outcomes with multitine electrodes
- Advantage of bipolar energy is that significantly higher temperatures are induced compared with those of monopolar devices

134. **The incidence of major urologic complications** with renal cryoablation and RFA is 4.9% and 6.0% respectively

Most common complication of cryoablation–bleeding

135. **Evidence of complete tissue destruction and treatment success**–complete loss of contrast enhancement on follow-up CT or MRI

136. **There is no significant difference** in the risk of local tumor recurrence, disease progression/metastasis, cancer specific survival, and overall survival between RFA and cryoablation.

❑❑

Chapter 13
ADRENALS

1. **Measurements**–5 cm in length by 3 cm in width and 1 cm thick.
   - **In the healthy adult, the glands weigh**–5 g each.
   - **Adrenal weight at birth**–5 to 10 g.
   - Right adrenal gland is **triangular** in shape while the left adrenal gland is **crescent shaped**
2. **Adrenal cortex** develops from mesoderm and **medulla** develops from neuroectoderm.
3. **Adrenal gland development** occurs normally in the absence of ipsilateral renal unit development, malrotation, or malascent.
4. **Adrenal cortex constitutes 90% of the gland.**
   - **Divided into three zones**–zona glomerulosa, zona fasciculata and zona reticularis.
   - **Zonation is complete by**–18 months, but adult configuration is not reached until the age of 10 to 12 years.
5. **The right adrenal**–bounded medially by the IVC and anteriorly by the liver

   Left adrenal gland–bounded medially by the aorta and anteriorly by the stomach, pancreas, and splenic vessels
6. **Arterial supply**
   - Superior adrenal arteries (branches from the inferior phrenic arteries)
   - Middle adrenal arteries (direct visceral branches from the aorta),
   - Inferior adrenal arteries (branches from the ipsilateral renal artery

   Venous supply
   - On the left, the adrenal vein is long compared with the right and is joined by the inferior phrenic vein prior to draining into the left renal vein
   - On the right adrenal vein drains directly into IVC

Lymphatic drainage

- Paracaval lymph nodes on the right
- Para-aortic lymph nodes on the left.

Nervous supply

The autonomic innervation of the adrenal glands includes

- Preganglionic sympathetic fibers to the chromaffin cells of the adrenal medulla
- Postganglionic fibers originating from the splanchnic ganglia provide innervation to the adrenal cortex.
- Parasympathetic innervations to the adrenal cortex and medulla is not well defined

7. **Primary effects of mineralocorticoids**
   - Increase in blood volume and blood pressure
   - Decrease in urine sodium and chloride
   - Increase in urine potassium and NH4
   - Increase in serum chloride and decrease in serum potassium
8. **The medulla secretes** epinephrine (80%), norepinephrine (19%), and dopamine (1%).
9. **Rate limiting step for the formation of all DHEA, and androstenedione is**–production of pregnenolone.
10. **Primary physiologic control of aldosterone secretion is**– angiotensin II.

    Second, less potent stimulus for aldosterone release is–potassium.
11. **Excessive production of glucocorticoids by the adrenal cortex is defined as Cushing syndrome**

    Causes of Cushing syndrome can be divided into

    (1) exogenous

    (2) ACTH-dependent

    (3) ACTH-independent
12. ACTH-dependent hypercortisolism accounts for 80% to 85% of endogenous Cushing syndrome.
    - 80% of ACTH-dependent disease is due to primary pituitary pathology and is known as **Cushing disease.** (The most common cause is a corticotropin-producing microadenoma)

- Ectopic ACTH production is the other main cause of ACTH-dependent hypercortisolism

13. **Most direct and reliable index of cortisol secretion**–24-hour excretion of cortisol in the urine.
14. **Ideal way to determine whether a patient has ACTH-dependent or ACTH-independent hypercortisolism is**–concurrent measurement of both plasma ACTH and cortisol.
15. **Ideal time to measure these hormones** is between midnight and 2 AM, when the concentrations are at the lowest.

    Highest level of cortisol is detected in the mornings, while nadir is observed at 11 PM.
16. **Most direct way to demonstrate pituitary hypersecretion of ACTH is**–to measure its level in the petrosal venous sinus and compare the level with the peripheral level.
17. **Gold standard approach for distinguishing ectopic ACTH production from Cushing disease**–Direct measurements of ACTH in the inferior petrosal sinus following CRH stimulation
    - High levels of ACTH in the inferior petrosal sinus, when compared to those in peripheral blood, indicate Cushing disease
    - Levels similar to peripheral plasma suggest an ectopic ACTH source
18. **ACTH secreting pituitary adenomas**
    - Current standard of care is transsphenoidal surgical resection.
    - Cure is seen in only 60% to 80% of patients
    - 25% of individuals relapse
    - Macroadenomas(> 1 cm) are resistant to neurosurgical treatment
19. **Adrenal carcinomas are often indistinguishable from adenomas :**
    - Larger size (>6 cm) are more common with carcinoma.
    - Necrosis and calcification are more common with adrenal carcinoma but are not diagnostic.
    - Mean attenuation on NCCT scan in adrenal carcinoma is 39 HU compared with adenomas (8 HU).
    - The majority of adrenal cortical carcinomas will be functional at the time of presentation
    - CT washout studies are considered the gold standard for adrenal imaging.

- Rapid loss of contrast enhancement can differentiate even lipid-poor adenomas from other lesions

20. Nelson's syndrome

- After bilateral adrenalectomy **10% to 20%** of patients develop pituitary tumors, usually chromophobe adenomas.
- Due to **lack of hypothalamic-pituitary feedback** and the high levels of ACTH.
- For prevention-patients should receive lifelong mineralocorticoid and glucocorticoid replacement
- Prophylactic pituitary radiotherapy is also an option.

21. Exploration of incidentally found adrenal mass

- Functional adrenal mass
- >5 cm on CT and solid
- <5 cm on CT, solid and high signal T2 on MRI
- Adrenal incidentaloma that grow >1 cm on follow-up imaging

22. Adrenal is site of metastasis in:

- 50% from patients with **melanomas and carcinomas of the breast and lung.**
- 40% from patients with renal cell carcinomas.
- Then, in order of frequency, carcinomas of the contralateral adrenal, bladder, colon, esophagus, gallbladder, liver, pancreas, prostate, stomach and uterus.

23. Weiss proposed nine histologic criteria
if >3 are present, the lesion is considered malignant.

Adrenocortical Carcinoma: Weiss Criteria

- High mitotic rate (>5/ 50 HPF).
- Atypical mitoses.
- Venous invasion.
- High nuclear grade (Fuhrman 34).
- Absence of cells with clear cytoplasm (<25% of cells).
- A diffuse growth pattern (more than one third of tumor).
- Necrosis.
- Sinusoidal invasion.
- Capsular invasion.

24. **Endothelial or lymphangiomatous cysts** account for 45% of adrenal cystic lesions and are usually small, measuring 0.1 to 1.5 cm in diameter.

- **Adrenal pseudocysts** that lack an epithelial lining are the next most common variety (39%).

25. **Myelolipoma**

- Rare, benign, metabolically silent lesions that arise primarily from the adrenal gland
- In all age groups
- Metabolically non-functional lesions.
- CT reveals a well-circumscribed adrenal lesion with varying amounts of mature adipose tissue (30 HU)
- The presence of macroscopic fat in an adrenal mass is virtually diagnostic of a myelolipoma.
- Asymptomatic myelolipomas are treated conservatively.
- Surgery is usually reserved for symptomatic lesions

26. **Ganglioneuromas**

Rare, benign tumors that tend to occur in the young and can grow to encase critical structures

27. **Chronic adrenal insufficiency**

- AR and associated with a deficiency in the enzyme 21-hydroxylase in over 95% of cases.
- Triad–hyponatremia, hyperkalemia and azotemia present in 50% to 60% of cases.

28. **Dexamathasone has longest** half life (36-54 hours) with **highest** anti-inflammatory potency

29. **Primary hyperaldosteronism (PAL) (Conn)**

- Hypertension, hypokalemia, hypernatremia, alkalosis, and periodic paralysis caused by an aldosterone-secreting adenoma.
- ↓ PRA and ↑ urine and plasma aldosterone levels. (In secondary aldosteronism- ↑ PRA)
- Unprovoked hypokalemia is the hallmark of hyperaldosteronism.
- Idiopathic hyperplasia and aldosterone-producing adenomas accounts for over 95% of cases

30. Surgically correctable PAL

- Aldosterone-producing adenoma
- Primary unilateral adrenal hyperplasia
- Ovarian aldosterone-secreting tumor
- Aldosterone-producing carcinoma

Surgically un-correctable PAL

- Bilateral adrenal hyperplasia
- Familial hyperaldosteronism type I
- Familial hyperaldosteronism type II

31. Screening test of choice for Conn syndrome is a morning plasma aldosterone (ng/dL) to renin (ng/mL/hr) ratio (ARR).

An ARR of 20 along with a concomitant aldosterone >15 ng/mL are indicative of Conn syndrome

32. The cornerstone of medical therapy in PAL caused by idiopathic hyperaldosteronism is a mineralocorticoid receptor antagonist (i.e., spironolactone, eplerenone).

33. Pheochromocytoma

- 10% are found in normotensive patients.
- 10% familial
- 10% pediatric
- 5% of all incidentalomas are pheochromocytomas.
- 25% of all pheochromocytomas are found incidentally.
- 10% to 20% are malignant. (malignancy can only be defined by the presence of clinical metastases)

34. Pheochromocytomas occur in MEN II–(triad includes pheochromocytoma, MCT and parathyroid adenomas).

35. Hereditary Forms of Pheochromocytoma

Syndrome	**Gene**	**Chromosome**
MEN type 2	RET oncogene	10q11
VHL type 2	VHL tumor	3p25
Neurofibromatosis type 1	NF1	17q11
Familial paraganglioma syndrome type 4	SDHB	1p36
Familial paraganglioma syndrome type 1	SDHD	11q23

36. **Classic hallmark of pheochromocytoma**–triad of headache, episodic sudden perspiration, and tachycardia

    Classic presenting symptom with pheochromocytoma–Paroxysmal hypertension

37. **Confirmation of the diagnosis**–increase in catecholamines in the blood or urine, occur in 95% to 99% of patients with pheochromocytoma.

    - >3 times elevation of catecholamines

      → MRI +ve → Pheochromo-cytoma

      → MRI–ve→Reconfirm with MIBG

    - >3 times elevation of catecholamines

      →MRI +ve→Pheochromocytoma

      →MRI –ve→Follow up.

38. **Imaging for pheochromocytoma**

    - CT- Attenuation of >10 HU on unenhanced CT. (because of rich vascularity and low lipid content)
    - MRI- Bright, **"light bulb"** image on T2–weighted study.
    - ^{123}I-MIBG, affords a high sensitivity (83% to 100%) and high specificity (95% to 100%)

39. **General anesthesia for pheochromocytoma patients include**–induction with an intravenous agent such as thiopental followed by isoflurane as the inhalation agent of choice.

    - For control of hypertension α blockade (phenoxybenzamine) should be started before β blockade

40. **Laparoscopic adrenalectomy**–standard of care for adrenal lesions with the exception of invasive adrenocortical carcinoma or adrenocortical carcinoma with caval thrombus.

❑❑

Chapter 14

URINE TRANSPORT STORAGE AND EMPTYING

1. **Mitochondria**–Perform nutritive functions of the cell.

   Endoplasmic reticulum–Ca^{2+} storage sites.

2. **Caspases**–promote ureteral bud branching.

   Angiotensin–act through the AII receptor and is involved in the recanalization process of ureter

3. **The RMP of the ureteral cell**–(–33 to 70) mV, (determined by **K^+ ions** across cell membrane)

4. **In excited state**–membrane loses its preferential permeability to **K+** and becomes more permeable to **Ca2+** ions that move inward across the cell membrane

5. **Plateau** is due to a persistent inward **Ca2+** current and to an influx of **Na+.**

   Repolarization of the membrane is due to a renewed increase in permeability to **K+.**

6. **"Pacemaker cells"**–Located near the pelvicalyceal border.

   Latent pacemaker cells–are present in all regions of the ureter.

7. **Conduction velocity** in the ureter 2 to 6 cm/sec.

   Baseline ureteral pressure–0 to 6 cm H_2O.

   Superimposed ureteral contractions–20 to 80 cm H_2O occur 2 to 6 times per minute.

8. **Cycle of smooth muscle shortening**

   - With excitation, increase in the **sarcoplasmic Ca2+** concentration
   - At higher concentration, Ca2+ forms an active complex with the Ca2+binding protein **calmodulin**
   - The Ca2+calmodulin complex activates, **myosin light-chain kinase**
   - The activated myosin light-chain kinase, catalyzes the **phosphorylation of myosin**

- Phosphorylation of the myosin light chain allows actin to activate myosin Mg2+-ATPase **activity**
- This leads to **hydrolysis of ATP** and the **development of smooth muscle tension or shortening**

9. ATP $\xrightarrow{\textbf{Mg}^{2+}\textbf{, GTP and adenyl cyclase}}$ cAMP.

10. cAMP $\xrightarrow{\textbf{Phosphodiesterase}}$ 5-AMP.

11. **Agents that increase cAMP levels and thus causes smooth muscle relaxation are**

- **Increase adenylyl cyclase activity,** such as the β-adrenergic agonist isoproterenol
- **Decrease phosphodiesterase activity,** such as theophylline and papaverine,

12. L-arginine $\xrightarrow{\textbf{NADPH and NOS}}$ NO and L-citrulline

Nitric oxide (NO) stimulates soluble guanylyl cyclase activity and causes **smooth muscle relaxation**

13. **There are three NOS isoforms.**

	Ca2 +	**NADPH**
Neuronal NOS (nNOS)	Dependent	Dependent
Endothelial NOS (eNOS),	Dependent	Dependent
Inducible NOS (iNOS)	Non dependent	Dependent

14. **Hysteresis**–Resting or contractile force developed at any given length depends on the direction in which the change in length is occurring and on the rate of length change.

Creep–As the obstruction persists, there is a gradual increase in ureteral length and diameter to considerable dimensions.

15. **Excitatory effect on ureteral and renal pelvic function** (increase the frequency and force of contractions).

- Cholinergic agonists.
- Anticholinesterases.
- Nicotinic agonists.
- αadrenergic agonist.
- Tachykinins.
- H_1 receptor.

- Capsaicin in high doses.
- Angiotensin.

Inhibitory effect on ureteral and renal pelvic function

- Nicotinic agonists.
- β-adrenergic agonist.
- H_2 receptors.
- CGRP.
- Capsaicin in low doses.
- Calcium antagonists
- Potassium channel openers.

16. **The ureter decompensate** when intravesical pressure approaches 40 cm H_2O.
17. **Two weeks of ureteric obstruction results in**
    - Increase in ureteral contractility but a decrease in contractile intraluminal pressures.
    - Decrease in the ability to generate an active intraluminal pressure and coaption of ureteral lumen thus impair urine transport in the obstructed ureter.
18. **Factors that affect the spontaneous passage of calculi are**
    (1) Size and shape of the stone
    (2) Intrinsic areas of narrowing within the ureter
    (3) Ureteral peristalsis
    (4) Hydrostatic pressure of the column of urine proximal to the calculus
    (5) Edema, inflammation, and spasm of the ureter at the site at which the stone is lodged
19. **Bladder compliance (C)** = change V/change P.
20. **Normal bladder compliance** should be <12.5 mL/cm H_2O.
21. **Pdet** = Pves–Pabd.
22. **Hydroureteronephrosis of pregnancy**
    - Begins in the second trimester of gestation
    - Subsides within the first month after parturition.
    - It is more severe on the right side

- Ureteral dilatation does not occur below the pelvic brim

23. Laplace law- Tension = Pves X Radius /2diameter

24. Musculature of bladder- rhabdosphinter +Lissosphincter + periuethral muscle

Lissosphincter includes

- Periureteric sheath
- Detrusor base
- Urethral smooth muscle

25. Urinary bladder is composed of 50% collagen and 2% elastin

26. Parameters abnormally elevated in patients with bladder disease compared with normal patients

- Percentage volume of connective tissue
- Ratio of connective tissue to smooth muscle
- Ratio of type III to type I collagen.

27. Umbrella cells forms the primary urine-plasma barrier and is unique in several ways.

- Ability to increase and to decrease considerably their surface area
- Multinucleate.
- Outer leaflet consisting of protein plaques and lipid and with a lipid inner leaflet.
- High gradient between the plasma and the urine in terms of water concentration, urea concentration, K+ concentration, osmolality, and pH

28. **Uroplakins**–primary attachment site of type 1 pili.

The primary function is to be part of the primary plasma-urine barrier.

29. **Striated muscle** within the distal urethra is composed primarily of slow-twitch myofibrils.

Periurethral striated muscles contain both fast-twitch and slow-twitch fibers.

Rhabdosphincter

- In the male–35% is fast-twitch and 65% is slow-twitch fibers.
- In the female–87% is slow-twitch and 13% is fast-twitch.

30. **Pelvic parasympathetic nerves**

- Arise at the sacral level of the spinal cord, excite the bladder and relax the urethra.

Lumbar sympathetic nerves

- Inhibit the bladder body and excite the bladder base and urethra (**mainly by β_3 adrenoceptor**).

Pudendal nerves excite the external urethral sphincter.

31. **Onuf's nucleus** is the external urethral sphincter motor neurons and are located along the lateral border of the ventral horn

32. **Bladder Afferent**

Fiber type	Location	Normal function	Inflammation effect
Aδ (finely myelinated axons)	Smooth muscle	Sense bladder fullness	Increase discharge at lower pressure threshold
C fiber (unmyelinated axons)	Mucosa Mucosa muscle	Respond to stretch Nociception to overdistention	Increase discharge at lower threshold Sensitive to irritants

Small myelinated Aδ fibers

- Normal sensations of bladder filling.

C-fiber

- Normally has high mechanical thresholds and do not respond to even high levels of intravesical pressure.
- In **the irritated state**, these fibers become responsive to low-pressure bladder distention like mechanoreceptive Aδ fibers.
- Fiber stimulation can than cause bladder pain and urge incontinence

33. **Excitatory transmitter**–Glutamic acid.
Inhibitory neurons–GABA and glycine.

34. **Micturition reflex** is normally mediated by a **spinobulbospinal reflex pathway**

- **Transections at any point above the colliculi**–facilitates micturition.
- **Transections at any point below the colliculi**–abolish micturition.

35. **Bladder ice-water test**

- Clinical demonstrations of reemergence of the primitive neonatal micturition reflex.
- Method to assess the C fiber–mediated micturition reflex.
- Way to differentiate "upper" from "lower" motor neuron lesions.

36. **Anticholinergics**

- Darifenacin is selective for the M3 subtype (30 folds as over M2)
- Darifenacin is not tissue selective, because salivary glands also contain M3 receptors.
- Solifenacin receptor selectivity for M3 receptors over M2 receptors (10-fold)
- Solifenacin is selective to the bladder over the salivary gland
- **M2 receptors predominate (M2 : M3 is 3:1)**
- **M3 receptors most important for contraction**

37. **Adrenergic receptors**

- The β3-adrenergic receptor is the most highly expressed subtype among α- and β-adrenoceptor subtypes
- α1a adrenoceptor is the major subtype in the prostate and urethra

38. **In decreasing order of potency,** PGF2α, PGE1, and PGE2 contract the human detrusor

    The predominant forms found in human urothelium are 6-oxo-PGF2α > PGE2 > PGF2α > thromboxane B2

39. **Capsaicin and its RTX are vanilloids**–stimulate and desensitize a specific population of sensory nerves (unmyelinated C fibers) to produce pain and release neuropeptides.

40. **Smooth sphincter**

- Smooth musculature of the bladder neck and proximal urethra
- Physiologic but not an anatomic sphincter
- Not under voluntary control.

Striated sphincter

- Part of the outer wall of the proximal urethra (**intrinsic or intramural striated sphincter or rhabdosphincter)**

- Surrounds the urethra at the level of the membranous portion in the male and primarily the middle segment in the female (**extrinsic or extramural striated sphincter**).
- The extramural portion is under voluntary control

41. **Genuine stress incontinence (GSI)**–hypermobility of the bladder outlet because of poor pelvic support and with an outlet that was competent at rest but lost its competence only during increases intra-abdominal pressure.

    Intrinsic sphincter deficiency (ISD)–poorly functional bladder neck and proximal urethra at rest.

42. **Neurogenic detrusor overactivity (detrusor hyperreflexia)**–Overactivity accompanied by a neurologic condition.

    Idiopathic detrusor overactivity (Detrusor instability)–Detrusor overactivity without concurrent neurologic etiology.

43. **Striated sphincter dyssynergia (DESD)** is most commonly seen after complete suprasacral spinal cord injury, following the period of spinal shock.

    Smooth sphincter dyssynergia is seen most classically in autonomic hyperreflexia

    Detrusor areflexia secondary to bladder muscle decompensation or to various conditions that produce inhibition at the level of the brainstem micturition center, the sacral spinal cord, bladder ganglia, or bladder smooth muscle.

44. **Sensory neurogenic bladder**–DM, tabes dorsalis and pernicious anemia

    Motor paralytic bladder–Extensive pelvic surgery, trauma and Herpes zoster.

45. **Zero reference level for uroflowmetry transducer is at** superior edge of the symphysis pubis.

46. **Physiologic filling rate** for cystometry = body weight (in kg)/4, expressed as mL/min.

47. **Detrusor Leak Pressure Point (DLPP)**

    - Lowest detrusor pressure at which urine leakage occurs in the absence of either a detrusor contraction or increased abdominal pressure.
    - The higher the DLPP, the higher the urethral resistance
    - **DLPP>40 cm H_2O**– higher risk for upper tract deterioration.

48. Abdominal /Valsalva Leak Pressure Point (ALPP/VLPP)

- Intravesical pressure at which urine leakage occurs because of increased abdominal pressure in the absence of a detrusor contraction.
- Measure of sphincter strength.
- There is **no normal ALPP** as patients without SUI do not leak at any physiologic abdominal pressure.
  - o A VLPP <60 cm H_2O–significant ISD.
  - o VLPP of 60 to 90 cm H_2O–equivocal, suggesting a combination of urethral hypermobility and some component of ISD.
  - o VLPP > 90 cm H_2O–urethral hypermobility and minimal ISD.

49. Maximum urethral closure pressure (MUCP)

- The maximum difference between the urethral pressure and the intravesical pressure.
- Normal MUCP is 40 to 60 cm H_2O.
- ISD is MUCP < 20 cm H_2O.

Functional profile length

- The length of the urethra along which the urethral pressure exceeds intravesical pressure in women.
- In continent women, the functional **urethral length is 3 cm.**
- **Continence point** in women is at midurethra.

50. Uroflowmetry

- Voided volumes >150 mL should only be interpreted.
- **In men**–Qmax >15 mL/sec–normal and < 10 mL/sec–abnormal.
  There is a decline in Qmax with age.
- **In women**–Qmax >30 mL/sec–normal
  Qmax in women is not dependent upon age.

51. Maximum cystometric capacity–volume includes both the amount voided and PVR.

Functional bladder capacity–volume voided as determined by a voiding diary.

Maximal anesthetic capacity–volume of the bladder after filling under anesthesia (general, spinal, epidural).

52. **Forty percent of patients** with urge incontinence do not have detrusor overactivity on a CMG.

53. **Bethanechol supersensitivity test**

- Distinguish the cause of detrusor underactivity as neurogenic or myogenic
- A positive test suggests an interruption in the afferent or efferent peripheral, or distal spinal innervation, of the bladder.

54. **Pressure flow studies-** differentiate between patients with low flow because of obstruction and those with poor bladder contractility.

It identify three voiding states

1. Low detrusor pressure and high flow rate (normal).
2. High detrusor pressure and low flow rate (obstructed).
3. Low detrusor pressure with low flow rate (impaired detrusor contractility).

55. **Detrusor opening pressure**

- Detrusor pressure at the onset of measured flow.
- Pressure >80 cm H_2O may indicate BOO.

Detrusor pressure at maximal flow

- Detrusor contraction at the time when the flow rate is at its maximum.
- Pressure > 100 cm H_2O, indicates BOO even if the flow rate is normal.

56. **Male generally voids** with a Pdet of 40 to 60 cm H_2O, and women typically void with lower pressures.

57. **AG number/Bladder outlet obstruction index (BOOI)** = PdetQmax–2 Qmax

- >40 obstruction.
- <20 no obstruction.
- 20 to 40 equivocal.

58. **Bladder contractibility index (BCI)** = PdetQmax + 5 Qmax.

- BCI >150 is strong.
- BCI <100 is weak.
- BCI of 100 to 150–normal contractility.

59. **Urodynamic study is recommended before surgery for urinary incontinence only if**
    - clinical suspicion of detrusor overactivity
    - history of previous surgery for stress incontinence or anterior compartment prolapse
    - symptoms are suggestive of voiding dysfunction
60. **The micturition reflex is normally under voluntary control** and is organized in the rostral brainstem (the pontine micturition center [PMC]).
61. **Causes of detrusor overactivity (DO)**

    Neurogenic detrusor overactivity
    - Supraspinal neurological lesions(parkinsonism, hydrocephalus, stoke)
    - Suprasacral spinal lesions(tumor, injury, multiple sclerosis)
    - DM

    Neurogenic detrusor overactivity
    - Infection
    - BOO
    - Bladder tumor
    - Bladder stones
62. **Absent or diminished detrusor activity**
    - Infrasacral lesions
    - Subdivided into cauda equina lesions (within the spinal canal) and peripheral lesions (outside the spinal canal)
63. **Causes of low bladder compliance**

    Neurogenic
    - Myelodysplasia
    - Suprasacral spinal cord injury/lesion
    - Radical hysterectomy
    - Abdominoperineal resection

    Non-Neurogenic (Increased Collagen)
    - Tuberculous or radiation cystitis

- Chronic indwelling catheter
- Bladder outlet obstruction

64. Male sphincter mechanism

- **Proximal "bladder neck mechanism"**
    - o Consist of bladder neck, prostate and prostatic urethra to the level of verumontanum
    - o This portion of the continence mechanism is removed during prostatectomy, leaving only the distal urethral sphincter mechanism to prevent urinary leakage.
- **Distal urethral mechanism**
    - o It is at the apex of the prostate.
    - o This extends from the verumontanum to the proximal bulb
    - o It is composed of the prostatomembranous urethra, cylindrical rhabdosphincter (external sphincter muscle) surrounding the prostatomembranous urethra, and extrinsic paraurethral musculature and connective tissue structures of the pelvis
    - o In damaged distal urethral sphincter (e.g., a pelvic fracture), continence can be maintained solely by the proximal bladder neck mechanism

65. Female sphincter mechanism

- Proximal bladder sphincter mechanism is weak
- Distal urethral mechanism
    - o Extend along the majority of the length of the female urethra and prone to the effect of exogenous influences such as pelvic floor weakness and damage or denervation consequent on childbirth

66. Causes of transient incontinence (DIAPPERS)

- **D**elerium
- **I**nfection (urinary tract infection)
- **A**trophic vaginitis/urethritis
- **P**sychologic (e.g., severe depression, neurosis)
- **P**harmacologic
- **E**xcess urine production
- **R**estricted mobility
- **S**tool impaction

67. Classification systems used to quantify Pelvic organ prolapse

Most widely used are the Baden-Walker classification and the Pelvic Organ Prolapse Quantification system, known as the "POP-Q"

In the POP-Q system, nine specific points of measurement are obtained in relation to the hymenal ring

68. The degree of urethral hypermobility–assessed by the **Q-tip test.**

- **Hypermobility**–resting or straining angle >30 degrees from the horizontal.

69. Pad weight–gain of >1.3 g over 24 hours is considered a "positive" test.

70. Video-urodynamics–most precise diagnostic tool for voiding dysfunction.

71. The Agency for Healthcare Policy and Research (AHCPR) suggests that PVR less than 50 mL represents **adequate emptying** and PVR greater than 200 mL represents **inadequate emptying**

72. Most common Patterns of Voiding Dysfunction Seen with Various Disease or Injury

Disorder	Detrusor activity	Compliance	Smooth sphincter	Striated sphincter	Other
CVAO(MC)	O	N	S	S	
Parkinson's disease	O	N	S	S Pseudodyssynergia	Bradykinesia TURP not contraindicated
SCI–Above T6	O	N	D	D	Autonomic hyperreflexia
SCI–T6 to S2	O	N	S	D	
SCI–Sacral	A	N/↓	CNR/O	F	
Myelodysplasia	A	N	O	F	
Disk disease	A	N	CNR	S	
Radical pelvic surgery	I/A	↓/N	O	F	
Diabetes	I,A,O	N	S	S	Sensory loss and motor neuropathy

- Detrusor activity–I, impaired; O, overactive; A, areflexia.
- Compliance–N, normal.

- Smooth sphincter–S, synergic; D, dyssynergic; O, open, incompetent at rest; CNR, competent nonrelaxing.
- Striated sphincter–S, synergic; D, dyssynergic; F, fixed tone.

73. **Most frequently involved with associated micturition dysfunction are**–superior aspects of the frontal lobe.
74. **Parkinson disease (PD)**
    - Neurodegenerative disorder of unknown cause that affects primarily the dopaminergic neurons of the substantia nigra
    - Asymmetry of symptoms and signs, resting tremor, and a good response to levodopa
    - Symptoms- urgency, frequency, nocturia, and urge incontinence.
    - 25% to 50% have "obstructive" symptoms or a combination.
    - The most common urodynamic finding is detrusor overactivity.
    - The smooth sphincter is synergic
    - Pseudodyssynergia as well as bradykinesia can occur at the onset of voluntary micturition.
    - TURP is not contraindicated in patients with PD
75. **The sacral spinal cord begins at**–spinal column level T12 to L1.
    - **The spinal cord terminates in the cauda equina at**–spinal column level of L2.
76. **Spinal shock**
    - Includes a suppression of autonomic activity, as well as somatic activity
    - Bladder is acontractile and areflexic.
    - Radiologically, the bladder has a smooth contour with no evidence of trabeculation.
    - The bladder neck is generally closed and competent
    - The smooth sphincter mechanism is functional.
    - MUCP is lower than normal but still maintained at the level of the external sphincter zone
    - Normal guarding reflex is absent and there is no voluntary control
77. **Autonomic hyperreflexia**
    - It is an acute massive disordered autonomic (primarily sympathetic) response to specific stimuli in patients with SCI above the cord level of T6 to T8 (the sympathetic outflow).

- It is more common in cervical (60%) than thoracic (20%) injuries.
- Onset after injury is variable- usually soon after spinal shock to years after injury.
- Distal cord viability is a prerequisite.
- Headache, hypertension, and flushing of the face and body above the level of the lesion with sweating.
- Bradycardia is a usual accompaniment, although tachycardia or arrhythmia may be present.
- The stimuli for this exaggerated response commonly arise from the bladder or rectum and generally involve distention
- Symptoms resolve quickly if the stimulus is withdrawn.
- Striated and striated sphincter dyssynergia occurs
- Sublingual nifedipine is capable of alleviating this syndrome when given during cystoscopy

78. **Diabeties mellitus**–impaired bladder sensation, increased cystometric capacity, decreased bladder contractility, impaired uroflow, and, later, increased residual urine volume.

79. **Sphincter dyssynergia**

   A. **Detrusor Sphincter Dyssynergia (DESD)**

- Involuntary contraction or lack of relaxation of striated sphincter.

   B. **Smooth sphincter dyssynergia (proximal urethral obstruction, primary bladder neck obstruction and dysfunctional bladder neck).**

- Involuntary contraction or lack of relaxation of smooth sphincter (the smooth muscle of the bladder neck and proximal urethra).
- Almost exclusively in young, anxious, and high-strung individuals.
- Normal DRE, a negligible PVR, and normal endoscopic bladder appearance.
- Evidence of BOO obtainable by urodynamic study.
- Treatment–Alpha adrenergic blocking agents / bladder neck incision.

80. **Trapped prostate**

- When prostatic enlargement develops with smooth sphincter dyssynergia double obstruction results.

81. Non-neurogenic neurogenic bladder (occult voiding dysfunction, occult neuropathic bladder, learned voiding dysfunction or Hinman syndrome).

- Involuntary obstruction at the striated sphincter level in absence of neurologic disease.

82. "Anxious bladder" or a "bashful bladder"

- Hesitancy when attempting to initiate micturition in the presence of others.

83. Fowler syndrome

- Syndrome of urinary retention in young women in the absence of overt neurologic disease.
- Bladder capacity > 1 liter with no sensation of urgency is necessary for the diagnosis.
- No neurologic or laboratory features to support a diagnosis of any neurologic disease.

84. Incidence of OAB

- Both genders have similar rates of OAB
- "OAB wet" is more prevalent in women and "OAB dry" is more prevalent in men

85.

	Painful bladder syndrome	Overactive bladder
Incontinence	Rare	Present with urgency
Voided volumes	Similar	Differ widely

86. Detrusor activity are of two types:

1. Phasic DO

- Contractions of increasing amplitude as the bladder volume increases
- This pattern seen in most idiopathic DO.

2. Terminal DO

- Single involuntary detrusor contraction occurring at cystometric capacity
- Causes incontinence, often resulting in complete bladder emptying.
- Seen in the elderly person with "precipitant voiding" such as elderly patients who have suffered cerebrovascular accident.

86. **Nomenclature**

- **Night-time frequency-** voids that occur after the individual has gone to bed but before he or she has gone to sleep and voids that occur in the early morning, which prevent the individual from getting back to sleep as he or she desires
- **Nocturnal enuresis-** loss of urine occurring during sleep
- **Polyuria-** 24-hour voided volume in excess of 2.8 L (>40 mL/kg).
- **Frequency-** number of voids recorded during waking hours including the last void before sleep and first void after waking and rising in the morning
- **Nocturia-** number of voids recorded during a night's sleep: each void is preceded and followed by sleep.
- **Nocturnal urine production-** adding the first morning void to the nocturnal voided volume
- **Nocturnal polyuria** is defined as nocturnal urine production exceeding 20% of 24-hour output in younger adults and 33% in older adults

87. **Drugs with grade A or level 1 recommendation** for detrusor overactivity is:

- Tolterodine (antimuscarinic drugs).
- Trospium.
- Solifenacin.
- Darifenacin.
- Fesoterodine
- Oxybutynin (mixed actions).
- Propiverine.

88. **Anticholinergics**

	Tertiary	**Quaternary**
Lipophilicity	Higher	Lower
Molecular size	Small	Large
Charge	Low	High
GIT	Well absorbed	Not well absorbed
CNS	Crosses easily	Does not cross
Drugs	Atropine, tolterodine, oxybutynin, propiverine, darifenacin and solifenacin	Trospium

89. Tolterodine

- Major active 5-hydroxymethyl metabolite (5-HMT) significantly contributes to the therapeutic effect of tolterodine
- No selectivity for muscarinic receptor subtypes
- Has functional selectivity for the bladder over the salivary glands

90. Oxybutynin

Well absorbed and undergoes extensive upper gastrointestinal and first-pass hepatic metabolism

The primary metabolite is *N*-desethyloxybutynin (DEO)

- It has pharmacologic properties similar to those of the parent compound
- It occurs in much higher concentrations after oral administration
- It has been implicated as the major cause of dry mouth

91. Trial on antimuscarinic drugs

- **OBJECT trial** compared oxybutynin extended-release (ER), 10 mg once daily, with tolterodine immediate-release (IR), 2 mg twice daily.
    - o **Conclusion**–Oxybutynin ER was more effective than tolterodine IR.
    - o Rates of dry mouth and other adverse events were similar in both treatment groups.
- **OPERA study** compared oxybutynin ER at 10 mg/day or tolterodine ER at 4 mg/day.
    - o **Conclusion**–Reductions in weekly urgency incontinence and total incontinence episodes were similar with the two drugs.
    - o Dry mouth was more common with oxybutynin ER, but tolerability was comparable, including adverse events involving the CNS.
- **ACET trial**–2 mg or 4 mg of once-daily tolterodine ER and in the other trial to 5 mg or 10 mg of oxybutynin ER.
    - o **Conclusion**–Patients treated with tolterodine ER 4 mg reported a significantly lower severity of dry mouth compared with oxybutynin ER 10 mg.

92. Duloxetine

- Combined serotonin-norepinephrine reuptake inhibitor.
- Stimulation of the pudendal nerve at the level of Onuf's nucleus in the sacral cord, causing increased urethral sphincter tone.
- At a dose of 40 mg twice daily, duloxetine decreased incontinence episodes by about 51% versus 33% for placebo.
- Only drug used in treatment of SUI with grade A recommendation.
- Side effects include nausea (most common) and dry mouth.
- Increased risk of suicidal thinking and behavior in patients taking antidepressants
- Withdrawn from the U.S. FDA for the treatment of SUI

93. Capsaicin

- Capsaicin exerts a biphasic effect: initial excitation is followed by a long-lasting blockade
- In sufficiently high concentrations, capsaicin causes "desensitization" initially by releasing and emptying the stores of neuropeptides and then by blocking further release
- Resiniferatoxin (RTX) is an analogue of capsaicin, approximately 1000 times more potent for desensitization than capsaicin but only a few hundred times more potent for excitation

94. Botulinum toxin

- Types A and B are in clinical use in urology, but mostly BTX-A.
- Commercially available products of type A (Botox and Dysport).
- The toxin blocks the release of acetylcholine.
- Positive outcomes in DESD, pelvic floor spasticity, and possibly BPH and interstitial cystitis.
- A good response rate appears to occur within 1 week and last for 6 to 9 months before reinjection is necessary.

95. Both estrogen and estrogen plus progesterone causes worsening of preexisting urinary incontinence (both stress and urgency) and an increased new incidence of urinary incontinence

96. Desmopressin (DDAVP)

- Synthetic vasopressin analog with a pronounced antidiuretic effect but practically lacking vasopressor actions.

- The dose–20 μg intranasally at bedtime.
- Drug is orally active, even if the bioavailability is low (<1% compared with 2% to 10% after intranasal administration).
- Risk of water retention and hyponatremia.
- Effective in pediatric nocturnal enuresis and also in adults with nocturia of polyuric origin.

97. Bethanechol

- It exhibits a relatively selective in-vitro action on the urinary bladder and gut with little or no nicotinic action
- It is cholinesterase resistant and causes an in-vitro contraction of smooth muscle from all areas of the bladder

98. Agents that decrease outlet resistance

At the level of smooth sphincter

- α-adrenergic receptor agonist
- NO

At the level of smooth sphincter

- Benzodiazepines
- Baclofen
- Dantrolene
- Botulinum toxin

99. Urinary incontinence

- **Stress**–Involuntary leakage on exertion or on sneezing or coughing.
- **Urge**–Involuntary leakage accompanied by or immediately proceeded by **urgency.**
- **Mixed**–Involuntary leakage of urine associated with urgency and also with exertion, effort, sneezing or coughing.

100. Urinary incontinence

- **Unconscious (unaware) incontinence**–involuntary loss of urine that is unaccompanied by either urge or stress.
- **Overflow (paradoxical) incontinence** is–not a symptom or condition but rather a term used to describe leakage of urine associated with urinary retention.

- **Extraurethral incontinence** is–the observation of urine leakage through channels other than the urethra (e.g., fistula or ectopic ureter).

101. **Most important zone of continence**–midurethra supported anteriorly by the pubourethral ligaments.

102. **Bulbocavernosus reflex**
   - Checked by
     (1) Suddenly squeezing the glans penis or clitoris and feeling the anal sphincter and perineal muscles contract.
     (2) Suddenly pulling the balloon of the Foley catheter against the bladder neck.
   - The absence of this reflex in men is almost always associated with a neurologic lesion, but the reflex is not detectable in upto 30% of otherwise normal women.

103. **For women with SUI (Efficacy):**
   - PFMT = duloxetine.
   - PFMT > electrical stimulation and bladder training
   - PFMT and surgery are both effective therapies but PFMT is better as a first-line treatment because it is less invasive

   For women with SUI or mixed UI:

   PFMT > vaginal cones

   PFMT> phenylpropanolamine or clenbuterol because of the side effects with the medications

   For women with UUI or mixed UI:

   PFMT and bladder training are both effective first-line therapy

   PFMT > oxybutynin

104. **High-frequency stimulation (50 to 200 Hz)** has been used with vaginal or anal electrodes for SUI

   Low-frequency stimulation (5 to 20 Hz) is intended to activate inhibitory bladder reflexes and reduce detrusor overactivity.

105. **EGGS–Expectations, Goal setting, Goal achievement, and Satisfaction–**

   It is the process in which the patient's perspective is explored to develop an individualized treatment plan

106. Pessary usage

- Pessaries used for prolapse only should be fitted with an empty bladder.
- Pessaries intended for use in SUI should be fitted with the bladder at a comfortable fullness.

107. Patients are classified into three groups based on the assessment of pelvic floor muscle strength at baseline examination :

(1) those with no or minimal ability to isolate and contract the levator muscles

(2) those who can isolate the correct muscles with poor strength, and

(3) those with good pelvic floor muscle strength and isolation on the initial examination

- **First group**–these patients need some form of teaching/ biofeedback (or passive stimulation) just to get started
- **Second group**–these patients require some form of pelvic muscle rehabilitation
- **Third category**–If these patients have significant UI there is generally severe urethral incompetence and severe bladder dysfunction; and they require more aggressive treatment

108. Sacral Nerve Responses

Sacral nerve	Motor and sensory response
S2	Motor: Plantar flexion of the entire foot clamp movement of the anal sphincter
	Sensory: Sensations in the leg and buttock
S3	Motor: Dorsiflexion of the great toe and a bellows reflex (anal wink)
	Sensory: Paresthesias or sensation of pulling in the rectum, scrotum or vagina
S4	Motor: Bellows reflex only
	Sensory: Sensation of pulling in the rectum only

109. For optimal bladder emptying to be achieved–sacral anterior root stimulation with posterior rhizotomies of S2, S3, and S4 would be required

110. The Brindley device–most commonly used for electrical stimulation.

111. The detrusor–innervated primarily by S3 and to a smaller extent by S2 or S4.

Rectal stimulation–by all three roots equally (S2, S3 and S4).

Erectile stimulation–by S2 with a small contribution from S3 and none from S4.

112. Surgical methods for SUI

- Open retropubic colposuspension
- Laparoscopic retropubic colposuspension
- Suburethral sling procedure
- Needle suspension
- Periurethral injection
- Artificial sphincter
- Vaginal anterior repair (anterior colporrhaphy

113. Retropubic suspension surgery

Indication–correction of anatomic SUI.

1. For a patient undergoing a laparotomy for concomitant abdominal surgery that cannot be performed vaginally.
2. Where there is limited vaginal access.

Contraindication

1. When SUI exists solely due to ISD.
2. Panpelvic floor weakness
3. When there is an inadequate vaginal length or mobility of the vaginal tissues, for example, after prior vaginal surgery or radiotherapy

114. Recommendation from the ICI committee (grade A)

- Anterior colporrhaphy should not be used in the management of SUI alone
- MMK procedure is not advised for the treatment of SUI
- Open colposuspension is as effective as any other procedure in primary or secondary surgery at curing SUI with proven long-term success
- Paravaginal defect repair is not recommended for the treatment of SUI alone
- Laparoscopic colposuspension is not recommended for the routine surgical treatment of SUI in women

- Endoscopic and nonendoscopic bladder neck needle suspension procedures, with and without bone anchors, are not recommended for the treatment of SUI

115. Sutures used in:

- MMK procedure(chromic catgut).
- Burch procedure(chromic catgut).
- VOS procedure(polyglycolic acid or polydioxanone).
- Paravaginal repair(silicon-coated Dacron).

116. No significant difference in cure rates–**between retropubic suspensions** and **pubovaginal approach**

117. TVT appears to be at least equivalent to the **Burch colposuspension.**

118. Retropubic suspensions are more effective than either **needle suspensions or anterior colporrhaphies.**

119. Two types of absorbable meshes are available:

Polyglycolic acid (Dexon) takes 90 days for absorption.

Polyglactin 910 (Vicryl) hydrolyze by 21 days and loses its mechanical support by 30 days

120. Most desirable synthetic for pelvic floor reconstruction are monofilament, macroporous mesh, most commonly polypropylene mesh.

121. The pubococcygeus can be palpated during physical examination of the pelvis as a bulky muscular ridge on both right and left lateral side walls of the vagina.

122. After hysterectomy, the vaginal cuff will have dimples at the 3 and 9 o'clock areas, at the locations of the cardinal uterosacral ligament attachments.

123. Nomenclature

- **Colpocleisis**: obliteration of vaginal lumen.
- **Colporrhaphy**: repair of vaginal wall.
- **Colpectomy**: resection of vagina.
- **Colpopexy**: suspension of vaginal wall.
- **Culdotomy**: incision into (posterior) cul-de-sac (pouch of Douglas).
- **Culdoplasty**: surgical obliteration of cul-de-sac.

124. Summary of Principal Risks and Benefits of Vaginal Apical Repairs

Procedure	Major risks	Major benefits
Sacrospinous ligament Fixation	• Postoperative anterior prolapse • Injury to pudendal and inferior gluteal arteries and pudendal and sciatic nerves • Ligament may be atrophied in elderly • More difficult to teach and learn	• No ureteral injury; rectal injury rare
Uterosacral ligament suspension	• Possible bowel and ureteral injuries • Ligaments may not be apparent or usable	• Normal vaginal supports; resultant vaginal axis may be most physiologic
Iliococcygeus suspension	• Possible shortened vagina	• No vital structures nearby

125. The ideal material for sling is

- Sterile, biocompatible, noncarcinogenic, and consistent in quality.
- The implanted material is incorporated into the host with minimal tissue reaction and provides long-lasting suburethral support with minimal complications.

126. Type of graft

- **Autologous graft** is the gold standard, associated with no tissue reaction and negligible urethral erosion.
- **Allografts** can lead to transfer of infection, and also, the type of processing technique may disrupt the microstructure and affect strength properties.
- **Xenografts** have less tensile strength than allograft in situ and have the highest propensity to encapsulate.

127. Type 1 mesh

- A synthetic polypropylene monofilament mesh.
- Pore size under 150 μm.
- Allows optimal migration of host inflammatory components and is optimal for inciting fibrous tissue ingrowth.

128. For TOT tape insertion

- Cystoscopy is performed to exclude needle penetration of the lower urinary tract.
- The use of a 70-degree lens is essential, as is complete distention of the bladder with irrigant to exclude subtle tangential injury.

129. TOT

- Never penetrates the adductor longus muscle.
- Implanted material traverse adductor magnus, adductor brevis, and gracilis muscles during its path into the pelvis.
- At the level of the obturator foramen, the tape traverse both the obturator externus and internus muscles as well as the obturator membrane.
- More medially, the tape entered the anterior compartment of the ischiorectal fascia.
- The tape remained outside the pelvic space and did not penetrate the levator ani muscular group.

130. Comparing TOT with TVT procedures–no significant difference in postoperative voiding dysfunction, complications, or overall continence.

131. The ideal injectable agent

- Should be easily injectable and conserve its volume over time.
- It should also be biocompatible, nonantigenic, noncarcinogenic, and nonmigratory
- Agent should cause little or no inflammatory reaction or fibrotic ingrowth
- The components of the bulking agent should not separate or dissociate on injection
- If the substance used is not successful it should not interfere with subsequent surgical intervention

132. Types of injectable material for SUI

Biologic

BULKING–Homologous: bovine collagen, porcine collagen

FUNCTIONAL–Autologous muscle stem cells

Synthetic

Carbon-coated zirconium beads (Durasphere), polydimethylsiloxane (Macroplastique), hyaluronic acid, dextranomer (Deflux), polyacrylamide hydrogel (Bulkamid), calcium hydroxyapatite (Coaptite)

Balloons

Adjustable balloons (ACT, ProACT)

133. Indicators of ISD

- MUCP of less than or equal to 20 cm H2O
- ALPP of less than or equal to 60 cm H2O

134. Stamey incontinence grading system

- Grade 0–Continent
- Grade 1–Patient loses urine with sudden increases in abdominal pressure but not while supine
- Grade 2–Patient loses urine with physical stress (walking; changing from a reclining to a standing position;sitting up in bed)
- Grade 3–Patient with total incontinence; urine loss unrelated to physical activity and/or position

135. Bulking agents

- Patients with isolated ISD are the **best candidates for injection.**
- Injectable agents may provide a rapid response for some patients and are an option for those who do not wish to undergo more invasive procedures.
- The efficacy and duration are inferior to surgery, and follow-up injections may be required.
- Those with detrusor overactivity or impaired contractility of the bladder may be more prone to complication.

136. Agent is implanted within the urethral wall, preferably into the submucosa or lamina propria.

137. Males and females are injected by either transurethral or periurethral approach (The transurethral approach is much more commonly reported than the periurethral approach.)

138.

	Periurethral	**Transurethral**
Bleeding	Less	More
Learning curve	Longer	Shorter
Volume of injected material	Higher	Lower
Rate of urinary retention	Higher	Lower

139. Patients rendered dry or socially continent are considered as a treatment success in evaluation of results.

Type of surgery		Success rate
Sling surgery	–	81% to 98%
Sphincter surgery (abdominal or transvaginal approach)	–	90%
PTFE	–	70% to 95%
GAX Collagen	–	64% to 95%
Fat	–	70% to 90%
Silicone macrospheres	–	70% to 82%

140. In postprostatectomy urethra

- Most male patients undergoing injection therapy for mild postprostatectomy incontinence require four to five injections with reinjections every 6 to 12 months to maintain dryness.
- If material extravasation occurs in all quadrants during injection, the procedure should be terminated and rescheduled after 4 weeks

141. In bladder overdistension–potential complications include bladder rupture (5% to 10%), hematuria and retention.

142. Denervation

- Central denervation appears to be more suitable for patients with SCI or neurogenic DO but may cause a wide range of unintended side effects.
- Peripheral denervation is relatively bladder selective and more suitable for DO, with fewer neurologic side effects
- Denervation may be achieved by sectioning anterior (motor), posterior (sensory) or both sacral roots, converting an overactive bladder into an areflexic one

143. The anterior S3 nerve root is the dominant motor innervations of the human bladder

144. Clean intermittent catheterization (CIC)

- **Lapides** popularised CIC.
- For adult patients, catheterization is performed at a minimum of **every 4 to 6 hours** to minimize bacterial dwell time.
- **12- to 16-Fr soft catheter** is used

- Any patient requiring intermittent catheterization may obtain up to **200 sterile catheters per month** for one-time use

145. **The long-term risk of** carcinoma in the SCI patient with a chronic catheter has been estimated to be 8% to 10%

146. **In males, the benefits of an indwelling suprapubic catheter** over urethral catheterization include a lower incidence of epididymitis and urethral stricture disease with preservation of sexual function

147. **Condom catheter**
    - The most common male external collection device is the condom catheter.
    - Perceived as more comfortable than indwelling catheters; however, the device can be unacceptable due to its visibility and potential for foul odors.
    - Associated with pressure-related injuries, especially when used by patients with impaired sensation or cognition.
    - Associated with a lower incidence of complications than indwelling catheters, but higher complication rates than if no devices or products are used at all.

148. **For decreasing outlet obstruction surgical sphincterotomy is done at 12-o'clock sphincterotomy,**
    - The anatomy of the striated sphincter is such that its main bulk is anteromedial.
    - 12-o'clock incision is least likely to cause hemorrhage, with reported rates of 5% to 20%.
    - The rate of postoperative erectile dysfunction with this incision is approximately 5%

149. **Pharmacologic sphincterotomy can be attempted with** botulinum toxin for the treatment of DESD

150. **Young-Dees principle**
    - Construction of a neourethra from the **posterior** surface of the bladder wall and trigone.
    - In the male, the prostatic urethra affords additional substance for closure and increase in outlet resistance.

    Leadbetter modification
    - Proximal reimplantation of the ureters to allow more extensive tubularization of the trigone.

Tanagho principle

- Used **anterior** bladder neck to create a functioning neourethral sphincter.

151. **"Trigger voiding"**–induced by pulling the skin or hair of the pubis, scrotum, or thigh; by squeezing the clitoris; or by digital rectal stimulation.

152. **To facilitate bladder emptying**

- Bladder neck incision at the 5 and/or 7 o'clock position: a single full-thickness incision extending from the bladder base down to the level of the verumontanum.
- **DLPP as the most reliable urodynamic parameter** to predict the risk of upper tract complications after sphincterotomy.

153. **Changes in bladder physiology due to age**

- Bladder capacity does not change
- Bladder sensation, contractility, and the ability to postpone voiding decline in both sexes
- Urethral length and maximum closure pressure, as well as striated muscle cells in the rhabdosphincter and urogenital diaphragm, decline with age in women

154. **Principles of indwelling catheter**

- Infection prophylaxis, as well as treatment of asymptomatic bacteriuria, is not recommended
- Surveillance cultures are unnecessary
- If symptomatic urinary tract infection (UTI) develops, change the catheter before obtaining a culture specimen
- If catheter obstruction occurs frequently, and urine cultures reveal Providencia stuartii or Proteus mirabilis, antibiotic treatment may reduce the frequency of obstruction
- For long-term need, a silicone or silicone hydroge–lcoated catheter should be considered.

155. **Detrusor hyperactivity with impaired contractility (DHIC)** is the most common form of detrusor overactivity in the elderly.

156. **Most common type of acquired fistula of the urinary tract**–VVF.

157. **In the industrialized world, the most common cause (>75%) of VVF**–injury to the bladder at the time of gynecologic, urologic, or other pelvic surgery.

- After **abdominal hysterectomy rate of iatrogenic bladder injury is**–0.5% and 1.0% and **fistula** is 0.1% to 0.2%.
- **Post-hysterectomy VVFs are thought to result most commonly** from an incidental unrecognized iatrogenic cystotomy near the vaginal cuff.
- Bladder injuries are at least three times more common during **abdominal hysterectomy compared with vaginal hysterectomy**

158. In developing world, VVF most commonly results from– prolonged obstructed labor.

Obstetric fistulae tend to be larger, located distally in the vagina, and may involve large portions of the bladder neck and proximal urethra

159. Radiation

- Higher radiation doses–greater risk for morbidity as well as with fistula formation.
- Median interval from completion of radiation therapy to presentation of VVF–8.7 months.

160. Postsurgical VVFs have an associated ureteral injury or ureterovaginal fistula in–12%.

161. Investigations for VVF

- Upper urinary tract evaluation is important and **IVU** is sufficient for this purpose.
- **An endoscopic examination and MCU** should be performed.

162. Uncomplicated postgynecological urinary tract fistulas repaired–as soon as identified.

- **VVF resulting from obstructed labor**–3- to 6-month delay before definitive repair.
- **Radiation-induced fistulas**–6 to 12 months delay before repair.

163. Abdominal versus Transvaginal Repair of Vesicovaginal Fistula

	Abdominal	**Transvaginal**
Timing of repair	Often delayed 3-6 months	Can be done inmediately
Exposure	Fistula low on bladder neck may be difficult to expose transabdominally	Fistula high at the vaginal cuff may be difficult to expose transvaginally

Location of ureters	Fistula near ureteral orifice may necessitate reimplantation	Reimplantation may not be necessary even if fistula track is near ureteral orifice
Sexual function	No change in vaginal depth	Risk of vaginal shortening
Use of adjunctive	Omentum, peritoneal flap, rectus abdominis flap gluteal skin or gracilis	Martius fat pad, peritoneal flap, flaps myocutaneous flap
Relative indications	Large fistulas • Location high in a deep narrow vagina • Radiation fistulas • Failed transvaginal approach, Small-capacity bladder requiring augmentation, need for ureteral reimplantation • Inability to place patient in the lithotomy position	Uncomplicated fistulas • Low fistulas

164. Transvaginal approach–Raz, Latzko, Webster.

Transabdominal approach–O'Conor (Suprapubic Intraperitoneal-Extraperitoneal), GilVernet (transvesical).

165. The blood supply to the martius flap is provided

- **Inferiorly**–posterior labial vessels (off the internal pudendal artery).
- **Superiorly**–external pudendal artery.
- **Laterally**–obturator artery.
- **The lateral blood supply is sacrificed** during mobilization of the flap.
- In cases where mobilizing and then tunneling the Martius flap to reach certain location compromise its blood supply and viability, **a peritoneal flap is preferred**

166. Most common etiology of ureterovaginal fistula is–surgical injury to the distal ureter, with gynecologic procedures being most common cause.

- **Most ureterovaginal fistulas** occur during procedures for benign as opposed to malignant indications.
- **The incidence of iatrogenic ureteral injury** during major gynecologic surgery is estimated to be about 0.5% to 2.5%.

167. **Large VVF**–continuous urine leakage.

168. **Ureterovaginal fistula**–urine leakage with normal voiding habits as bladder filling is maintained from the contralateral kidney (Similar pattern of voiding in ectopic ureter also).

169. **Course of pelvic ureter**

In the deep pelvis, the ureter passes at the lateral edge of the uterosacral ligament and ventral to the uterine artery, and then passes just lateral to the cervix and fornix of the vagina

170. **Vesicouterine fistula**

- Caesarean section is by far the most common cause
- This may or may not present with constant urinary incontinence owing to the sphincter-like activity of the cervix.

171. **Youssef's syndrome**

- Complex of vesicouterine fistula.
- Menouria.
- Cyclic hematuria with associated apparent amenorrhea.
- Infertility.
- Urinary continence in a patient who has undergone prior LSCS.

172. **Diagnosis of a urethrovaginal fistula**–micturating cystourethrogram.

173. **Colovesical fistula**

- **Diverticulitis** accounting for approximately 70% of cases.
- **Gouverneur's syndrome**–The classic presentation of vesicoenteric fistula is–suprapubic pain, urinary frequency, dysuria and tenesmus.
- **Triad of findings on CT** that are suggestive of colovesical fistula consists of:
  1. Bladder wall thickening adjacent to a loop of thickened colon.
  2. Air in the bladder.
  3. Presence of colonic diverticula.
- **CT is now generally considered to be the most sensitive and specific modality.**
- **The Bourne test**–useful adjunctive study in the evaluation of colovesical fistula.

174. Uroenteric fistulas

- Most likely to occur in the setting of inflammatory bowel disease such as **Crohn's disease.**
- The segment of bowel most likely to be involved is the **terminal ileum.**
- Most cases of ureteroenteric fistula are **unilateral and right sided.**

175. Bladder diverticula

Congenital diverticula	**Acquired diverticula**
Childhood	After 60 years
Solitary and exclusive in boys	Multiple and more common in men
Lateral and posterior to the ureteral orifice	At the ureterovesical hiatus
Congenital weakness at the level of the UV junction	BOO or neurogenic vesicourethral dysfunction
Smooth walled	Trabeculated

176. Hutch diverticulum–If the diverticulum encompasses the ureteral orifice in the setting of a neurogenic bladder and vesicoureteral reflux.

177. In relation to size

Diverticula > saccules > Cellules

178. Most common histologic type of malignant neoplasia seen within bladder diverticula is–transitional cell carcinoma.

179. Bladder diverticulectomy

Is not indicated in all cases.

Surgical treatment should be reserved for

Chronic relapsing UTI, stones within the diverticulum, carcinoma or premalignant change, and, upper urinary tract deterioration as a result of obstruction or reflux

180. Urethral diverticula

- The urethropelvic ligament is composed of two layers of fused pelvic fascia that extend toward the pelvic sidewall bilaterally.
- Within and between these two leaves of fascia lies the urethra and urethral diverticula.
- **Tubuloalveolar glands** exist over the entire length of the urethra posterolaterally.

- Majority of the glands drains into the distal third of the urethra. (**Skene's glands** are the largest and most distal of these glands).
- **Urethral diverticula are thought to originate** from pathologic processes involving the periurethral glands.
- **The most common surgical approach to urethral diverticula-excision and reconstruction.**

181. Skene's gland abscesses and cysts

	Urethral diverticula	**Skene gland abnormalities**
Location	Proximal and mid urethra	Distal urethra
Drainage	Drain into distal urethra	Do not communicate with urethral lumen

182. Most common malignant pathologic process in urethral diverticula is–adenocarcinoma.

183. Male Perineal Sling and Artificial Urinary Sphincter

- Function by addressing the underactive outlet and (inadequate resistance of the sphincter) by increasing the resistance to urinary flow during the storage phase.
- Pathophysiology of the underactive outlet in the male is ISD.
- Not for uncontrolled overactive bladder, elevated storage pressures secondary to detrusor contractions, or decreased compliance and/or VUR.

184. Most frequently utilized male sling is the–bone-anchored perineal sling.

185. Cuff placement

- **In men with post-prostatectomy incontinence**–the bulbous urethra is the classic route of implantation of AUS through a perineal incision.
- **In the male patient with SUI who has not had previous radical prostatectomy**–cuff placed around the bladder neck through a transabdominal incision.
- **AUS cuff in children and women** is–placed at the bladder neck and is typically 6 to 8 cm in circumference.

❑❑

Chapter 15

BLADDER, LOWER GENITOURINARY CALCULI AND TRAUMA

1. **Benign tumor of bladder includes**
   - Epithelial metaplasia
   - Leukoplakia
   - Inverted papilloma
   - Papilloma
   - Nephrogenic adenoma
   - Cystitis cystica and glandularis
   - Leiomyoma (most common nonepithelial benign tumor of the bladder)
2. **Incidence of bladder cancer**
   - Three to four times more common in men than in women.
   - In men–fourth most common cancer after prostate, lung and colorectal cancers.
   - In women–ninth most common cancer.
3. **Males have higher 5-year survival** rates than women.
4. **Bladder cancer rarely been found** incidentally at autopsy.
5. **The median age of bladder cancer**–70 years

   Incidence and mortality from bladder cancer increases with age.
6. Bladder cancer is less common in African-Americans than in **whites**

   Death rate from bladder cancer is higher in **African-Americans** than in whites.
7. **Relative risk associated with urothelial cancer formation** is maximum with rubber workers and bus drivers
8. **Relative risk of bladder cancer with chronic UTI** –14 to 16 times
9. **Urothelial cancer formation after radiation**
   - Not age related

- Latency period is 15 to 30 years.
- Increased risk in patients with prostate or cervical cancer who are treated with radiation.

Chemotherapeutic agent that has been proven to cause bladder cancer– cyclophosphamide

10. **Characterstics of high grade papillary carcinoma is**
    - Fused branching papillae
    - Disordered organisation of cells
    - Enlarged nuclear size
    - Marked pleomorphism
    - Marked variation of nuclear chromatin
    - Multiple prominent nucleoli
    - Frequent mitosis
    - Absent umbrella cells
11. **In adolescents and in adults younger than 30 to 40 years:**
    - More favorable prognosis.
    - Present more frequently with superficial, low-grade tumors.
    - Risk for disease progression is the same, grade-for-grade, in younger patients as in older ones.
12.

	PUNLMP	LOW GRADE	HIGH GRADE
Recurrence (%)	27-47	48-71	55-58
Stage progression (%)	0-4	2-12	27-61
Survival (%)	93-100	82-96	74-90

13. **Hallmark of low grade nonmuscle-invasive disease**–alterations in the *FGFR-3* and deletions of chromosome regions 9p and 9q

    The main genetic changes that separate noninvasive from invasive disease–high *FGFR-3* and low *TP53* mutation rates and general genetic stability.
14. **The genetic abnormalities associated with CIS include alterations to**–*RB, TP53,* and *PTEN* (all these genes carry poor prognosis)
15. CIS

    Primary CIS–is not associated with papillary or invasive lesion, has TP53 overexpression but lacks deletion of chromosome 9.

Secondary CIS–is associated with papillary lesions, can display alterations in chromosome 9

16. **Causes of gross hematuria**
    - Only 50% have a demonstrable cause
    - 20% will have a urological malignancy
    - 12% will have a bladder tumor
    - 10% of patients with recurrent gross hematuria will have prostate cancer.
17. **A full hematuria evaluation for bladder cancer includes-**
    - Cystoscopy
    - Urine cytology
    - Upper-tract imaging (primarily a CT scan of the abdomen and pelvis)
    - PSA blood test.
18. **Oncogenes associated with bladder cancer**–*RAS* gene family.
19. **Tumor suppressor gene associated with bladder cancer**
    - *TP53* (chromosome 17p) **(most frequently altered gene in human cancers).**
    - *RB* (chromosome 13q) **(in aggressive TCCs).**
    - 9q loss **(early event in the development of low-grade superficial tumors).**
20. **Prognostic factors**
    - **Receptor for EGF**–increased expression is associated with more aggressive biologic behaviour.
    - **Tissue expression and urinary excretion of MMP9**–increased in all patients with bladder cancer and that levels reflect tumor grade and stage.
    - **Ecadherin**–important barrier against invasion that can become disrupted in invasive tumors.
    - **Urokinase plasminogen activator**–facilitate invasion of urothelial cancer cells.
    - **VEGF, bFGF**–stimulate angiogenesis.
    - **PCNA and/or Ki 67**–increased expression associated with worse prognosis.

- **Survivin**–inhibitor for apoptosis, is upregulated in urothelial cancer.
- **DNA triploid to tetraploid chromosome**–unfavorable pathologic characteristics and patients have a poor prognosis.

21. Most bladder carcinogens are aromatic amines

- **Cigarette smokers**–four fold higher incidence of bladder cancer than non-smokers (4-aminobiphenyl).
- **Phenacetin**–associated with an increased risk for TCC of the renal pelvis and bladder.
- **Chronic cystitis in the presence of indwelling catheters or calculi**–increased risk for squamous cell carcinoma (SCC) of the bladder.
- **2-10% of paraplegics** with long-term indwelling catheters develop bladder cancer, 80% of which are SCCs.
- **Schistosoma haematobium cystitis**–related to SCC.
- **HPV**–2%-35% of human bladder cancers are infected by HPV DNA.
- **Women treated with radiation for carcinoma of the uterine cervix or ovary**–twofold to fourfold increased risk of developing bladder cancer.
- **Cyclophosphamide**–nine fold increased risk of developing bladder cancer (mesna may reduce the risk of bladder cancer).

22. TCC was slightly elevated in relatives–greater among 2nd and 3rd–than 1st-degree relatives.

- This argues strongly against a straight–forward genetic mechanism being responsible.

23. Definition

- **Epithelial hyperplasia**–increase in the number of cell layers.
- **Urothelial metaplasia**–bladder lining, in focal areas, demonstrating a nontransitional epithelial appearance.
- **Von Brunn's nests**–islands of benign–appearing urothelium situated in the lamina propria.
- **Cystitis cystica**–von Brunn's nests in which urothelium in the center of the nest has undergone eosinophilic liquefaction.

- **Cystitis glandularis**–similar to cystitis cystica except that the transitional cells have undergone glandular metaplasia. Cystitis glandularis may be a precursor of adenocarcinoma.
- **Atypical hyperplasia**–similar to epithelial hyperplasia, except that there are also nuclear abnormalities and partial derangement of the umbrella cell layer.
- **Dysplasia**–epithelial changes that is intermediate between normal urothelium and carcinoma in situ.
- **Inverted papilloma**–benign proliferative lesion associated with chronic inflammation or bladder outlet obstruction.
- **Leukoplakia**–squamous metaplasia with marked keratinization, downward growth of rete pegs (acanthosis), cellular atypia and dysplasia.
- **Carcinoma in situ**–velvety patch of erythematous mucosa, endoscopically invisible. Histologically, it consists of poorly differentiated TCC confined to the urothelium.

24. **In carcinoma in situ (CIS)**–Urine cytopathology is positive in 80% to 90%.
25. **CIS**
    - Present in 25% or more of patients with high grade superficial tumors.
    - Between 40% and 83% progress to muscle-invasive cancer.
26. **According to the new WHO and ISUP system**
    - **Well-differentiated tumors (grade 1)**–papillary urothelial tumors of low malignant potential (PUNLMP).
    - **Moderately differentiated tumors (grade 2)**–low-grade urothelial carcinomas.
    - **Poorly differentiated tumors (grade 3)**–high-grade urothelial carcinoma.
27. **Bilharzial SCC**
    - 10 to 20 years younger than patients with TCC.
    - Exophytic, nodular, fungating lesions and well differentiated.
    - Low incidence of LN and distant metastases.
28. **Nonbilharzial SCC caused by**
    - Chronic irritation from urinary calculi.

- Long-term indwelling catheters.
- Chronic urinary infections.
- Bladder diverticula.

29. **Primary vesical adenocarcinoma**
    - Arise in the bladder base area or in the dome.
    - Most common type of cancer in exstrophic bladders.
    - Develop in response to chronic inflammation and irritation.
    - Poor prognosis.
30. **Urachal carcinomas**
    - Arise outside the bladder, and they are usually adenocarcinomas.
    - Tumors exhibit wider and deeper infiltration of the bladder wall than expected, compromising the results of partial cystectomy.
31. **Metastatic adenocarcinoma**–the primary sites for these tumors include the rectum, stomach, endometrium, breast, prostate and ovary.
32. **Tumor spread**
    - **Most common is en bloc spread,** which occurs in about 60% of tumor.
    - Tentacle-like invasion occurs in about 25% of tumors.
    - Lateral spread occurs in only about 10%.
33. **Newly diagnosed bladder cancers**

    Stage
    - 70% are nonmuscle invasive (Ta, T1 and CIS) at presentation.
    - 70% present as stage Ta, 20% as T1, and 10% as CIS

    Grade
    - 55%-60% are–**well differentiated or moderately differentiated, superficial papillary TCCs.**
    - 40%-45% are–**high-grade lesions.**
    - **Half of high grade are muscle invading (20%)** at the time of diagnosis.
    - **Half of patients with muscle invasive bladder cancer (10%)** already have occult distant metastases.
34. **Most important risk factor for progression is grade**, not stage

35. **Patients receiving BCG therapy who had lower urinary fibronectin levels** before the initiation of treatment (but after TUR) had a much higher likelihood of tumor free at 1 year.

36. **Most common presenting symptom** of bladder cancer is painless hematuria.

37. **Urine cytology**
    - **Falsely negative cytology**–even in 20% of patients with high grade tumor.
    - **False-positive cytology**–may occur in 1% to 12% of patients and is usually due to urothelial atypia, inflammation, or changes caused by radiation therapy or chemotherapy.
    - **Cytology should be performed on fresh urine** with adequate fixation.
    - Morning urine is not suitable because of the frequent presence of cytolysis.

38. **Location of bladder tumor**
    - **Tumors encroaching on the ureteral orifices**–resected without regard for the orifice.
    - **Tumors on the lateral bladder wall**–stimulation of the obturator nerve during resection (resulting in violent contraction of the adductor muscle of the thigh).
    - **Tumors arising in bladder diverticula** often should be sampled rather than resected.

39. **ALA**
    - **When administered intravesically in conjunction with fluorescent cystoscopy using blue light at 375 to 440 nm,** can enable detection of lesions invisible with white light cystoscopy.
    - **Under blue light they emit red fluorescence,** which can help in the diagnosis of unidentified malignant lesions.

40. **Transurethral ultrasonic assessment using 5.5-MHz** is helpful in distinguishing infiltration of superficial versus deep muscle and extravesical spread.

41. **CT in bladder tumor**
    - Can detect only gross extravesical tumor extension, LN and liver metastases that is >1 cm.
    - It fails to detect nodal metastases in upto 40% to 70% of patients.

42. **MRI** is more sensitive than CT or, radionuclide bone scans for determining the presence of bone metastases.

43. **2009, TNM Staging**

Ta	Papillary, epithelium confined
Tis	Flat carcinoma in situ
T1	Tumor invades subepithelial connective tissue
T2a	Superficial muscularis propria invasion
T2b	Deep muscularis propria invasion
T3a	Microscopic extension into perivesical fat
T3b	Macroscopic extension into perivesical fat
T4a	Cancer invading pelvic viscera (e.g., prostatic stroma, vaginal wall, rectum, uterus)
T4b	Extension to pelvic sidewalls, abdominal walls or bony pelvis
N1	Metastasis in single LN in true pelvis (IILN, EILN, presacral and obturator)
N2	Metastasis in multiple LN in true pelvis (IILN, EILN, presacral and obturator)
N3	Common iliac LN involvement
M1	Distant metastases documented

44. **Patients receiving the megadose vitamin**

- (40,000 units Vitamin A, 100 mg Vitamin B_6, 2000 mg Vitamin C, 400 units of Vitamin E and 90 mg zinc) regimen did significantly better, with projected 5-year recurrences.

45. **Carcinosarcomas** are highly malignant tumors containing malignant mesenchymal and epithelial elements.

46. **Most common primary sites for bladder secondaries are**–prostate, ovary, uterus, colon and rectum, lung, breast, kidney and stomach; primary melanoma, lymphoma and leukemia may also involve the bladder.

47. **Most common histologic subtype of sarcoma in bladder**–Leiomyosarcoma

    Active chemotherapeutic agents for bladder sarcomas are–doxorubicin, ifosphamide, and cisplatin

48. **Secondary prostatic urethral involvement in patients with a history of urothelial cancer is**

- 15% at 5 years and 30% at 15 years

- It is uniformly associated with extensive intravesical therapy

49. **For patients with noninvasive prostatic urethral cancer, or with prostatic ductal disease, treatment is**–complete TURP and BCG therapy.

50. **Bladder pheochromocytoma**
    - <1% of all bladder tumors.
    - <1% of all pheochromocytoma.
    - 10% of pheochromocytoma are malignant.
    - Arise from paraganglionic cells within the bladder wall, usually in trigone.
    - No sex predilection.
    - Peak age of incidence–2nd to 4th decades.
    - Hematuria–only about half of patients.
    - Treatment of choice–partial cystectomy with excision of the tumor.
    - TUR is generally contraindicated because it may precipitate a hypertensive crisis.

51. **Low risk**–Low-grade Ta lesion only, **whereas all high-grade and T1 lesions (including CIS) are high risk.**

52. **Low-grade Ta lesions recur**–50% to 70% **and progress**–5% of cases.

53. **High-grade T1 lesions recur in**–80% **and progress**–50% of cases.

54. **Prognosis depends on** tumor size, multiplicity, papillary versus sessile configuration, presence or absence of lymphovascular invasion, and status of the remaining urothelium.

55. **TUR can be performed in** sterile water. Saline solutions conduct electricity and disperse energy from the monopolar cautery cutting loop.

56. **Risk of obturator reflux can be decreased by:**
    1. Bipolar electroresection (TURIS).
    2. Laser resection.
    3. The use of general anaesthesia with muscle–paralyzing agents.
    4. Direct injection of 20 to 30 ml of lidocaine into the obturator nerve and its canal.

57. **Management of perforation**
    - **Extraperitoneal perforation**–prolonged urethral catheter drainage.

- **Intraperitoneal perforation**–often requires open or laparoscopic surgical repair.

58. ReTURBT

1. **Indication**–Patients with pT1 and high-grade Ta tumors.
2. **Repeat TUR** can demonstrate worse prognostic findings in upto 25% of specimens.
3. **The efficacy of BCG** in preventing progression appears to be higher in patients with high-grade papillary tumors and CIS if a restaging TURBT was performed before instillation of BCG.

59. Random biopsies are indicated only in the setting of multiple tumors or positive cytology.

Biopsy of the prostatic urethra is recommended for cases of:

- Bladder neck tumor.
- When bladder CIS is present or suspected.
- When there is positive cytology without evidence of tumor in the bladder.
- When abnormalities of the prostatic urethra are visible.

60. Mitomycin C (MMC)

- **Most effective adjuvant intravesical chemotherapeutic** agent perioperatively.
- Single dose administered within 6 hours lessens recurrence rates, whereas a dose 24 hours later does not, and maintenance therapy does not reduce the risk further.

61. Laser therapy

- **Advantages**–bleeding is negligible and there is no risk of obturator reflex.
- **Disadvantages**–costly, can result in perforation of a hollow, viscous organ and also no tissue available for pathologic inspection

62. The carbon dioxide laser is completely absorbed by fluid so is not appropriate for use in the treatment of bladder cancer.

63. BCG mode of action

- The initial step–direct binding to fibronectin, preferential upregulation of interferon-γ, IL-2 and activation of cell-mediated cytotoxic mechanisms.
- Treatment begun after 2 to 4 weeks of tumor resection.

- After instillation, the patient should retain the solution for 2 hours.

64. BCG efficacy

- **In CIS** the initial tumor-free response rate is as high as 80%.
- Can effectively treat **residual** papillary lesions (60%) after TURBT.
- Can decreased tumor **recurrence** of 30% when a 6-week course of BCG was administered after recovery from TURBT.
- Reduces the risk of **progression** by 23% to 27%.

65. **If the initial treatment of chemotherapy fails,** a course of BCG should be undertaken. BCG has demonstrated 20% disease-free survival in this setting.

66. BCG failure

- **If initial 6 weekly BCG induction course fails** than additional response to a second induction course is 25%
- **Further courses of BCG or chemotherapy beyond two** are not recommended routinely, as they will fail 80% of the time.
- Failure to respond to an initial course of intravesical therapy is occasion to reconsider cystectomy.
- Failure to respond to a second course is an indication for immediate cystectomy

67. Cleveland clinic approach to management of BCG Toxicity

- **Moderate symptoms (Grade 1)**–Anti-cholinergics, topical anti-spasmodics, analgesics, nonsteroidal anti-inflammatory drugs.
- **Severe symptoms (Grade 2)**–Grade 1 treatment + Dose reduction to ½ to $^1/_3$. Isoniazid 300 mg/day and rifampin 600 mg/day, orally until symptom resolution.
- **Serious complication (Grade 3)**–Grade 1 and grade 2 treatment + Isoniazid, 300 mg/day, rifampin 600 mg/day, ethambutol, 15 mg/kg/day single daily dose for 3 to 6 months (If solid organ involvement).

68. Contraindications to BCG Therapy

Absolute

1. Immunosuppressed and immunocompromised patients.
2. Immediately after transurethral resection.
3. Personal history of bacillus Calmette-Guérin (BCG) sepsis.

4. Gross hematuria.
5. Traumatic catheterisation.
6. Total incontinence.

Relative

1. UTI.
2. Liver disease.
3. Personal history of tuberculosis.
4. Poor overall performance status.

69. **Agents for perioperative use**–doxorubicin, epirubicin, mitomycin, thiopeta and gemcitabine.

    Agents not used (BCG and interferon).

70. **BCG**–only intravesical agent used for high risk group.
71. **Valrubicin**–semisynthetic analog of doxorubicin that has been approved by the FDA for treatment of BCG refractory CIS in patients who cannot tolerate cystectomy.
72. **Thiotepa**–only chemotherapeutic agent approved by the FDA specifically for the intravesical treatment of papillary bladder cancer.
73. **Persistent disease after BCG therapy can be categorized as:**
    - **BCG-refractory** (nonimproving or worsening disease despite BCG).
    - **BCG-resistant** (recurrence or persistence of lesser degree, stage, or grade after an initial course, which then resolves with further BCG).
    - **BCG-relapsing** (recurrence after initial resolution with BCG).
74. **Patients who undergo immediate cystectomy for pathologic T1 tumors**–10-year DFS of 92%, compared with 64% with those with clinical T1 tumors.
    - **Term early cystectomy** is based on the fact that it is performed before the traditional surgical indication of documented T2 but actually it should be more correctly termed as **timely cystectomy.**
75. **Prognostic factors on which stratification of recurrence and progression groups are divided (EAU Guidelines 2012):**
    1. Number of tumor.
    2. Tumor diameter.
    3. Recurrence rate.

4. Stage (Ta/T1).
5. CIS.
6. Grade.

76. Treatment recommendation

Small-Volume, Low-Grade Ta

Single dose of postoperative intravesical chemotherapy

Multifocal or Large Low-Grade Ta, or Recurrent Low-Grade Ta

Intravesical BCG or MMC

High-Grade Ta, T1, or CIS

(If T1 disease, but no muscularis in specimen, repeat resection).

Recommendation: Intravesical BCG with maintenance therapy

Option: Consider cystectomy for selected patients

High-Grade Ta, T1, and/or CIS Following Prior Intravesical Therapy

Consider cystectomy as therapeutic alternative

77. Radical cystectomy should be strongly considered for patients with:

- Muscle invasive bladder cancer.
- Non-muscle invasive bladder cancers that are: **(EAU Guidelines 2012)**
    - o T1HG.
    - o Associated with diffuse CIS.
    - o In diverticula.
    - o Multifocal.
    - o Substantially involve the distal ureters or prostatic urethra.
    - o Refractory to initial therapy.
    - o Too large or anatomically inaccessible to remove endoscopically.

78. Commercially Available Markers

Marker	Sensitivity (%)	Specificity (%)
Cytology	48	96
Hematuria dipstick	68	68
NMP22 Bladder Chek	55.7	85.7
BTA stat	68	74
ImmunoCyt	74(2nd maximum)	80
UroVysion	77(Maximum)	98 (Maximum)

79. Surveillance Strategies (EAU Guidelines 2012)

Ta or T1	CPE/Cytology	Upper tract imaging
Low risk for recurrence and progression	**CPE at 3 Months if negative** 9 Months later and than annually for 5 years	–
High risk of progression	**CPE and urine cytology at 3 Months, if negative** 3 months for a period of 2 years Then every 6 months thereafter until 5 years Then yearly	**Yearly**
Intermediate risk of progression	**In-between follow-up scheme using cystoscopy and cytology**	–

80. Site of the highest concentration of prostatic ducts is–midprostate (or bladder neck in shorter prostates) to the mid to distal verumontanum and 5 and 7 o'clock adjacent to the verumontanum.

81. Standard radical cystectomy includes:

Bilateral pelvic lymphadenectomy and

- In Male patients–removal of the prostate and bladder en bloc.
- In Female patients–anterior exenteration requires removal of the uterus, fallopian tubes, ovaries, bladder, urethra and a segment of the anterior vaginal wall.

82. Candidates for orthotopic reconstruction

Final decision to use residual urethra cannot be made until frozen-section analysis demonstrates a tumor-free distal urethral margin.

83. Follow-up after radical cystectomy

- Patients with pT1 disease–Annual screening with physical examination, serum chemistry and CXR.
- Patients with pT2 disease–Semiannual evaluation.
- Patients with pT3 disease–Quarterly evaluation and semiannual CT scan.

84. The management of patients with grossly involved lymph nodes includes

- **If disease is recognized on preoperative imaging** and outside the true pelvis, a CT-guided biopsy is performed to establish histology- if it is positive, then chemotherapy is initiated and followed by RC
- **When adenopathy is encountered at the time of a RC**, a frozen section biopsy is undertaken to confirm the presence of metastasis, and extended lymph node dissection and RC are performed.
- **Cystectomy is not performed when**
  (1) Lymph node metastases are unresectable because of bulk or proximal extent above the common iliac vessels
  (2) There is evidence of extensive periureteral disease
  (3) The bladder is fixed to the pelvic sidewall
  (4) Tumor is invading the rectosigmoid colon

85. Neoadjuvant cisplatin-based combination chemotherapy–modest improvement in overall survival of 5% to 6% among patients with locally advanced disease (Advanced Bladder Cancer Meta-analysis Collaboration, 2003).

- Neoadjuvant cisplatin-containing combination chemotherapy improves overall survival **(EAU Guidelines 2012).**
- Pre-operative radiotherapy is not recommended to improve survival **(EAU Guidelines 2012).**
- **Adjuvant chemotherapy**–9% improvement in survival at 3 years for patients who received chemotherapy compared with controls (Advanced Bladder Cancer Meta-analysis Collaboration, 2005).
- Adjuvant chemotherapy is advised within clinical trials, but not as a routine therapeutic option **(EAU Guidelines 2012).**

86. Bladder preservation can be attempted in patients with

(1) initial occurrence of bladder cancer
(2) no CIS
(3) size < 3 cm
(4) stage T2 (no palpable mass)
(5) not in the dome or high posterior wall because of the risk of bowel injury.

Patients with T3b tumors are not candidates for complete TUR, and those with T4 tumors are not eligible because, by definition, the tumors are invading surrounding structures

87. **For metastatic TCC**

- **Gemcitabine+ cisplatin (GC)** provides a survival advantage similar to that of MVAC with a better safety profile and tolerability.
- **Most significant toxic effects** with GC–thrombocytopenia and neutropenia.
- **First line treatment in cisplatin ineligible patients** ('unfit') with either PS 2 or impaired renal function–carboplatin-containing combination chemo-therapy, preferably with gemcitabine/ carboplatin **(EAU Guidelines 2012).**

88. **In patients with confirmed muscle invasive bladder cancer**–CT of the chest, abdomen and pelvis is the optimal form of staging, including CT urography for complete examination of the upper urinary tracts.

- A chest CT is obtained routinely in patients with muscle-invasive disease or N+ disease in whom the risk of visceral metastasis is greatest.
- Bone scintigraphy is obtained in these highest-risk patients and in patients with an elevated alkaline phosphatase or new-onset bone pain.

89. **The "standard" LN dissection**

- Lateral limit–Genitofemoral nerve.
- Medially- IIA
- Cephalad limit–Bifurcation of CIA.
- Caudal limit–Endopelvic fascia (cooper ligament).

90. **The "extended" LN dissection**–includes the tissue along the common iliacs upto the aortic bifurcation.

- The extended lymphadenectomy has been shown to improve survival in patients with both LN-negative and limited LN metastatic disease.

91. **If a continent orthotopic diversion is being considered in females**–pubourethral ligaments are not divided, and only the bladder neck and the initial 1 cm of urethra are removed.

92. **Partial cystectomy**

Indication

- Normally functioning bladder with good capacity, a first-time tumor recurrence with a solitary tumor, and a tumor location in an area that allows a 1 to 2cm margin of resection, such as at the dome.

- Urachal adenocarcinoma.
- Tumor within a bladder diverticulum.

Absolute contraindications

- CIS elsewhere in the bladder and multifocal tumors.

Relative contraindications

- High-grade tumors.
- Tumors located at the trigone or the bladder neck.
- Tumors that would require ureteral reimplantation.

93. **Patients who have undergone partial cystectomy** .ould have:

- Cystoscopy and urinary cytologic examination every 3 months for at least 2 years.
- Regular CT scans of the pelvis and abdomen are recommended.

94. **Prostate and seminal vesicle-sparing laparoscopic RC**

Indication

- Continent young men with low-volume, pTa, pT1, pT2 TCC of the bladder, >1 cm proximal to the bladder neck without concomitant prostate or urethral disease.

Thorough evaluation to exclude concomitant prostate cancer prior to procedure in:

- Patients with abnormal findings on DRE, PSA > 3 ng/mL, <12% of PSA, or hypoechoic nodule on TRUS.

95. **Whole-gut irrigation is contraindicated in patients with**

- Unstable cardiovascular system
- Cirrhosis
- Severe renal disease
- Congestive heart failure
- Obstructed bowel

96. **Celiac plexus**

- Left gastric artery.
- Hepatic artery.
  - o Right gastric artery.
  - o Gastroduodenal artery→Right gastroepiploic artery.

- Splenic artery
  - o Short gastric artery.
  - o Left gastroepiploic artery.

97. **Stomach for urinary diversion**

Advantages

- Thick seromuscular layer that can easily be separated from the mucosa (submucosal ureteral reimplantation becomes easier).
- Less permeable to urinary solutes, it has a net excretion of chloride and protons rather than a net absorption of them.
- Produces less mucus.

Disadvantages

- Hypochloremic, hypokalemic metabolic alkalosis.
- Hematuria-dysuria syndrome with respiratory distress in some patients.

98. **Segments of small bowel that** may be exposed to pelvic irradiation and pelvic disease:

- Last 2 inches of the terminal ileum.
- 5 feet of small bowel beginning approximately 6 feet from the ligament of Treitz.

99. **Sudeck's critical point**—Located between the junction of the **sigmoid and superior hemorrhoidal arteries.**

100. **Basic surgical principles for all the anastomoses are-**

- Only as much ureter as needed should be mobilized so that there is no redundancy or tension on the anastomosis.
- Mobilization should not strip the ureter of its periadventitial tissue
- The ureterointestinal anastomosis must be performed with fine absorbable sutures
- The bowel should be brought to the ureter and not vice versa
- At the completion of the anastomosis, the bowel should be fixed to the abdominal cavity,
- Anastomosis should be retroperitonealized

101. **Ureterocolonic anastomosis**

- Nonrefluxing
  - o Leadbetter and Clark.

  - o Goodwin.
  - o Strickler.
  - o Pagano (**Least stricture rate).**
- Refluxing
  - o Nesbit.

102. Uretersmall bowel anastomoses

- Refluxing
  - o Bicker–end-to-side ureter–small bowel anastomosis.
  - o Wallace–end-to-end ureter–small bowel anastomosis (**Best result in relation of stricture formation and leakage).**
- Nonrefluxing
  - o Nipple.
  - o Serosal tunnel.
  - o Le Duc (**Lowest incidence of stricture and highest success rates in preventing reflux).**

103. Urinary fistulas following urteroilleal anastomosis

- Occur within the first 7 to 10 days postoperatively
- Incidence of 3% to 9%
- The incidence of urinary intestinal leak is markedly reduced by the use of soft Silastic stents

104. Renal deterioration

- 18% of patients who have ileal conduits versus 13% who have nonrefluxing colon conduit
- The most common cause of death in patients who have had a ureterosigmoidostomy for more than 15 years is acquired renal disease (i.e., sepsis or renal failure)

105. Patient may be considered for a retentive diversion

- Urine pH of 5.8 or less after an ammonium chloride load.
- Urine osmolality of >600 mOsm/kg in response to water deprivation.
- GFR >35 mL/min.
- Minimal protein in the urine.

106. Most common late complication of illeal conduit-Pyelonephritis (17%).

107. Electrolyte imbalance

- **Stomach**–Hypochloremic, hypokalemic metabolic alkalosis with increase aldosterone
- **Jejunum**–Hypochloremia, hyperkalemia, hyponatremic metabolic acidosis with increase renin and angiotensin
- **Ileum and colon**–Hyperchloremia, hypokalemia, hypocalcemia and metabolic acidosis

108. Alteration of the sensorium following diversion procedure is due to

- Magnesium deficiency
- Drug intoxication
- Abnormalities in ammonia metabolism

109. Osteomalacia in urinary intestinal diversion may be due to

- Persistent acidosis
- Vitamin D resistance
- Excessive calcium loss by the kidney

110. Deterioration of the upper tracts is more likely when the culture of **pure Proteus or Pseudomonas** is detected and should be treated.

Mixed cultures may generally be observed, provided they are not symptomatic.

111. Following renal diversion procedure most susceptible to development of renal calculi are patients with

- Hyperchloremic metabolic acidosis
- Pre-existing pyelonephritis,
- UTI with a urea-splitting organism

Majority of stones formed are composed of calcium, magnesium and ammonium phosphate.

112. Configuration that has the most volume for the least surface area is- sphere

113. Splitting the bowel wall on its antimesenteric border and reconfiguring it–coordinated activity fronts, restarts after period of 3 months

114. The MAINZ pouch is mixed augmentation with ileum 'n' cecum

Sigma rectum or the Mainz II pouch, creates a low-pressure rectosigmoid reservoir of increased capacity

115. **Most technologically demanding of all the continence mechanisms, and associated with the highest complication and reoperation rates**–nipple valves

116. **Appendiceal tunneling techniques** are the simple continent urinary diversion to perform but disadvantages are:
    - Appendix may be unavailable in some patients because of prior appendicectomy.
    - Appendiceal stump may be too short to reach the anterior abdominal wall or umbilicus.
    - The large amount of mucus cannot be easily emptied through the catheter that would be admitted through an appendiceal stump (14 to 16 Fr).

117. **Most reliable of all catheterizable reservoirs**–Indiana pouch.
    - It is among the easiest to construct, and it has very low short-term and long-term complications.

118. **The Penn pouch was the first continent diversion employing the** Mitrofanoff principle in which the appendix served as the continence mechanism.

119. **The use of the stomach to create a urinary reservoir has following advantages**
    - Reservoir for individuals with pre-existing metabolic acidosis or renal insufficiency.
    - Hyperchloremic acidosis does not occurs
    - In patients in whom shortening of the bowel may be expected to lead to some degree of malabsorption, the use of stomach is an attractive alternative.
    - The acid pH of the urine may also reduce the risk of bacterial colonization.
    - When the entire lower bowel has been irradiated, stomach tissue may provide alternative

120. **Single strongest pathologic predictor in males** of subsequent recurrence of urethral tumor after radical cystectomy (RC) for bladder cancer is–prostatic stromal invasion.

121. **Most significantly associated with secondary urethral tumor in women after RC for bladder cancer is**–Bladder neck involvement.

122. **Accurate assessment of the urethra and application for orthotopic diversion** is determined by–intraoperative frozen-

section analysis of the distal surgical margin in men (apical prostatic urethra) and women (proximal urethra).

123. **The risk of a urethral recurrence and local pelvic recurrence** of 10% is seen in patients undergoing RC for bladder cancer.

124. **The innervation of the striated urethral rhabdosphincter** arises from the branches of the pudendal nerve and is most important to maintain continence in patients with an orthotopic neobladder

The striated rhabdosphincter muscle fibers are concentrated anterior and lateral to the proximal urethra

125. Length and location of segment isolated to form **neobladder** by various techniques is:

- **Camey**–A total of 65 cm of ileum is isolated, with an area of the ileum identified to reach to the region of the urethra in a tension-free manner.
- **Hautmann neobladder**–A segment of terminal ileum of 70 cm is selected.
- **Studer**–A portion of terminal ileum 54 to 60 cm long is isolated, 25 cm proximal to the ileocecal valve.
- **T pouch** is constructed from 44 cm of distal ileum placed in an inverted V configuration.
- **Le Bag**–A 20-cm segment of ascending colon and a corresponding length of terminal ileum are isolated, and bowel continuity is restored.

126. **Continence following neobladder**

- Failure to empty or urinary retention- 4% to 25% of patients and tends to be more common in females.
- Day-time continence develops gradually over 3 to 6 months and is ultimately achieved in 80% to 90% of both male and female patients.
- Persistent nocturnal incontinence is common, observed in 20% to 50% of patients.
- Nocturnal continence may continue to improve beyond 12 months from surgery.
- Factors influencing continence rates include age, intestinal segment used, and possibly the application of a nerve sparing technique.

127. **Penile fracture**–Tunica albuginea resist rupture until intracavernous pressures rise to more than 1500 mm Hg. Tunical tear is usually transverse and 1 to 2 cm in length.

128. **Penile trauma**

- **If Buck's fascia remains intact**, the penile hematoma remains contained between the skin and tunica, resulting in a typical eggplant deformity.
- **If Buck's fascia is disrupted**, hematoma can extend to the scrotum, perineum, and suprapubic regions. A blood clot directly against the fracture site can be palpated; the "rolling sign".

129. **MRI** is a noninvasive and highly accurate means of demonstrating disruption of the tunica albuginea.

130. Successful **penile reimplantation** is possible within 16 hours of cold ischemia time or 6 hours of warm ischemia.

131. **Degree of hematoma does not correlate with the severity of testicular injury**, absence does not entirely rule out testis rupture, and contusion without fracture can present with significant bleeding.

132. **Thick** (0.010- to 0.015-inch), **nonmeshed, split-thickness skin grafts** are preferred for extensive penile reconstruction.

133. **Meshed split-thickness skin grafts** are employed for scrotal reconstruction.

134. **Pelvic fracture are associated with 83% to 95% of bladder injuries**. Conversely, bladder injury has been reported to occur in only 5% to 10% of pelvic fractures.

135. **Indicators of bladder injury**

- Suprapubic pain or tenderness
- Free intraperitoneal fluid on CT or ultrasound examination
- Inability to void or low urine output
- Clots in urine or clots noted in bladder on CT
- Enlarged scrotum with ecchymosis
- Abdominal distention or ileus

136. **Immediate cystography**

Absolute indication

- Blunt external trauma with gross hematuria associated with pelvic fracture.

Relative indications

- Blunt trauma with:
  - o Gross hematuria without a pelvic fracture.
  - o Microhematuria with or without pelvic fracture.
- Penetrating injuries of the buttock, pelvis, or lower abdomen with any degree of hematuria.

137. **Bladder injury**
   - Nearly **100% accurate for bladder injury**–Retrograde or stress cystography.
   - **Three-film technique** is recommended, including an image before administration of the contrast agent, a full bladder AP film, and a drainage film.
   - Dense, flame-shaped collection of contrast material in the pelvis is **characteristic of extraperitoneal extravasation.**
138. **CT cystography** is as accurate and reliable as plain film cystography to evaluate suspected bladder injury as long as the bladder is filled in retrograde fashion with contrast material diluted to 2% to 4% (6:1 with saline) to a volume of 350 to 400 mL.
139. **Indications for immediate repair of bladder injury:**
   - Intraperitoneal injury.
   - Penetrating injury.
   - Bladder neck/vaginal or rectal injury.
   - Open pelvic fracture.
   - Pelvic fracture requiring ORIF.
   - Undergoing laparotomy for some other reason.
140. If bladder is repaired, a **cystogram is obtained** 7 to 10 days after surgery.
141. Because the posterior urethra is fixed at both the urogenital diaphragm and the puboprostatic ligaments, **the bulbomembranous junction is more vulnerable to injury during pelvic fracture urethral distraction (PFUDD).**
   - **In children**, injuries are more likely to extend proximally to the bladder neck because of the rudimentary nature of the prostate.
142. **Urethral disruption** is heralded by the triad of blood at the meatus, inability to urinate and palpable full bladder.

143. **When blood at the urethral meatus is present,** an immediate gentle RGU should be performed to rule out urethral injury.

144. **Direct-vision internal urethrotomy** are best reserved for selected short urethral strictures.

145. **Open posterior urethroplasty through a perineal anastomotic approach is the** treatment of choice for most urethral distraction injuries.

146. **Endemic bladder calculi are:**

- **Most commonly composed of**–ammonium acid urate alone or in combination with calcium oxalate.
- Occurs in the absence of obstruction, local disease, neurologic lesion, or known primary infection.
- Children **younger than 10 years** are typically affected.
- Male-to-female ratio of 10:1.
- Usually solitary and **rarely recurs once removed.**
- Mixed cereal diet with milk supplements reduces the incidence of endemic bladder calculi.

147. **Incomplete bladder emptying** is identified as the greatest single factor in vesical stone formation, and BPH is the most commonly condition causing incomplete emptying.

148. Bladder calculi are associated with urinary tract infection, **most common with Proteus.**

149. Increased risk for development of a bladder stone compared with patients who were **catheter free and had continent bladder control** within the first year after injury is:

- Patients managed with a **PUC or SPC**–ninefold increased risk.
- Patients using **CIC or a condom** catheter–fourfold increased risk.

150. **Cystoscopy is the single most accurate examination** to document the presence of a bladder calculus.

151. **Cystolitholapaxy**

- Crushing of the calculus with irrigation of the fragments from the bladder.
- Contraindications include small-capacity bladders, multiple stones or calculi larger than 2 cm that cannot be engaged, hard stones, bladder calculi in children and small-caliber urethras.

152. Percutaneous cystolithotomy

Indications

- Pediatric patients with narrow urethras and in patients with large stone burdens or multiple calculi with anticipated prolonged operative times.

Contraindications

- History of bladder malignant disease, prior abdominal or pelvic surgeries, prior pelvic radiotherapy, active urinary or abdominal wall infection and pelvic prosthetic devices.

153. Prostatic calculi

- Depositions of **calcified material on corpora amylacea.**
- Primarily composed of **calcium phosphate trihydrate and carbonate.**
- Most commonly seen in men older than 50 years with BPH.
- Usually **asymptomatic.**
- No treatment is indicated for asymptomatic prostatic stones.
- In symptomatic, transurethral resection can unroof and remove the calculus.

❑❑

Chapter 16
PROSTATE

1. **Wolffian ducts develop into**–seminal vesicles, epididymis, vas deferens, ampulla and ejaculatory duct.
   - Developmental growth of this group of glands is stimulated by **fetal testosterone.**
   - The developmental **growth is completed by the 13th week.**
2. **Urogenital sinus develop into**–prostate.
   - Development is directed primarily by **DHT.**
   - The prostate first appears by 3rd month and is well differentiated by **4 months of fetal development.**
3. The prostatic epithelium in the human is **composed of two major cell types–epithelial cells and stromal cells.**
   - The epithelium cell types include mature secretory and terminally differentiated cells, neuroendocrine cells, transit-amplifying cells and basal/stem cells.
4. **Prostate Zones**

   Anterior fibromuscular–30% of prostate mass, no glandular elements, smooth muscle

   Peripheral–Largest zone, 75% of prostate glandular elements, site of carcinomas

   Central–25% of prostate glandular elements; surrounds ejaculatory ducts

   Transitional–Smallest zone , surrounds upper urethra complex sphincter, 5% of prostate glandular elements, site of BPH.
5. **Testosterone (T) is converted by 5α-reductase into DHT** or converted **by aromatase into estrogens**, in leydig cells and the process is irreversible.
6. **The estrogen causes a negative feedback on LH release** that reduces the serum signal for testicular production; therefore, estrogen acts as an effective "chemical castration".
7. **Testosterone (T)**
   - **Testosterone blood production rate**–6 to 7 mg/day in the human.

- **Plasma half-life of T is only 10 to 20 minutes** (man undergoing bilateral simple orchiectomy is functionally castrate within 1 to 2 hours of surgery)
- **Testosterone plasma concentration is**–611 ng/100 mL ± 186.
- Only **2% of the total serum T is unbound (free testosterone)** in the plasma.

8. **DHT**

Plasma concentration is–56 ± 20 ng/100 mL.

In comparison to testosterone:

- DHT is a potent androgen (1.5 to 2.5 times as potent as T).
- 90% of total prostatic androgen is in the form of DHT, principally derived from testicular androgens.
- DHT is a more potent androgen than testosterone because of its higher affinity for the AR
- Its has low plasma concentration and binds tightly to plasma proteins

It is the major form of androgen found within the prostate gland and is 5 times higher than T.

9. **Administration of T** → ↓TeBG levels in the plasma.

Administration of estrogen →↑ TeBG →↑binding of T→↓free T plasma concentration.

10. **Properties and Distribution of 5α-Reductase Types I and II**

	Type I	**Type II**
Chromosome localization	5	2
5αReductase deficiency	Normal	Mutated
Prostate cells		
Luminal epithelial	+	–
Basal epithelial	–	+
Stromal	+	+
Skin	+	–
Finasteride	Inhibits	
Dutasteride	Inhibits	Inhibits

– → Absent + → Present

11. Cell adhesion molecules

1. **Integrins**–link the cell to the basement membrane and extracellular matrix components through heterodimer interactions.
2. **Cadherins**–link the cell to neighboring cells through homotypic polymers.
3. **Selectins**–link the cell to carbohydrate moieties primarily on the vascular system.
4. **Immunoglobulin**–superfamily adhesion molecules.

12. The androgen receptor gene is on the long arm of the X chromosome at position Xq11.2q12.

13. Citric acid

- One of the major anions in human seminal plasma is citrate
- The concentration of citrate in the ejaculate is 500 to 1000 times higher than that in the plasma.
- Prostate secretory epithelial cells form citrate from aspartic acid and glucose.

14. Major source of citric acid, polyamines, zinc is prostate
Major source of fructose and prostaglandins is seminal vesicles

15.

bFGF	Basic fibroblast growth factor (prostate growth factor, endothelial growth factor tumor angiogenesis factor, osteoblastic factor)	• Potent mitogen working on the stromal cells • Involved in angiogenesis and cellular chemotaxis • Is a weak epithelial mitogen • Elevated in BPH
EGF	Epidermal growth factor; urogastrone	• Controversial in normal human prostate but elevated in cancer
TGF-α	Transforming growth factor α	• Low levels in human prostate
TGF-β	Transforming growth factor β	• Negatively regulates prostate epithelial cell growth • Positive factor in stimulating stromal cell growth and fibroblast growth • Elevated in BPH

16. Human seminal fluid contains the highest concentration of **endothelins.**

Endothelins are the most potent vasoconstrictors.

17. **Castration causes**–90% loss in prostatic epithelial cells and 40% loss in stromal cells.

18. **Mitosis can be divided into four phases:**

- **Prophase** (chromosomes are duplicated).
- **Metaphase** (chromosomes are aligned along a central axis or plate).
- **Anaphase** (pairs of duplicated chromosomes separate).
- **Telophase** (separation of nucleus and cytoplasm).

19. **Volume of the normal human ejaculate**–3 ml.

- **Two components: spermatozoa and seminal plasma.**
- Spermatozoa<1% of the total ejaculate, are present in the range of 100 million/ml.
- **Contribution**—Seminal vesicle–(1.5 to 2 mL), prostate–(0.5 mL), and Cowper's gland and glands of Littre–(0.1 to 0.2 mL).
- **First fraction of human ejaculate**- originates from Cowper's gland and the prostate and contains the liquefaction factors.
- **Final fraction of the ejaculate**- originates from seminal vesicle and is responsible for the coagulation of the ejaculate

20. **The source of fructose is**–seminal vesicles.

- Patients with congenital absence of the seminal vesicles also have an associated absence of fructose in their ejaculates.

21. **The richest sources of prostaglandins**–seminal vesicles.

22. **PSA** (*hKLK3*)

- **It is a glycoprotein acting as a serine protease of MW 33,000.**
- **Contains 7% carbohydrate.**
- Found almost exclusively in the **epithelial cells of the prostate.**
- The PSA gene (*hKLK3*) are located on **chromosome 19.**
- **It lyse the clot** in the ejaculate.
- **It is an organ-specific** but not a cancer-specific marker.

23. **PSA**

- **Complexed to α_1-antichymotrypsin** (PSA-ACT). This form of complexed PSA (PSA-ACT) is enzymatically inactive yet has immunoreactivity.
- **Free PSA**, found in lower concentrations than complexed PSA (PSA-ACT), is also enzymatically inactive, yet also has immunoreactivity.
- PSA is also **complexed to α_2-macroglobulin** (PSA-A2M) but is not immunoreactive.

24. Major function of semenogelin involves **capacitation**

(series of changes in that sperm undergo as they traverse the female urogenital tract to reach the zona pellucida and fertilize the egg)

25. **Prostate acid phosphatise (PAP)**

- Activity > 200 times more abundant in prostate tissue than in any other tissue.
- Osteoclasts are also a rich source of tartrate-insensitive acid phosphatase (TRAP).
- It is a glycoprotein dimer of molecular weight 102,000 and contains 7% carbohydrate.

26. **Human ejaculates**

- First fraction–from Cowper's gland and the prostate (liquefaction factors).
- Final fraction–enriched in seminal vesicle secretions (coagulation of the ejaculate).

27. **pH**

- **pH of prostate secretions** ranges from 6 to 8, with a mean value of 6.6.
- **With prostatic inflammation,** the pH tended to be 7 or higher.
- **pH of freshly ejaculated human semen** is slightly alkaline (pH 7.3 to 7.7).
- **On standing,** semen first becomes alkaline with the loss of carbon dioxide and then later acidic owing to accumulation of lactic acid.

28. The prostate, maintains its ability to **respond to androgens throughout life.**

Aging prostate maintains a **high level of DHT as well as a high level of AR.**

29. BPH first develops in the periurethral transition zone of the prostate.

30. Neither symptoms nor flow rate nor prostate volume **measures can predict presence and degree of obstruction reliably.**

31. BPH–true hyperplastic process.

Histopathologically BPH is characterized by an increased number of epithelial and stromal cells in periurethral area of the prostate

32. Only other species known to develop naturally occurring BPH–**dog (but does not develop symptoms of outlet obstruction because of lack of capsule in dogs)**

33. α1a is the most abundant adrenoreceptor subtype present in the human prostate.

34. Changes that lead to detrusor instability or decreased compliance are associated with–frequency and urgency.

Changes associated with decreased detrusor contractility are associated with–deterioration in the force of the urinary stream, hesitancy, intermittency, increased residual urine

35. No men younger than 30 years had evidence of BPH.

36. Paul Abrams coined the term lower urinary tract symptoms to replace the old and inappropriate term prostatism.

37. Determination of size of prostate

- **DRE tends to underestimate prostate size.**
- Magnitude of the underestimation increases with increasing prostate size from 25% to 50%.
- **TRUS volume measurements** using the prolate ellipsoid volume formula are **the most widely accepted measure of prostate volume.**
- **If accurate measurement of prostate volume** is needed to determine whether to perform open prostatectomy rather than TURP, ultrasound (transabdominal or transrectal) is more accurate than cysto-urethroscopy.

38. The Proscar Long-Term Efficacy and Safety Study (PLESS)

- 3000 men with moderate symptoms and enlarged prostate glands randomly assigned to treatment with finasteride 5 mg daily versus placebo over 4 years.
- **Episode of AUR**–incidence rate of 1.8 per 100 person–years.
- **Risk of AUR** increases with increasing serum PSA as well as prostate volume.

PLESS represents the **longest-duration** multicenter, randomized, double-blind, placebo-controlled study reported to date in the medical therapy of BPH literature.

- The cumulative incidences **of AUR** at 4 years in the finasteride and placebo groups were 7% and 3%, respectively **(57% risk reduction).**
- The cumulative risk of undergoing **BPH-related surgery** was 10% and 5% in the placebo and finasteride groups, respectively **(55% risk reduction).**
- The detection of prostate cancer was not significantly different in the placebo and finasteride group, suggesting that **finasteride does not mask the diagnosis of prostate cancer**

39. The Medical Therapy of Prostatic Symptoms (MTOPS)

- 3045 men treated with placebo versus doxazosin versus finasteride versus combination therapy for 4 to 5 years and was designed as a progression study.
- **Endpoint**–worsening of 4 points on the I-PSS score verified twice within 4 weeks, AUR, socially unacceptable incontinence, recurrent UTI, or renal insufficiency related to BPH.
- 14% of placebo-treated patients experienced **4 points worsening** in the I-PSS over 4 years of follow-up.
- There was not a single case of **renal insufficiency** related to BPH.
- **Incidence rate of AUR** was 0.6 per 100 patient years.
- **AUR increased** with increasing prostate volume as well as increasing baseline serum PSA
- **Invasive therapy and AUR risk** were significantly reduced by finasteride and combination therapy (finasteride and doxazocin) only.
- **All treatment regimens (placebo, doxazosin, finasteride and combination)** brought about a **significant improvement in AUA symptom score and Qmax at 4 years.**

- **AUASI score and PFR improved significantly more in the combination** therapy group compared with the monotherapy groups
- **The number needed to treat to prevent a case of BPH progression** as defined in MTOPS in the overall population was 8.4 for the combination therapy group and 13.7 and 15.0, respectively, for the doxazosin- and finasteride-treated patients

40. On the basis of TRUS, the growth of the prostate in the men 40 to 79 years old was estimated to be about **0.6 mL per year or 6 mL per decade of life.**

41. **Complications of BPH**

- Prevalence of **bladder stones** was eight times higher in diagnosis of BPH.
- **UTI** constitutes the main indication for surgical intervention in about 12%.
- **Bladder decompensation.**
- **Urinary incontinence.**
- **Upper urinary tract deterioration and azotemia**–patients in renal failure have an increased risk for complications following TURP compared with patients with normal renal function (25% versus 17%).
- **Hematuria**–2.5%.
- **Acute Urinary Retention**–25% and 30% of men who underwent TURP had AUR as their main indication.

42.

	Spontaneous AUR	**Precipitated AUR**
Another episode of AUR	15%	9%
Need for surgery	75%	26%

43. **The risk of AUR and need for surgery is predictable from:**

- Advancing age.
- Increased prostate size.
- Higher serum PSA levels.

44. **Olmsted County study**–men with moderate to severe LUTS, impaired flow rates, or enlarged prostates are more likely to undergo treatment, with increases in risk of similar magnitude to those associated with AUR.

- The cumulative risk of developing AUR in an unselected group of men between the ages of 40 and 79 years over a 50M follow-up was 6.8 events per 1000 person–years.

45. Recommendations for assessment of LUTS: (EAU Guidelines 2012)

- I-PSS (mild symptoms (0 to 7), moderate (8 to 19) or severe (20 to 35) symptoms).
- Assess the upper urinary tract function with Cr measurement and/or an USG.
- DRE.
- Uroflowmetry and PVR.
- The measurement of PSA is recommended when a diagnosis of prostatic carcinoma will change the decision.

46. Imaging of the upper urinary tract is recommended in: (EAU Guidelines 2012)

- History of recurrent UTI.
- History of urolithiasis.
- History of urinary tract surgery.
- History of urothelial tumor (including IVU).
- Haematuria (including IVU).
- Urinary retention.

47. Pressure-flow studies should be considered for patients prior to surgical treatment in: (EAU Guidelines 2012)

- Qmax > 15 mL/s.
- < 50 or > 80 years of age.
- Can void but have PVR > 300 mL.
- Suspicious of having neurogenic bladder dysfunction.
- Have bilateral hydronephrosis.
- Had radical pelvic surgery.
- Had previous unsuccessful (invasive) treatment.

48. CT and MRI currently have no place in the routine imaging: **(EAU Guidelines 2012)**

- **Routine imaging of the urinary bladder and urethra** cannot be recommended as a diagnostic test in the work-up of patients with LUTS.
- **Endoscopy** is recommended as a guideline at the time of surgical treatment only.

49. **Uroflowmetry**

- Flow rate measurements are inaccurate if the voided volume is <125 to 150 mL.
- Flow rate recording is the **single best noninvasive urodynamic test** to detect lower urinary tract obstruction.
- Qmax more specifically identifies patients with BPH than does the Qave.
- Qmax > 15 mL/s appear to have somewhat poorer treatment outcomes after prostatectomy than patients with a Qmax < 15 mL/s.
- A Qmax <15 mL/s does not differentiate between obstruction and bladder decompensation.

50. **Post void residue (PVR)**

- Large PVR may predict a slightly higher failure rate with a strategy of watchful waiting.
- It is uncertain whether PVR predicts the outcome of surgical treatment.
- It is uncertain whether PVR volume indicates impending bladder or renal damage.
- Men with significant PVR amounts should certainly be monitored more closely if they elect nonsurgical therapy,

51. **Indication of urethrocystoscopy**

- History of microscopic or gross hematuria
- Urethral stricture disease
- Bladder cancer or suspicion of carcinoma in-situ
- Prior lower urinary tract surgery (especially prior TURP).

52. **The definition of bladder overactivity (detrusor instability)** is the development of a detrusor contraction exceeding 15 cm H_2O at a bladder volume less than 300 ml.

53. **Retention** (Mitchell)

- **Acute retention**–Painful inability to void with PVR < 800 ml.
- **Chronic retention**–PVR >500ml + upper tract dilation in a patient who is still able to void spontaneously.
- **Acute on chronic retention**–Painful inability to void with PVR > 800 ml.

54. Selecting candidates for medical therapy: (EAU Guidelines 2012)

- The ideal candidate for medical therapy should have bothersome symptoms and negatively affecting QOL.
- Medical therapy should not be offered to individuals presenting with absolute indications for surgical intervention.
- Men with mild symptoms are suitable for watchful waiting.
- **α_1-blockers** should be offered to men with moderate-to-severe LUTS.
- **5α-reductase inhibitors** should be offered to men who have moderate-to-severe LUTS and enlarged prostates (> 40 mL) or elevated PSA (> 1.4-1.6 µg/L).
- **PDE5–inhibitors** reduce moderate to severe male LUTS.

55. Absolute indication of surgery

- If the patient has refractory urinary retention (failing at least one attempt of catheter removal).
- Secondary to BPH
  - o Recurrent UTI.
  - o Recurrent gross hematuria.
  - o Bladder stones.
  - o Renal insufficiency.
  - o Large bladder diverticula.

56. Classification of α-Adrenergic Blockers and Recommended Doses

Class of α Blocker	Dose
Non–selective	
Phenoxybenzamine	10 mg
α_1 selective	
Prazosin	2 mg
Long-Acting α_1	
Terazosin	5 mg or 10 mg
Doxazosin	4 mg or 8 mg
Alfuzosin SR	10 mg
Subtype Selective α_{1a}	
Tamsulosin	0.4 mg
Silodosin	8 mg
Naftopidil	

57. **α_1a AR and α_1b AR** are predominant in the human stroma and epithelium, respectively.

58. **Terazosin**–most extensively investigated α_1 blockers for BPH.

Hytrin Community Assessment Trial (HYCAT)–The treatment-related improvement (terazosin minus placebo) in the AUA symptom score and urinary PFR was 3.9 symptom units and 1.4 mL/sec respectively.

The ability to treat two common coexisting conditions (BPH and hypertension) is a potentially desirable feature of the drug.

59. **Doxazosin is a long-acting α_1 blocker**. The half-life of doxazosin is longer than that of terazosin (22 vs. 12 hours).

60. **Tamsulosin is the most potent available α_1 antagonist** indicated for the treatment of BPH.

Tamsulosin dose does not have to be titrated.

61. **SR alfuzosin**–new formulation allows for a once daily dosing regimen without dose titration.

- In **ALFUS study** the QOL index improved by 18% in active group compared with 8% in the placebo arm.
- In **ALFORTI trial** there was a 35% improvement from baseline of QOL.
- Because of the lack of adverse effects and BP changes, **alfuzosin has been described as a uroselective drug.**

62. **Alfuzosin,** when administered for 2 consecutive days in patients with AUR, was associated with a significantly higher rate of successful voiding after catheter removal than with placebo (55% vs 29%).

63. **Alfuzosin in Acute Urinary Retention (ALFAUR) study**

- Alfuzosin 10 mg once daily significantly increased the rate of success of a trial without catheter (TWOC), compared with placebo (62% vs 48%).
- Elderly patients (> 65 years) and patients with a bladder volume of > 1 liter at the time of AUR had a significantly greater risk of TWOC failure.

64. Silodosin

- α 1_a subtype selective
- Shown to increase urine flow in 2 to 6 hours after the initial dose.
- The most common drug-related side effect was retrograde ejaculation followed by dizziness
- No reported events of symptomatic orthostatic hypotension or dizziness when administered with a single dose

65. Naftopidil

Relative selective α1d-adrenergic receptor antagonist

66. AntiHypertensive and Lipid Lowering Treatment to Prevent Heart Attack Trial (ALLHAT)–there was no significant increase in CHF between doxazosin and the other antihypertensive agents.

67. α1-Adrenergic-mediated dizziness and asthenia are likely due to effects at **the level of the CNS.**

68. Intraoperative floppy iris syndrome (IFIS)

- The clinical manifestations are poor preoperative pupil dilation, iris billowing and prolapse, and progressive intraoperative miosis.
- Association with the α1-adrenergic antagonist tamsulosin has become well established
- α1a is the predominant receptor subtype in the iris dilator muscle as well.
- Occur until patients have been on tamsulosin therapy for 4 to 6 months.
- IFIS can also occur up to several years after discontinuation of tamsulosin.

69. Alpha-blocker therapy: (EAU Guidelines 2012)

- Can result in a rapid improvement in symptoms by a factor of 20%-50% and an improvement in the flow rate of 20%-30%.
- If a patient does not experience an improvement in symptoms after an 8-week trial, treatment should be discontinued.

70. Zanoterone is a steroidal competitive AR antagonist.

71. Flutamide is an orally administered nonsteroidal antiandrogen that inhibits the binding of androgen to its receptor

72. **Cetrorelix** is a gonadotropin-releasing hormone antagonist that has been investigated for BPH.

A potential advantage over the LHRH agonists in the treatment of BPH is the ability to titrate at the level of androgen suppression.

73. **5-alpha reductase inhibitors**

- Reduces prostate volume approximately 20%.
- Finasteride is effective in the management of gross hematuria associated with BPH.
- Maximum benefits are seen at a mean period after 6 months.
- Men with small prostates (< 40 mL) are less likely to benefit from finasteride.

74. **The Veterans Affairs (VA) study** unequivocally demonstrated the superiority of α-adrenergic blockade over androgen suppression for the treatment of clinical BPH over a 1-year interval.

75. **CombAT study.**

- In men with a pretreatment PSA between 1.5 and 10 ng/mL, combination of dutasteride and tamsulosin was more effective than either drug alone.
- In men with larger prostates, although the tamsulosin effect was rapid, over time dutasteride was the more effective agent.
- Superiority of combination therapy versus dutasteride was seen from month 3 and versus tamsulosin from month 9

76. **Prospective European Doxazosin and Combination Therapy Trial (PREDICT)**–the improvement in IPSS was not significantly different in the alfuzosin versus combination groups, questioning the lack of effectiveness of finasteride in the short term (1 year).

77. **ED is commonly found in the male population who are at risk for LUTS**

The common mechanisms include the following:

1. Pelvic atherosclerosis
2. Autonomic hyperactivity
3. The calcium-independent Rho-kinase activation pathway

4. Reduced nitric oxide (NO) levels, which is probably the best explored process so far

Role of PDEIs in patients with LUTS

- PDEIs (phosphodiesterase inhibitor) improve urinary symptoms scores but do not improve flow rates.
- The combination of α-adrenergic blockers and PDEIs may lead to a synergistic benefit, thereby improving LUTS.
- The combination of α-adrenergic blockers and PDEIs may lead to symptomatic hypotension.
- Combination of α-adrenergic blockers and PDEIs may be of value in therapy for men with both ED and LUTS

78. Suggested mechanism of phytotherapy

- Inhibition of 5α-reductase
- Antiandrogenic
- Estrogenic
- Inhibition of aromatase
- Decrease of sex hormone–binding globulin
- Action on α-adrenergic receptors

79. Analysis of large studies such as the PLESS, MTOPS, and the CombAT study indicate that following factors increases the risk of AUR

- Increasing age
- Presence of LUTS
- Low PFR
- Prostatic enlargement
- Raised PSA

80. Prostate stents

Temporary stents

- First generation–Urospiral and ProstaKath.
- Second generation–MemoKath and ProstaCoil.
- Polyurethane- intraurethral catheter, Barnes, Trestle and Spanner
- Biodegradable- Polyglycolic acid

Permanent stents

- Urolume and Memotherm.
- The ASI stent- It is introduced on a balloon, which was then inflated, thus expanding the stent.
- The Ultraflex stent is made of nickel-titanium alloy

81. Prostatic stents: (EAU Guidelines 2012)

- Alternative to catheterisation for men unfit for surgery.
- Temporary relief of benign prostatic obstruction (BPO) after minimally invasive treatment.

82. Transurethral needle ablation: (TUNA) (EAU Guidelines 2012)

- The generator produces a monopolar RF signal of 490 kHz, which allows excellent penetration and uniform tissue distribution. (The aim is to increase prostatic temperature to in excess of 60° C.)
- Nitric oxide synthase receptors are found to be most vulnerable to thermal damage, which occurred earliest, with damage to the α-adrenergic receptors maximal at 1 to 2 weeks.
- An average improvement in the mean symptom score of 13.1 symptom units and in the mean PFR of 6 mL/sec to be expected at 12 months
- It is an alternative to TURP for patients who wish to avoid complications of TURP, but patients should be aware of significant re-treatment rates and less improvement in symptoms and QOL.

83. Transurethral microwave therapy: (TUMT) (EAU Guidelines 2012)

- Prostatron device is used.
- It achieves symptom improvement comparable to TURP, but is associated with decreased morbidity and lower flow improvements.

84. TUMT VS TUNA

Microwaves treat a broad area and can penetrate tissue more deeply than RF.

In microwave central temperature is lower than with RF

Treatment with microwaves takes longer than RF to produce coagulative necrosis.

85. LASER: (EAU Guidelines 2012)

- Light amplification by the stimulated emission of radiation.
- HoLEP and KTP of the prostate are minimally-invasive alternatives to TURP in men with LUTS secondary to BPO which lead to **immediate, objective and subjective improvements comparable to TURP.**
- With regard to intra-operative safety, KTP is superior to TURP and **should be considered in patients receiving anticoagulant medication or with a high CVS risk.**

86.

	Wavelength (nm)	Penetration	Absorption	Properties
(Nd:YAG)	**1060**	**5-10mm**	Not absorbed by hemoglobin or water	Good hemostatic and cutting properties
CO_2	**10600**	**0.1mm**	**Highly absorbed with water**	Only small vessels < 0.5 mm coagulated effectively
(KTP)	**532**	**0.8mm**	Highly absorbed by hemoglobin	Used for incisions, resection, and ablation and can be passed through an endoscopic instruments
Ho : YAG	**2140(pulsed mode)**	**1-2mm**	**Highly absorbed with water**	Provides good hemostasis when used in a pulsed mode at low pulse repetition rate. At higher repetition rates, it may also be used for incisions

87. TUR syndrome

- Occur in 2% of the patients.
- Mental confusion, vomiting, hypertension, bradycardia and visual disturbance.

- Patients symptomatic-serum sodium concentration should be raised to >125 mEq/dL.
- The risk is increased if the gland is >45 g and the resection time is >90 minutes.
- Ammonium intoxication has been suggested as a possible cause.
- It is **secondary to dilutional hyponatremia.**
- Corrected by giving 200 mL of 3% saline solution very slowly over a period of time.

88. Monopolar TURP

- It is the current surgical standard procedure for men with prostate sizes of 30-80 mL and moderate-to-severe LUTS secondary to BPO.
- It provides subjective and objective improvement rates superior to medical or minimally invasive treatments **(EAU Guidelines 2012).**

89. Bipolar TURP achieves short-term results comparable to monopolar TURP **(EAU Guidelines 2012).**

90. Trans-urethral incision of prostate (TUIP)

- Using a Colling's knife, an incision is made at the 5 and 7 O'clock positions.
- It starts just distal to the ureteral orifice and ends just proximal to the verumontanum.
- It is the surgical therapy of choice for men with LUTS secondary to benign prostatic obstruction (BPO) and prostate sizes < 30 mL without middle lobes **(EAU Guidelines 2012).**

91. Intraprostatic botulinum toxin and intraprostatic ethanol injections for LUTS due to BPO or urinary retention are still experimental **(EAU Guidelines 2012).**

92. Open prostatectomy is the first choice of surgical treatment in men with drug-refractory LUTS secondary to BPO and prostate sizes > 80-100 mL **in the absence of Holmium lasers (EAU Guidelines 2012).**

93.

	TURP	**Open prostatectomy**
Retreatment rate	Higher	Lower
TUR syndrome	Present	Absent
Perioperative hemorrhage	Less	More
Hospital stay	Shorter	Longer
Removal of prostate	Not complete	Complete

94. Open Prostatectomy Advantages of Various Approaches:

Retropubic (Millin)	Suprapubic (Freyer's)
• Excellent anatomical exposure	• Direct access to the bladder is achieved (bladder stone and diverticula can be dealt)
• Clear visualization to control bleeding	• Preferred in patients with large median lobe protruding into the bladder
• No surgical trauma to the urinary bladder	
• Ensure complete removal	
• Prostate urinary continence	

95. Open prostatectomy should be preferred over TURP in:

- Weigh more than 75 g.
- Prostatectomy and diverticulectomy should be performed concurrently.
- Large bladder calculi.
- Ankylosis of the hip, preventing proper positioning for TUR.
- In men with recurrent or complex urethral conditions, such as urethral stricture or previous hypospadias repair, to avoid the urethral trauma associated with TURP.
- Association of an inguinal hernia with an enlarged prostate suggests an open procedure, as the hernia may be repaired through the same lower abdominal incision.

96. Contraindications to open prostatectomy include:

- Small fibrous gland.
- Presence of prostate cancer.
- Previous prostatectomy or pelvic surgery that may obliterate access to the prostate gland.

97. Following open prostatectomy–postoperative:

- Day 1–Clear liquid diet.
- Day 2–PUC removed and SPC clamped to allow a voiding trial.
- Day 3–Drain removed if < 75 mL per day.
- Day 5–Remove SPC and discharge.

98. **The estimated lifetime risk of prostate cancer is 16.72%, with a lifetime risk of death at 2.57%.**

Prostate cancer (PCa) is the **fourth most common male malignant** neoplasm worldwide.

PCa is currently the **second most common cause of cancer death in men (EAU Guidelines 2012).**

99. **The CONCORD study-**

- Worldwide population study based on analysis of cancer survival in five continents. It recenty analyzed international differences in survival for breast, colorectal, and prostate cancer
- Using data from cancer registries, age-standardized 5-year survival rates were found to vary greatly, ranging from 80% or higher in the United States (92%), Australia, and Canada, to less than 40% in Denmark, Poland, and Algeria.

100. **Lowest yearly incidence rates**–Asia.

- **Highest**–North America and Scandinavia, especially in African Americans.
- **Mortality is highest**–Sweden.
- **Lowest**–Asia (Singapore, Japan and China).

101. **Prostate cancer is rarely diagnosed in men <50 years**–<0.1% of all patients.

- 85% diagnosed > 65 years.
- Non-palpable cancers account for 75% of newly diagnosed disease.

102. **Familial prostate cancer** is defined as cancer in a man with one or more affected relatives.

Hereditary prostate cancer is a subset of the familial form and has been defined as:

- o Nuclear families with three or more affected members.
- o Cancer in three successive generations.
- o Two affected individuals diagnosed with cancer <55 years.

103. **Risk factors**

- Significant associations of prostate cancer with a **history of sexually transmitted infection or prostatitis**

- **Exposure of the prostate to androgens**–plays important role in prostate carcinogenesis.
- **Shortened CAG trinucleotide repeat length** in exon-associated with advanced, hormone-refractory disease.
- A **polymorphism of CYP3A4**–associated with locally advanced and poorly differentiated tumors.
- **Estrogens**–decrease risk by inhibition of prostate epithelial cell growth. Increase risk by eliciting inflammation or by the production of mutagenic metabolites.
- **IGF1 level** and prostate cancer–positive association is present.
- **Leptin** has been shown to stimulate proliferation of the androgen independent prostate cancer cell lines.
- **Very high calcium intake** above daily recommendation may modestly increase risk.
- **Polymorphisms resulting in a vitamin D receptor** with lower activity have been associated with increased risk for prostate cancer
- **High levels of dietary fat** stimulate proliferation of prostate cancer cells.
- **Obesity** was associated with a lower risk of low grade disease but a greater risk of high-grade disease

104. Etiology

- Loss of **NKX3-1** alleles is common in prostate lesions as they progress from PIN to local, metastatic and androgen-independent tumors.
- **PTEN on chromosome 10q23**–play a role in both initiation and progression of prostate cancer.
- Genetic alterations in the **tumor suppressor genes RB1 and TP53** are commonly present in metastatic or hormone refractory disease.
- Both increased **telomerase expression** and (paradoxically) shortened telomere length in high-grade PIN and invasive cancers.
- Expression of **GSTP1,** is absent in about 70% of PIN and virtually all cases of prostate cancer.
- **Loss of heterozygosity for p27** in 50% of patients with metastatic prostate cancer.

- **VEGF**-mediator of tumor angiogenesis and expressed in a majority of prostate cancers.
- **E-cadherin** expression is reduced in a significant percentage of poorly differentiated tumors.
- **β-MethylacylCoA racemase** is upregulated in virtually all prostate cancer.
- **Overexpression of PSMA** is observed after androgen withdrawal and in hormone–refractory disease.
- **EGF and EGFR** is important in prostate cancer.

105. The main findings of the prostate cancer prevention trial (PCPT) are as follows:

- **Prevalence of prostate cancer was reduced** by 24.8% in those randomized to finasteride compared with placebo.
- **Prevalence of Gleason grade 7 to 10 tumors was higher** in the finasteride group than in the placebo group.
- The risk reductions associated with finasteride among **risk groups defined by age, family history, race and PSA were of the same general magnitude.**
- **Sexual side effects were more common** with finasteride, whereas urinary symptoms were more common with placebo.

106. Baseline 5:1 benefit-to-risk ratio as defined by the number of cancers prevented for each excess high-grade cancer in those taking finasteride.

107. Chemoprevention by:

- Isoflavone components of soy, including genistein.
- Lycopene.
- Green tea.
- NSAIDS.

Neither selenium nor vitamin E should be used for preventing prostate or other cancers (SELECT study)

108. Prostatic intraepithelial neoplasia (PIN)

- Architecturally benign prostatic acini or ducts lined by **cytologically atypical cells.**
- **Low-grade PIN should not be commented in diagnostic reports.**
- **High-grade PIN is a precursor to some prostate carcinomas.**

109.

	Atypical needle biopsy	Prostatic intraepithelial neoplasia (PIN)
Incidence	High grade PIN-7.6%	5.2%
Mean risk of cancer	26.4%	42% to 49%
Need for repeat biopsy	No	Yes
Correlation with PSA or DRE findings	No	No

110. Prostate cancer–**85% of tumor mass is peripheral in location.**

- **Multifocal** in more than 85%.
- Extraprostatic extension preferentially occurs **posteriorly and posterolaterally.**

111. **The most common route of seminal vesicle invasion**–tumor penetration out of the prostate at the base of the gland, with growth and extension into the peri-seminal vesicle soft tissue and eventually into the seminal vesicles.

112. Following in frequency after lymph nodes, bones, and lung, the next most common **regions of spread of prostate cancer at** autopsy are bladder, liver and adrenal gland.

113. **The Gleason system**

- Based on the glandular pattern of the tumor as identified at **low magnification.**
- Gleason scores range from 2 (1 + 1 = 2), well differentiated to **10 (5+5=10), totally undifferentiated tumors.**
- **Gleason score 2 to 4** on needle biopsy is never assigned.
- Gleason score 4 + 3 = 7 have a worse prognosis than with Gleason score 3 + 4 = 7.

114. Only 25% of men with seminal vesicle invasion and none with LN metastases are **biochemically progression-free at 10 years after radical prostatectomy.**

115. **Independent predictors of progression of prostate cancer**– gleason grade, extraprostatic extension, and margins of resection

116. **Tumor volume** does not independently predict post-radical prostatectomy progression.

117. **Mucinous adenocarcinoma of the prostate**

- Propensity to develop bone metastases.
- Increased serum acid phosphatase and PSA levels with advanced disease.

118. Small cell carcinomas of the prostate

- 50% of the cases, the tumors are mixed small cell carcinoma and adenocarcinoma of the prostate.
- Majority of prostatic tumors with clinically evident ACTH or ADH production.
- The average survival of patients with small cell carcinoma of the prostate is <1 year.

119. Prostatic duct adenocarcinomas

- Tumors arising in the peripheral prostatic ducts present like ordinary (acinar) adenocarcinoma of the prostate and may be diagnosed on needle biopsy.
- Underestimated clinically because DRE and serum PSA levels may be normal.
- Most are advanced stage at presentation and have an aggressive course.

120. Pure primary squamous carcinoma of the prostate

- Associated with poor survival.
- Develop osteolytic metastases.
- Do not respond to estrogen therapy.
- Do not develop elevated serum acid phosphatase levels with metastatic disease.

121. Most common mesenchymal tumor within the prostate and is seen almost exclusively in childhood–**Rhabdomyosarcoma.**

Most common sarcomas involving the prostate in adults–**leiomyosarcomas.**

122. Transitional cell carcinoma (TCC)

1. Primary TCC of the prostate

- Accounts for 1% to 4% of all prostate carcinomas.
- More than 50% of the patients present with stage T3 or T4 tumors.
- Bone metastases tend to be osteolytic.

2. **TCC involving prostatic ducts and acini**
   - Seen in patients with a history of flat transitional cell CIS of the bladder who have been treated for a period of months to years with intravesical topical chemotherapy.
3. **Direct invasion from bladder TCC into the stroma of the prostate.**

123. **Differentiation between prostate adenocarcinoma and TCC**

	Prostate adenocarcinoma	**Transitional cell carcinoma**
PSA and PAP	Positive	Negative
HMW-cytokeratin (34βE12)	Negative	**57% to 70%**
CK-7	19% to 35%	**70% to 100%**
CK-20	2% to 72%	15% to 71%

124. The most common form of leukemic involvement of prostate is–**chronic lymphocytic leukemia.**

125. Calcifications along the surgical capsule known as **"corpora amylacea" highlight the plane between the PZ and TZ.**

126.

TRUS	**4 MHZ**	**7 MHZ**
Resolution	Lower resolution	High resolution image
Focal length	2–8 cm	1–4 cm
Volume measurements	Increase accuracy	Less accurate
Internal architecture visualization	Poor	Good

127. **Formula to calculate prostate size** - ($\pi/6 \times$ transverse diameter $\times$ AP diameter $\times$ longitudinal diameter),

128. **Average prostate is between 20 and 25 g and remains constant until about age 50**

129. **Androgen ablation with LHRH analogs will cause**–30% volume decrease with androgen deprivation in prostates with and without cancer

130. **For patients with a serum PSA value between 4.0 and 10.0 ng/ml**
   - Use percentage of free PSA thresholds of <25%
   - This will allow detection of 95% of cancers while eliminating 20% unnecessary biopsies

131. On conventional gray-scale TRUS

- 39% of all prostate cancers are isoechoic.
- 1% of cancers may be hyperechoic.
- 17% to 57% of cancers may be hypoechoic.

132. Indications of TRUS-Directed Biopsy

- Diagnosis of suspected symptomatic prostate cancer (i.e., bone metastasis, cord compression)
- Screening for prostate cancer in asymptomatic patient > age 50 with > 10-year life expectancy
- Prostate nodule regardless of PSA level
- PSA > 4.0 ng/dL regardless of age
- In men at age 40-60 years if PSA > 2.5 ng/dL
- In men at age 40 years if PSA > 0.6 ng/dL
- Increased PSA velocity (>0.75 ng/dL/year)
- Free PSA in considering initial biopsy with PSA < 10 ng/mL–<15%

133. Preparation before biopsy

- All **anticoagulant therapy** (warfarin, clopidogrel, aspirin/ NSAIDs, herbal supplements) should be stopped 7 to 10 days before prostate biopsy.
- **Oral fluoroquinolone** is given 30 to 60 minutes before biopsy and continue therapy for 2 to 3 days.
- Patients should self-administer a **cleansing enema** at home before biopsy.
- **Infiltration anesthesia** around the nerve bundles with local anesthetic may provide excellent pain control.
- Patients are placed in the **left lateral decubitus position** with knees and hips flexed 90 degrees.

134. The original sextant biopsy scheme includes one core from the base, mid and apex bilaterally.

135. Repeat prostate biopsy

- **Second prostate biopsy** in all cases of a negative finding on initial biopsy appears justified.
- **Third and fourth repeat biopsies** should only be obtained in very selected patients with high suspicion of cancer and/or poor prognostic factors on the first or second biopsy.

136. **Most common complication seen after prostate biopsy**–bleeding.

137. **Although PSA (hK3)** is less expressed in prostate cancer, **hK2** levels have been shown to be elevated in poorly differentiated prostate cancer.

138. **PSA is organ specific**, primarily produced by the prostatic luminal epithelial cells

 Although it is organ specific, **PSA is not cancer specific**

139. **The serum half-life of PSA**, is 2 to 3 days.

140. **Uncomplexed PSA** is cleared from the serum within 2 to 3 hours and is excreted by the kidney.

141. **Prostate cancer cells do not make more PSA** but rather make less PSA than normal prostatic tissue.

142. **In men without BPH, the rate of change in PSA** is 0.04 ng/mL per year, compared with 0.07 to 0.27 ng/mL per year in men with BPH.

143. **Prostatic trauma after prostatic biopsy**–4 weeks for PSA to return to baseline values.

 - **DRE** can lead to increases in serum PSA (Clinically insignificant).
 - **Ejaculation** can lead to increase in PSA.

144. **Finasteride (5 mg)** lowers PSA levels by an average of 50% after 6 months of treatment.

145. **Suggestive of malignancy**

 - **PSAD** > 0.15 ng/ml of per gram of prostate level
 - **PSA velocity** > 0.75 ng/mL per year.
 - **Free/total PSA** < 0.18.

146. **PCA-3**

 - Expression of the DD3–PCA-3 protein has been localized to prostatic tissue
 - It has been found in 95% of prostate cancer and prostate metastasis specimens.
 - 66-fold upregulation of this protein in cancerous tissues compared with normal control tissues.
 - Furthermore, DD3 was detected from specimens containing as little as 10% cancer

- This test was capable of finding cancer within a large background of normal cells.

147. The α-methylacyl coenzyme A racemase (AMACR) gene, located on chromosome 5, is upregulated in prostate cancer tissues

148. Quebec prospective randomized controlled trial

- No role of screening in Prostate cancer.

149. Most useful first-line test for assessing the risk of prostate cancer–combination of DRE and serum PSA (TRUS is not recommended as a first-line screening).

150. The first elevated PSA level should not prompt an immediate biopsy.

The PSA level should be verified after a few weeks by the same assay under standardized conditions.

151. PSA and DRE for detection of prostate cancer

- In 18% of all patients, PCa is detected by **DRE alone**, irrespective of the PSA level.
- The pathologic features of prostate cancers detected with PSA testing **are more favorable** than those of cancers detected without PSA testing.
- Addition of PSA testing to DRE leads to detection of a greater proportion of **pathologically confined cancers** compared with cancer detection by DRE alone.
- When a PSA cutoff of 4 ng/mL and an abnormal DRE were used together as screening criteria for prostate cancer, **pathologically organ-confined disease was found in 71% of men** who underwent surgery for prostate cancer.

152. The American Cancer Society and the American Urological Association recommend that prostate cancer screening be offered annually beginning at age 50 years and earlier for those at higher risk (family history of disease, black).

153. The National Comprehensive Cancer Network has recommended that all men be offered baseline PSA screening at age 40 years and that the frequency of follow-up testing should depend on PSA test results.

154. The upper age limit for enrolment in current randomized screening trials of prostate cancer is **74 years.**

155. The PLCO–concluded that (prostate cancer) PCa related mortality was very low and not significantly different between screened and non screened group.

ERSPC–concluded that PSA-based screening reduced the rate of death from PCa by 20%, but was associated with a high risk of over-diagnosis.

- Based on the results of these two large, randomised trials, urological societies conclude that at present **widespread mass screening for PCa is not appropriate (EAU Guidelines 2012).**

156. 2009 Carcinoma prostate staging

T–Primary tumor

- T1–clinically inapparent tumor not palpable or visible by imaging.
- T1–a Tumor incidental histological finding in 5% or less of tissue resected.
- T1–b Tumor incidental histological finding in more than 5% of tissue resected.
- T1–c Tumor identified by needle biopsy (e.g. because of elevated PSA).
- T2 –Tumor confined within the prostate.
- T2a–Tumor involves one half of one lobe or less.
- T2b–Tumor involves more than half of one lobe, but not both lobes.
- T2c–Tumor involves both lobes.
- T3–Tumor extends through the prostatic capsule.
- T3a–Extracapsular extension (unilateral or bilateral) including microscopic bladder neck involvement.
- T3b–Tumor invades seminal vesicle(s).
- T4–Tumor is fixed or invades adjacent structures other than seminal vesicles: external sphincter, rectum, levator muscles, and/or pelvic wall.
- N1–Regional lymph node metastasis.
- M1a–Non-regional lymph node(s).
- M1b–Bone.
- M1c–Other sites.

157. D'Amico demonstrated that stratification into

- Low-risk (clinical stage T1 to 2a, PSA 10 ng/mL or less **and** Gleason score 6 or less)
- Intermediate-risk (stage T2b, PSA greater than 10 but less than **20** ng/mL or Gleason score 7)
- High-risk disease (stage T2c, PSA greater than 20 ng/mL **or** Gleason score 8 to 10)

158. CAPRA–Cancer of the Prostate Risk Assessment score

159. Partin Tables–Combination of PSA, Clinical Stage and Gleason Score is used to predict pathologic stage of localized prostate cancer.

160. For tumor staging: (EAU Guidelines 2012)

- **MRI** demonstrates higher accuracy for the assessment of uni or bilobar disease (T2), extraprostatic extension and seminal vesicle invasion (T3).
- Overall accuracy of PET in defining local tumor stage (pT2 and pT3a4) has been 70%.
- PET tends to understage PCa, and has a limited value in clinically localised PCa.

For nodal staging

- CT and MRI perform similarly in the detection of pelvic LN, although **CT** seems to be slightly superior.

For bone metastasis

- Radionuclide bone scan (bone scintigraphy) is the **most sensitive modality** for the detection of skeletal metastases.
- Bone survey films **(skeletal radiography), require >50% of the bone density to be replaced** with tumor before they can identify distant spread.

161. Monoclonal antibody radioimmunoscintigraphy (radiolabeled monoclonal antibody scan) have been used for identification of microscopic cancer deposits in regional and distant sites.

The ProstaScint scan uses this technology but has had limited accuracy in the detection of lymph node metastases

162. Laparoscopic pelvic lymphadenectomy prior to treatment is reserved for patients with

- Gleason score greater than 8

- Extraprostatic extension on DRE
- PSA greater than 20 ng/ml
- Suspicion of enlarged lymph nodes on radiologic evaluation

< 10% likelihood of having node metastases and can be spared nodal evaluation are patients with **(EAU Guidelines 2012)**

- Stage T2 or less.
- PSA <20 ng/Ml.
- Gleason score <6.

163. Radionuclide bone scan, abdominal-pelvic CT scan, and MRI scan are not indicated if the tumor has a:

- Gleason sum of <7.
- Serum PSA level is <10 ng/Ml.
- Biopsy findings do not reveal an extensive or highly aggressive cancer

164. The feasibility of performing nerve-sparing surgery is questionable when:

- Extensive cancer in the biopsy specimens.
- Palpable extraprostatic tumor extension.
- Serum PSA level >10 ng/ml.
- Biopsy Gleason score > 7.
- Poor–quality erections preoperatively, current and future lack of a sexual relationship.
- Other medical conditions that may adversely affect erections.

165. Median time from **PSA failure to the development of metastases** after RP is 8 years

Median time from **metastases to death** is 5 years

Thus the median time from diagnosis to death is more than 13 years.

166. An ideal candidate for radical prostatectomy

- Patient with life expectancy of at least 10 years, and his tumor would be deemed to be biologically significant and completely resectable.

167. Radical prostatectomy approach

	Perineal	**Retropubic**
Blood loss	Less	More
Operative time	Short	Long
Pelvic LND	Not possible	Possible
Rectal injury	High	Low
Postoperative fecal incontinence	High	Low
Positive surgical margins	High	Low

168. Laparoscopic prostatectomy vs open RP

- Incontinence and anastomotic stricture rates are same as of open surgery.
- Nerve sparing is equivalent or even better with laparoscopic surgery
- Rates of positive surgical margins have been higher with laparoscopic prostatectomy

169. A rising serum PSA level is usually the **earliest evidence of tumor recurrence** after radical prostatectomy.

170. The return of erectile function after radical retropubic prostatectomy correlates with:

- Age of the patient.
- Preoperative potency status.
- Extent of nerve-sparing surgery.
- Era of surgery.

171. Relative contraindication to brachytherapy and external beam radiation therapy (EBRT).

- Prior TURP.
- Severe LUTS.
- Inflammatory bowel disease.

172. PSA "bounce"

- Inflammation in the prostate gland can produce transient PSA elevations.
- It occurs during the first 2 years after treatment and is less common with EBRT than with brachytherapy.

173. American Society of Therapeutic Radiology and Oncology (ASTRO) definition

- It requires three consecutive PSA increases measured 6 months apart and back-dates the time of cancer progression to halfway between the PSA nadir and the first rising PSA level.

Phoenix definition–PSA level to rise by 2 ng/ml.

174. After RP–patient is considered to have progressed if the PSA level is >0.4 ng/mL, 8 weeks after the procedure.

175. The radiation doses delivered to the prostate are approximately **145 Gy for iodine** and **125 Gy for palladium**, which are substantially higher than those with EBRT.

176. Adverse effects:

	Brachytherapy	**EBRT**
Urinary symptoms	More	Less
Proctitis	Less	More
Rectal injury	Less	More
Erectile dysfunction	More	Less

177. Patients with detectable PSA (>0.1 ng/mL) after RP usually have persistent cancer, although some have only retained benign prostatic tissue causing the PSA elevation.

178. If salvage radiotherapy is planned, it should be initiated before the PSA level rises above **0.5 ng/mL.**

179. Management of localised carcinoma prostate.

	Active Surveillance (AS)	**Watchful Waiting (WW)**
Aim	To individualize treatment	To avoid treatment
Patient characteristics	Fit for radical treatment with life expectancy > 15 yr	Life expectancy < 15 yr
Tumor characteristics	**T1T2, PSA < 15 ng/mL, GS ≤ 7**	**Any T stage, any PSA, GS ≤ 7**
Monitoring	Frequent PSA testing and biopsies	PSA and repeat biopsies unimportant
Indications for treatment	Short PSADT or ↑stage on biopsy	Symptomatic progression
Treatment timing	Early	Delayed
Treatment intent	Radical	Palliative

180. Active Surveillance (AS)

- **It may be a feasible alternative** to initial curative treatment in patients with favorable, localized prostate cancer.
- About half of these patients remain free of progression at 10 years, and definitive treatment appeared effective in those with progression.
- **PSADT (PSA doubling time) is a predictor of cancer progression** for men on AS.

181. Watchful Waiting (WW)

Scandinavian Prostate Cancer Group Study Number 4 (SPCG-4)

- Randomised patients with clinical stage T1-T2 to WW or radical prostatectomy.
- After a median follow-up of 12.8 years, this study showed a significant decrease in CSM, overall mortality, metastatic risk progression and local progression in patients treated with RP versus WW.

182. Kattan nomogram includes:

- Pre treatment PSA.
- Clinical stage.
- Primary gleason grade.
- Secondary gleason grade.
- Ultrasound volume.
- Mm of cancer.
- Mm of non-cancer.

(EAU Guidelines 2012)

183. Point system for evaluating progression in patients treated with deferred therapy

	1 point	2 point	3 point
Gleason score	1	>1	Any new Gleason pattern 4 or 5
PSA velocity		>0.75 during 12 months	>0.75/yr during 24 months
DRE/TRUS	Increasing old lesion	New lesion not biopsy proven	New biopsy-proven lesion
Biosy specimen		Bilateral or multifocal cancer	>4 cores with cancer

Patients with three or more points were classified as having objective progression.

184. The lead time in PSA screening is about 10 years.

185. Role of active surveillance

- In patients with the lowest risk of cancer progression: cT12a, PSA < 10 ng/mL, biopsy Gleason score < 6 (at least 10 cores), < 2 positive biopsies, minimal biopsy core involvement (< 50% cancer per biopsy).
- Follow-up is based on DRE, PSA and repeated biopsies. The optimal timing for followup is still unclear (yearly or every 2 years).
- The trigger for active treatment is based mainly on grade progression on repeated biopsies or at the patient's request.

186. Role of RP

- **RP is the only treatment for localised PCa** to show a benefit for CSS, compared with conservative management.
- **Low-risk, localised prostate cancer (cT1–T2a and GS 2-6 and PSA < 10 ng/ml)**
  - o Patients should be informed about retropubic RP versus WW (survival benefit is similar).
  - o No role of eLND.
- **Intermediate-risk, localised prostate cancer (cT2b–T2c or GS = 7 or PSA 10-20 ng/ml)**
  - o Patients should be informed about retropubic RP versus WW (survival benefit is similar).
  - o eLND should be performed if risk of positive LN exceeds 5%.
- **High-risk, localised prostate cancer: cT3a or GS 8-10 or PSA > 20 ng/ml**
  - o RP is a reasonable treatment option in selected patients with cT3a PCa, GS 8-10 or PSA > 20.
  - o Furthermore, RP is optional in highly selected patients with cT3b–cT4 N0 or any cT N1 PCa in the context of a multimodality approach.
  - o eLND is perfomed in all cases.

187. Role of extended (eLND)

- Role in the treatment of a subset of **intermediate-risk cases with**

> 5% nomogram predicted risk of positive lymph nodes, and in **all high-risk cases.**

- It includes removal of the nodes overlying the external iliac artery and vein, the nodes within the obturator fossa located cranially and caudally to the obturator nerve, and the nodes medial and lateral to the internal iliac artery.
- It may increase staging accuracy and influence decision making with respect to adjuvant therapy. The number of lymph nodes removed correlates with time to progression.
- Recent literature has shown **improvement in CSS and OS in favour of completed RP** versus abandoned RP in patients who were found to be N+ at the time of surgery.

  (Previous belief was to abandon RP for clinical N+ disease, or cancel surgery if a frozen section shows LN invasion.)

188. The deep dorsal vein leaves the penis under Buck's fascia between the corpora cavernosa and penetrates the urogenital diaphragm.

189. The prostate receives arterial blood supply from the inferior vesical artery

- The artery terminates in two large groups: the urethral and capsular groups.
- Urethral vessels enter the prostate at the posterolateral vesicoprostatic junction and supply the vesical neck and periurethral portion of the gland.
- Capsular branches run posterolateral to the prostate and supply the outer portion of the prostate.
- Capsular vessels provide macroscopic landmark to aid in the identification of NVB.

190. The autonomic innervation of the pelvic organs and external genitalia arises from the pelvic plexus, which is formed by:

- Parasympathetic, visceral, efferent, preganglionic fibers that arise from S2 to S4.
- Sympathetic fibers via the hypogastric nerve from the thoracolumbar center.

191. The NVB are located in the lateral pelvic fascia between the prostatic fascia and the levator fascia.

192. **Pudendal nerve**–major nerve supply to the striated sphincter and levator ani.

193. **RP is deferred**–6 to 8 weeks after needle biopsy of prostate and 12 weeks after TURP.

194. **High anterior release of NVB at the apex before division of DVC**

- To speed up the recovery of sexual function and continence.
- Risk of positive surgical margins may be increased by this approach.
- This approach should be used only in men who are likely to have organ-confined disease and who are candidates for bilateral nerve sparing.

195. **Neurovascular bundles (NVB) should not be preserved**

- If induration is palpable in the lateral pelvic fascia.
- If NVB appears to be fixed to the prostate at the time it is being released.
- If there appears to be inadequate tissue over the posterolateral surface after the prostate has been removed.

196. **If there is troublesome bleeding from the DVC at any point**–completely divide the dorsal vein complex over the urethra and oversew the end.

197. **Bladder neck contractures**

- Occur in 0.5% to 10% of patients after radical prostatectomy.
- Due to inadequate approximation of mucosal surfaces at the time of surgery, urinary extravasation, or distraction of the bladder neck from a hematoma.
- Treatment–cold-knife incision of the bladder neck at 3, 6 and 9O'clock followed by CIC.

198. **Salvage prostatectomy**

- Offered only to men who at initial presentation had clinically localized prostate cancer.
- The procedure is reserved for patients with excellent health and LE > 15 years.
- Prostate biopsy, histologic grade, clinical examination findings, and serum PSA levels must suggest localized disease with no evidence of metastatic disease.

199. **In retrograde technique**–DVC is divided early in the operation and the prostatic pedicles late, there is potentially a greater risk of ongoing bleeding with this as compare to antegrade technique.

200. An extraperitoneal approach for laparoscopic RP or robot assisted RP helps **confine any urine leak but provides a smaller operative working space.**

201. **Advantage of brachytherapy**–very rapid dose falloff because of the very low energy of the radioactive sources used–(only 21 and 28 keV for palladium 103 and iodine 125, respectively).

- Higher activity seeds are required for ^{103}Pd versus ^{125}I to deliver a similar tumoricidal dose.

202. **Failure Pattern According to PSA Nadir, Time to Nadir and PSA Doubling Time**

	PSA Nadir (ng/mL)	Time to Nadir (months)	PSA Doubling Time (months)
No E/o Disease	0.4-0.5	22-33	NA
Local failure	1.0-2.0	12-18	11-13
Distant failure	>2.0	<12	36

203. **Radiographic factors that warrant consideration of prophylactic surgical fixation include:**

- An intramedullary lytic lesion ≥ 50% of the cross-sectional diameter of the bone.
- A lytic lesion involving a length of cortex ≥ than the cross-sectional diameter of the bone or > 2.5 cm in axial length.

204. **When the diagnosis of cord compression** is made or even suspected, all patients should receive steroid therapy.

205. **Strontium 89**

- Toxicity is mainly hematologic
- Platelet drop by 20% to 50%
- Response rate is 60% to 90%
- Response duration is 6 months

206. **Role of RT in prostate cancer (EAU Guidelines 2012)**

Role of EBRT

- In **T1c–T2c N0 M0**, 3D-CRT with or without IMRT is recommended, even for young patients who refuse surgical intervention.

- In **T3-4 N0 M0**, concomitant and adjuvant hormonal therapy for a total duration of 3 years, with EBRT, is recommended because it improves overall survival.
- In **T2c–T3 N0-X** and a Gleason score of 2-6, short-term ADT before and during radiotherapy can be recommended because it may favourably influence overall survival.
- In **c-pN1 M0** with no severe co-morbidity, pelvic external irradiation and immediate long-term adjuvant hormonal treatment is recommended because it will improve overall survival, disease-specific failure, metastatic failure and biochemical control.

Role of adjuvant RT

- In **pT3 N0 M0**, immediate post-operative EBRT after RP may improve overall survival and biochemical and clinical disease-free survival with the highest impact in cases of positive margins.

Role of brachytherapy

- In **cT1–T2a,** Gleason score < 7 (or 3 + 4), PSA < 10 ng/mL, prostate volume < 50 mL, without a previous TURP and with a good IPSS, transperineal interstitial brachytherapy with permanent implants can be an alternative.

Role of salvage RT

- In **pT2-3N0M0,** salvage irradiation is indicated in case of persisting PSA or biochemical failure, but before the PSA level > 0.5 ng/mL.

207. (EAU Guidelines 2012)

In patients who are unfit for surgery, or with a life expectancy < 10 years **cryosurgery** has evolved from an investigational therapy to a **possible alternative treatment for PCa.**

All other minimally invasive treatment options–such as HIFU microwave and electrosurgery are still experimental or investigational.

208. A tissue temperature of **–40°C to–50°C**, is lethal for cells.

209. Primary cryotherapy is suitable for patients with clinical stage T1c–T3 disease of any tumor grade who are not potent or not interested in maintaining their potency.

210. Salvage cryotherapy is contraindicated for PSA >10 ng/mL and GS of the recurrent cancer ≥9.

211. HIFU

- Strong ultrasound waves 10,000 times stronger than diagnostic ultrasound are generated by a transducer with a parabolic configuration
- The focal point is located 3 to 4 cm
- Ultrasound energy is concentrated, is absorbed by the tissue, and generates temperatures that can exceed 80° C, resulting in coagulative necrosis and the destruction of tissue

212. (EAU Guidelines 2012)

Role of neoadjuvant hormone therapy (NHT)

- NHT before RP does not provide a significant OS or DFS advantage over RP alone.
- NHT before RP does substantially improve local pathological variables such as organ-confined rates, pathological down-staging, positive surgical margins, and rate of lymph node involvement.

Role of adjuvant hormone therapy (HT)

- Adjuvant HT following RP shows no survival advantage at 10 years but DFS is highly significantly in favour of the HT arm.

213. Role of intermittent androgen therapy

- The initial (induction) cycle must last between 6 and 9 months.
- Treatment is stopped only if no clinical progression, PSA < 4 ng/mL in metastatic disease, or 0.5 ng/mL in relapsing disease.
- Treatment is resumed when the patient reaches either a clinical progression. This is usually 4-10 ng/mL in non-metastatic situations or 10-15 ng/mL in metastatic patients.
- It is better tolerated and sometimes benefits sexual functioning.

214. Androgen block

- **Combined**–Orchidectomy/LHRH agonist + nonsteroidal antiandrogen.
- **Minimal**–Finasteride + nonsteroidal antiandrogen.

- **Triple**–Orchidectomy/LHRH agonist + finasteride + nonsteroidal antiandrogen.

215. The standard castrate level of testosterone is **< 50 ng/dL.**

216. Androgen deprivation therapies

- **Bilateral orchidectomy**–Quickest way to achieve a castration level, usually <12 hours.
- **LHRH agonists**–transient rise in LH and FSH release.
  - This then elevates T production (known as the **'flare-up'** phenomenon).
  - It begins about 2-3 days after the first injection and lasts for 1 week.
  - Chronic exposure to LHRH agonists suppresses pituitary LH and FSH secretion and testosterone production.
  - Castration levels usually within 2-4 weeks.
- **LHRH antagonists (abarelix)** bind immediately and competitively to LHRH receptors in the pituitary gland. The effect is a rapid decrease in LH, FSH and testosterone levels **without any flare**.
- **Diethylstilboesterol (DES)** is one of the classic forms of hormonal therapy. Its efficacy is comparable to that of bilateral orchiectomy.
  - Significant cardiovascular side-effects of DES, even at lower dosages.
- **Antiandrogen**
  - Steroidal, e.g., cyproterone acetate (CPA), megestrol acetate and medroxyprogesterone acetate.
  - Non-steroidal, e.g., nilutamide, flutamide and bicalutamide.
  - Bicalutamide, 150 mg once daily, achieved a similar PSA response to castration, while maintaining a good tolerability profile.
  - Bicalutamide monotherapy should be avoided in patients with localised PCa.
  - High-dose bicalutamide has emerged as an alternative to castration for patients with locally advanced (M0) if PFS is the target, and in highly selected, well-informed cases of M1 PCa with a low PSA.

- **Inhibition of androgen synthesis**
  - o **Aminoglutethimide**–Aminoglutethimide inhibits the conversion of cholesterol to pregnenolone
  - o **Ketoconazole**–interferes with two cytochrome P450–dependent pathways:
    - Blocks conversion of lanosterol to cholesterol.
    - Blocks 17,20-desmolase, impacting on the conversion of C21 to C19 steroids.
  - o **Abiraterone**-abiraterone inhibits 17α-hydrolase and C17,20-lyase

    It has gained FDA approval for the treatment of patients with metastatic CRPC who have previously received docetaxel chemotherapy

217. Results of combined androgen blockade (Prostate Cancer Trialists' Collaborative Group)

- In these studies, 88% of patients had metastatic disease; the remainder had locally advanced disease.
- **Studies included the steroidal antiandrogen cyproterone acetate**
  - o 5-year survival with combined androgen blockade was 25.4% compared with 23.4% with standard ADT **(nonsignificant gain in favor of ADT of 1.8%)**
- **When nonsteroidal antiandrogens flutamide or nilutamide were considered**
  - o 5-year survival improved from 24.7% (standard ADT) to 27.6% for combined androgen blockade.

    (2.9% improvement was significant)

218. (EAU Guidelines 2012)

Role of hormonal therapy in advanced PCa

- ADT delays progression, prevents potentially catastrophic complications, and palliates symptoms effectively, but does not prolong survival.
- All forms of castration used as monotherapy (e.g. orchiectomy, LHRH and DES) have equivalent efficacy.
- Non-steroidal anti-androgen monotherapy (e.g. bicalutamide) is an alternative to castration.

Timing of ADT

- Immediate ADT (given at diagnosis) significantly reduces disease progression, as well as the complication rate due to progression itself, compared with deferred ADT (delivered at symptomatic progression). However, the survival benefit is at marginal and not related to CSS.

Metastatic PCa

- Addition of a non-steroidal anti-androgen to castration (CAB) results in a small advantage in OS over castration alone, but is associated with increased adverse events, reduced QoL, and high costs.

219. **Bisphosphonates**, such as pamidronate, alendronate or zoledronic acid, have been shown to **increase BMD** in the hip and spine by up to 7% in 1 year. **Significant benefit in OS** has recently been demonstrated for biphosphonates in PCa in M1 patients.

220. Bone protection can be by **denosumab,** a fully human monoclonal antibody against **RANKL**, which is a key mediator for osteoclast function, activation and survival.

221. **Follow-up (EAU Guidelines 2012)**

- **In asymptomatic patients,** serum PSA and DRE are the recommended tests for routine follow-up. These should be performed at 3, 6 and 12 months after treatment, then every 6 months until 3 years, and then annually.
- **After radical prostatectomy,** a serum PSA level of >0.2 ng/mL can be associated with residual or recurrent disease.
- **After radiation therapy,** a rising PSA level over 2 ng/mL above the nadir PSA, rather than a specific threshold value, is the most reliable sign of persistent or recurrent disease.
- **After hormonal treatment** patients should be evaluated at 3 and 6 months after the initiation of treatment and tests should include serum PSA, DRE, serum testosterone and careful evaluation of symptoms in order to assess the treatment response and the side-effects of the treatments given.

222. Management of PSA relapse (EAU Guidelines 2012)

After RP

- Local recurrences are treated by salvage RT with 64-66 Gy at a PSA serum level <0.5 ng/mL.
- For patients with presumed local recurrence who are too unfit or unwilling to undergo radiation therapy, expectant management can be offered.
- PSA recurrence indicative of systemic relapse is best treated by early ADT.

After RT

- Local recurrences may be treated by salvage RP in carefully selected patients, who presumably demonstrate organ-confined disease, i.e. PSA < 10 ng/mL, PSA DT > 12 months and biopsy Gleason score <7.
- In patients with presumed systemic relapse, ADT may be offered.

223. Definition of castrate resistant prostate cancer (CRPC)

- Testosterone < 50 ng/dL or < 1.7 nmol/L.
- Three consecutive rises of PSA, 1 week apart, resulting in two 50% increases over the nadir, with a PSA > 2 ng/mL.
- Anti-androgen withdrawal for at least 6 weeks for bicalutamide.

224. Treatment of CRPC

- Docetaxel at 75 mg/m^2 every 3 weeks is the **drug of choice** since it has shown a significant survival benefit.
- After a median 20.7 months of follow-up, overall survival in the every 3-week docetaxel arm was 18.9 months with a pain response rate of 35% and a PSA response of 45%.
- More hematologic toxicity and neuropathy in the every 3-week arm but slightly lower rates of nausea and vomiting, fatigue, nail changes, hyperlacrimation, and diarrhea as compare to weekly arm.

225. In patients with relapse following first-line docetaxel chemotherapy–Cabazitaxel and Abiraterone is regarded as first-choice option for second-line treatment.

226. Sipuleucel-T (Provenge)

- Vaccine derived from CD54+ dendritic cells, the major antigen-presenting cells, which are apheresed from individuals and processed with the recombinant fusion protein PAP and GM-CSF.
- Sipuleucel-T is the first therapeutic vaccine to be FDA approved for the treatment of any cancer and is indicated for use in men with asymptomatic or minimally symptomatic metastatic CRPC.

227. Causes of Osteolytic metastasis

- Kidney (expansile)
- Thyroid
- Lung
- Breast
- GIT

Causes of Osteoblastic metastasis

- Prostate
- Breast
- Seminoma
- Carcinoid
- Neurogenic
- Uterus
- Ovary

❑❑

Chapter 17

PEDIATRIC UROLOGY

1. **Embryology of kidney**
   - **In order of their appearance**–the pronephros, the mesonephros and metanephros.
   - **All three kidneys develop from**–intermediate mesoderm
   - **The first two kidneys regress** in utero.
   - **The definitive kidney, or the metanephros** forms in the sacral region.
2. **Ureteric bud**
   - **Arises from the distal portion of the nephric duct.**
   - Comes in contact with the condensing blastema of metanephric mesenchyme on **28th day.**
   - Crucial role of the RET-GDNF-GFRα1 pathway in the ureteric bud outgrowth.
3. **Nephron**–(glomerulus, proximal tubule, loop of Henle and distal tubule) derived from **metanephric mesenchyme.**

   Collecting system–(collecting ducts, calyces, pelvis and ureter) derived from **ureteric bud.**
4. Although renal maturation continues to take place postnatally, **nephrogenesis is completed before birth.**
5. **Between the 6th and 9th weeks, the kidneys ascend to a lumbar site** just below the adrenal glands.
6. **In HSK during ascent, the fused lower pole becomes trapped under the inferior mesenteric artery.**
7. **Cell types that are involved in the control of renal development:** the ureteric bud tip cells, the condensed mesenchymal cells, and the stromal or interstitial mesenchymal cells
8. **Partition of cloaca into an anterior urogenital sinus and a posterior anorectal canal:**
   - Occurs by the midline fusion of two lateral ridges of the cloacal wall and by a descending urorectal septum.

- This process occur during the **5th and 6th week.**

9. **Entrance of the nephric duct into the primitive urogenital sinus** serves as a landmark distinguishing the cephalad vesicourethral canal from the caudal urogenital sinus.
   - **The vesicourethral canal** gives rise to–bladder and pelvic urethra.
   - **Caudal urogenital sinus** gives rise to–phallic urethra in males and distal vaginal, vestibule in females.

10. **Common excretory ducts**
    - It is the portion of **nephric ducts distal to the origin of ureteric buds.**
    - The right and left common excretory ducts fuse in the midline as a triangular area, forming the **primitive trigone.**

11. **Weigert–Meyer rule**
    - **Lateral lower pole ureteric orifice** may result from a ureteric bud arising too low on the nephric duct.
      - o In such a ureteric orifice, VUR is more likely to occur because of an inadequate intramural tunnel.
    - **Caudal upper pole ureteric orifice** may result from a ureteric bud arising too high on the nephric duct.
      - o It may drain at the bladder neck, verumontanum or at vas deferens.

12. **Ureter undergoes a transient luminal obstruction** between 37 and 40 days of gestation and subsequently recanalizes

    At 12 weeks of gestation

    – first signs of ureteral muscularization and development of elastic fibers occurs

    – urachus involutes to become a fibrous cord, which becomes median umbilical ligament.

13. **Infants born to mothers treated with ACE inhibitors during pregnancy**–have increased rate of fetal loss, oligohydramnios, hypotension and anuria.

14. **Embryologically, the bladder is composed of two regions**–Trigone and the bladder body.
    - The bladder body is derived from the endoderm-lined vesicourethral canal and the surrounding mesenchyme.
    - Trigone is derived from mesoderm.

15. During the sixth week the cells of the genital ridge invade the mesenchyme in the region of future gonads to form aggregates of supporting cells called the **primitive sex cords**

16. The genital ridge mesenchyme containing the primitive sex cords is divided into the cortical and medullary regions.

Both regions develop in all embryos, but after the 6th week, they pursue different fates in the male and female.

17. The male and female genital structures are virtually identical till the 7th week:

- In males, medullary sex cords become presumptive seminiferous tubules.
- In females, cortical sex cords invest the primordial germ cells and become the ovarian follicles.

18. As the developing Sertoli cells begin their differentiation in response to the SRY, they also secrete a glycoprotein hormone called **Müllerian-inhibiting substance (MIS).**

19. Between the 8th and 12th week, **testosterone** secretion by Leydig cells stimulates the nephric (Wolffian) ducts.

20. Embryology

Paramesonephric (Müllerian) ducts FEMALE	**Mesonephric (Wolffian duct) MALE**
Appendix testis (superior pole of testis)	Appendix epididymis
Prostatic utricle	Paradidymis (Inferior pole of testis)
Fallopian tube	Epoöphoron
Uterus	Paroöphoron
Upper vagina	Gartner's duct cysts

21. Seminal vesicles–Arises from–distal nephric ducts.

Prostate and bulbourethral glands originates from–urogenital sinus.

22. In female embryos

- Primitive sex cords do not contain the Y chromosome.
- Do not elaborate SRY protein, and therefore do not differentiate into Sertoli cells.

- MIS synthesis, Leydig cell differentiation, and androgen production do not occur.
- Mesonephric (Wolffian) ducts degenerate, and the paramesonephric (Müllerian) ducts give rise to the fallopian tubes, uterus, and upper two thirds of the vagina.

23. Paramesonephric ducts

- Ducts begin to fuse in a caudal to cranial direction, forming a tube with a single lumen.
- This tube, called the uterovaginal canal, becomes the superior portion of the vagina and the uterus.
- The unfused, superior portions of the ducts become the fallopian tubes.
- Funnel-shaped superior openings of the ducts become the infundibula.
- Sinovaginal bulbs give rise to the lower third of the vagina.

24.

	Male	**Female**
Urogenital folds	Penile shaft	Labia minora
Genital tubercle	Glans	Clitoris
Labioscrotal folds	Scrotum	Labia majora

25. The formation of the distal glanular urethra may occur by a combination of two separate processes:

- Fusion of urethral folds proximally and the ingrowth of ectodermal cells distally.
- Stratified squamous epithelium of the fossa navicularis results from an ingrowth of surface ectoderm as far proximally as the **valve of Guérin.**
- The **lacuna magna (also known as the sinus of Guérin),** can give symptoms of hematuria and dysuria in some boys and may form as a result of dorsal extension of this ectodermal ingrowth.

26. Prior to gonadal differentiation, the testicle lies near the developing kidney, loosely held in place by two ligamentous structures:

- Dorsal ligament is referred to as the cranial suspensory ligament.
- Ventral ligament later develops into the gubernaculum.

27. **Both gonads descend to pelvic location by the third month,** but the testis descends into the scrotum with the aid of the gubernaculum at about the seventh month

28. **Urine production in the human kidney**–begins around 10 to 12 weeks.

29. **GFR at birth is 10% to 15% of the normal adult value and doubles in first 2 weeks of birth**

30. **The fetus produces hypotonic urine** with high sodium and low potassium content and in large volumes.

31. **Hourly human fetal urine production**–increases from 5 mL/hr at 20 weeks gestation to **50 mL/hr at 40 weeks gestation.**

32. **Serum osmolality**–primary determinant of the normal distribution of water between the ECF and ICF in a 1 : 2 ratio

33. **Proteinuria**

- It is first detected by urinary dipstick testing, which primarily detects albumin
- The colorimetric reaction between albumin and tetra bromophenol blue results in variable shades of green
- Trace indicates 15 mg/dL; 1+, 30 mg/dL; 2+, 100 mg/dL; 3+, 300 mg/dL; and 4+, >2000 mg/dL
- False-positive urine protein levels may be caused by alkaline urine, antiseptic cleanser, radiocontrast agents, or a highly concentrated sample.
- False-negative urine protein levels may be found in very dilute urine.
- Quantification of the proteinuria is best performed from a 24-hour urine collection
- **Protein excretion rate > 4 mg/m^2/hr is abnormal, and >40 mg/m2/hr is nephrotic-range proteinuria**

34. **Most common form of nephrotic syndrome in infants**–Congenital nephrotic syndrome Finnish

(It is an AR disorder with a mutation of the gene coding for nephrin on chromosome 19q13.1).

Most prevalent lesion for NS throughout childhood–Minimal change nephrotic syndrome

(Most children with proteinuria between 1 and 10 years of age who respond to oral corticosteroids have minimal change disease).

Most common cause of acute glomerulonephritis in children–postinfectious glomerulonephritis

35. **Poor prognostic factors**
    - Fetal urine:
        - o **Sodium** >100 mEq/L.
        - o **Chloride** >90 mEq/L.
        - o **Osmolality** is >200 mOsm/L.
        - o High **cystatin C**, is a marker of tubular damage in the fetus.
        - o **Valine concentration** is increased in fetuses with bilateral renal dysplasia and fetal or neonatal death.
        - o **Total protein** >20 mg/dl.
        - o **β_2-microglobulin** >4 mg/L.
    - Increased **amniotic fluid (*N*-acetyl-β-D-glucosaminidase) NAG** has been correlated **with renal impairment of IUGR.**
    - **When fetal urine approaches the character of serum,** irreversible damage have been done to the developing kidney.

36. Every infant **should void within the first 24 hours of life** regardless of gestational age.
    - After the first 2 days of life, **oliguria is generally defined as a urine flow rate <1 mL/kg/hr.**

37. **Polyuria**–any infant or child excreting more than 2000 mL/1.73 m^2 daily urine output should be evaluated further.

    Pollakuria–increase in urine frequency.

38. **By 7 days** in the term infant–**PCr concentration is normally <0.5 mg/dL.**

39. **Predictor of long-term outcome of infants with renal dysplasia**–Estimation of GFR at 6 months of age.
    - Infants with GFR <15 mL/min/1.73 m^2 are at risk for early renal failure

40. **FENa = 100% (UNa × PCr)/(PNa × UCr)**
    - In the older infant or child, <1% is consistent with prerenal oliguria.
    - FENa is increased in renal sodium wasting, adrenal insufficiency, and the SIADH.

41. In RTA "anion gap" is in the normal range (5 to15 mEq/L) and is defined as:

    Anion gap = Na^+ - [Cl^- + HCO^-]

42. **Diagnosis of RTA**

- **Requires the presence of hyperchloremic metabolic acidosis**
- A urine pH <5.5 in the presence of a total CO_2 below normal suggests, **gastrointestinal bicarbonate loss or a Type II RTA.**
- Urine pH >5.5 is consistent with **distal or type I RTA.**
- Elevated serum K in the presence of normal renal function suggests **type IV RTA.**

43. **In children with normal renal function, GFR may fall by 50%** before producing an increase in creatinine concentration

    Most common form of acute kidney injury is prerenal

44. **The only absolute contraindication to peritoneal dialysis (PD) is an inadequate peritoneal cavity**

    Most common complication of PD–peritonitis

    Most common organisms are gram positive (50%), gram negative (20%), and fungal (2.3%).

45. **Investigation to be done in children with nephrolithiasis:**

- Serum levels of electrolytes, calcium, phosphorus, and PTH and thyroid function tests.
- A urinalysis should be performed to screen for glucosuria.
- In addition, the urine amino acid pattern may reveal diffuse aminoaciduria.
- A 24-hour urine collection should be obtained for calculation of creatinine clearance, protein excretion, calcium excretion, and tubular reabsorption of phosphorus.
- USG to evaluate regarding hydronephrosis, nephrocalcinosis or nephrolithiasis that can develop in children with type I RTA.

46. **A urine specific gravity >1.020** generally rules out a serious abnormality of urinary concentration.

47. **Most common cause of hypercalciuria**–in neonates is administration of calciuric drugs, such as furosemide and glucocorticoids.

48. **Most common cause of glucosuria**–in hospitalized infants is IV dextrose at rates exceeding the tubular reabsorptive threshold.

49. **Overhydration of the neonate**

- Opening of a symptomatic patent ductus arteriosus.
- Cerebral intraventricular hemorrhage.

- Necrotizing enterocolitis.

Underhydration of the neonate

- Hypoglycemia.
- Hyperbilirubinemia.
- Hyperosmolality.

50. **Atrial natriuretic peptide (ANP)**
    - Secreted by cardiac myocytes.
    - Increase in GFR.
    - Natriuresis.
    - Diuresis
    - Inhibition of renin and aldosterone release.
    - Vasorelaxation.
    - Increase in vascular permeability.
51. **Renal concentrating capacity** is <1000 mOsm/kg in the first 2 months of life.
    - After perinatal natriuresis, neonates remain in **positive sodium balance** for a number of months, which is necessary for normal growth.
    - The threshold for **renal bicarbonate reabsorption is diminished** in the neonate, and net acid excretion matures by the second month of life.
52. **Mediator of apoptosis**–TGF-β1, FAS, p53, caspases.

    Inhibitor of apoptosis–EGF, IGF-1, HGF, and heparin-bound EGF.
53. **Histologic hallmarks of renal dysplasia is**–the presence of fibromuscular collars around tubular structures, so-called **primitive ducts.**
54. **Expression of renal renin is** increased in the obstructed kidney and decreased in the contralateral one.
55. **The echolucent pyramids** should not be confused for dilated calyces.
    - First become evident at about **20 weeks.**
    - Absence later in gestation is abnormal.
56. Hydronephrosis +increased renal echogenicity = **dysplastic changes** (but this is variable unless there is profound hydronephrosis, often with decreasing amniotic fluid).

57. **The thickness of the parenchyma** in the setting of HDN is important finding **but does not clearly predict decreased function.** Often this thinning is simply due to stretching of the parenchyma around a dilated collecting system.

58. **Findings that is strongly suggestive of reflux**–variation in the degree of hydronephrosis.

59. **Cysts do not communicate** visibly with each other, in contrast to dilated calyces.

    A single upper pole cyst is probably not a cyst but a dilated upper pole.

60. In the absence of testes in the inguinal canals or scrotum, the **diagnosis of a male fetus should not be made.**

    A female fetus with bilateral renal obstruction and BOO suggest–cloacal anomaly

61. **AF** is predominantly a product of fetal urine–after 16 weeks and by **20 or 22 weeks most AF is fetal urine.**

    Oligohydramnios

    - Due to urinary tract obstruction (may become evident only after 18-20 weeks of gestation).
    - Due to abnormal renal development without obstruction (bilateral MCDK or ARPKD).

62. **Late-onset oligohydramnios (>30 weeks)** is usually not associated with pulmonary insufficiency.

63. **Distended bladder and dilated upper tracts**

    - PUV.
    - Bilateral megaureters.
    - Bilateral reflux.

64. **PUV**

    - Dilated posterior urethra and fetal bladder.
    - Perinephric urinomata.
    - Increased renal parenchymal echogenicity, and occasionally a thick-walled bladder.
    - Bilateral hydroureteronephrosis.
    - Oligohydramnios.

65. **Possibility of a ureterocele** is suspected if there is presence of upper pole HDN (or cystic dysplastic upper pole) + dilated ureter that may be traced to the bladder + intravesical, thin-walled cystic structure associated with the base of the bladder.

66. **Ectopic ureter**–Upper pole HDN in the absence of an intravesical cystic structure.

- **Wall thickness of the ectopic ureter is much greater** than that of the ureterocele, as the latter is made up only of attenuated ureteral wall and the ectopic ureter impression includes both the ureter and bladder walls.

67. **USG appearance of an MCDK**–nonreniform structure, with multiple noncommunicating fluid-filled cystic spaces, no central large cyst, and minimal to no recognizable renal parenchyma.

68. **USG appearance of severely HDN kidneys**–presence of a central cystic structure that is medial.

These are usually of similar size and seen to communicate with the central cystic structure.

69. **ARPKD**–characterized by large uniformly echogenic kidneys without recognizable cysts.

70. **Congenital multilocular cystic nephroma**–macrocysts of varied sizes detectable on US.

71. **Bilateral renal agenesis**

- Progressive absence of AF after 16 to 18 weeks.
- Kidneys not detectable and no bladder filling seen.
- Adrenal glands may be visible in their normal position but with a linear appearance, the so-called **lying down adrenal.**
- Classical appearance of Potter's syndrome.

72. **Classical bladder exstrophy**–absence of bladder filling on repeated examinations, low-set umbilical cord, and abnormal-appearing external genitalia.

73. **Congenital mesoblastic nephroma**

- **Most common renal masses in the fetal urinary tract.**
- This benign tumor replaces the entire kidney with a homogeneous round mass.
- It may be associated with polyhydramnios.

- Considered potentially malignant and early postnatal removal is recommended.

74. **The diagnosis of an upper pole renal cyst in a fetus indicates**– presence of a duplication anomaly with hydronephrosis rather than a cyst.
75. **UPJ obstruction–largest single entity producing hydronephrosis,** followed by reflux, valves and megaureter.
76. **When severe bilateral hydronephrosis is present, with a suspicion of BOO, follow-up is needed which includes:**
    - AF volume, renal echogenicity, and the presence of any extrarenal fluid collections.
77. **Indications for in utero urinary decompression**

Indices	**Comment**
Evidence of BOO	Dilated bladder, hydroureteronephrosis
Normal karyotype	By amniocentesis
No systemic anomalies	For example, central nervous system, cardiovascular
Male singleton fetus	
Oligohydramnios	Early onset: <25 weeks
Noncystic kidneys	Cysts are poor prognostic sign
Favorable urinary indices	**Na < 100, Cl < 110, Osm < 210, β2-microglobulin < 10**

78. The technique of fetal intervention for BOO is based upon placement of a double pigtail **vesicoamniotic shunt (Rodeck shunt).**
79. **Postnatal management scheme for hydronephrosis**

Prenatal Findings	**Imaging**	**Timing**	**Possible Diagnoses**	**Surgery**
Mild hydronephrosis	RUS	2 to 3 months	Mild UPJO Mild UVJO Reflux	Unlikely
Moderate to severe hydronephrosis	RUS VCUG	1 to 2 months	Moderate UPJO Moderate UVJO Reflux Valves	Unlikely
Severe unilateral hydronephrosis	RUS VCUG IVP/ MAG3	1 month	UPJO UVJO Reflux Valves (unusual)	Possible

Severe bilateral hydronephrosis	RUS VCUG	<1 week	Reflux Valves Bilat UPJO Bilat UVJO	Probable
Intravesical cystic structure	RUS	<1 month	Ureterocele	Likely

RUS-renal ultrasound,
VCUG-voiding cystourethrogram,
PUJO-pelvicureteric junction obstruction,
VUJO-vesicoureteric junction obstruction,
IVP-intravenous pyelogram.

80. **Megacystis-megaureter association**–massively dilated bladder, HDUN, and bilateral VUR.

    US appearance, both prenatally and postnatally, may mimic that of PUV, yet the bladders in these children are typically **thin walled and smooth.**

81. **With bilateral HUN in the absence of reflux or valves,** consider:
    - Bilateral obstructive megaureters.
    - Evaluate for a neurogenic cause.

82. **The appearance of a protuberant mass in the perineum of a newborn girl should suggest four principal diagnoses:**
    - Most common entity in a newborn is a **periurethral cyst.**
    - Imperforate hymen with resulting hydrocolpos.
    - Prolapse of an ectopic ureterocele.
    - Urethral prolapse.

83. **Abdominal mass in newborn**–most common site of origin is Urinary tract (>60%), with HDN and MCDK being the most frequent.
    - **Most common non-genitourinary cause of abdominal mass in newborns is**–neuroblastoma.

84. **Renal vein thrombosis (RVT)**
    - Neonate with enlarged kidneys, hematuria, anemia and thrombocytopenia, with a history of a prolonged delivery and prematurity.
    - 20% of infants with gross hematuria are found to have RVT.
    - 20% of neonates with RVT have bilateral involvement.

- Etiology is impaired RBF in neonate with normally low BP, polycythemia, and dehydration, including adrenal hyperplasia and salt wasting.
- Diagnosis is by USG, in which an enlarged kidney is seen and the thrombus may be visualized directly.

85. Adrenal hemorrhage

- Occur in about 1% to 2% of healthy infants.
- Predisposing factors include prolonged labor, birth trauma, and large birth weight.
- Anemia, shock and an abdominal mass. Gross hematuria is unusual.
- USG is the most efficient diagnostic measure revealing echogenic suprarenal mass.
- Peripheral **eggshell calcifications** in contrast to stippled calcifications of neuroblastoma.

86. Renal artery thrombosis

- Hypertension and hematuria in a neonate.
- **Most common cause**–Umbilical artery catheterization.
- Associated with renal insufficiency, proteinuria and CHF.
- Thrombotic involvement of the aorta may be present.
- USG reveals the diagnosis and the extent of the thrombus.
- Unilateral involvement–expectant management, although thrombolytic therapy may be appropriate.
- Occasionally requires removal of a nonfunctional kidney.

87. Emergent (as soon as possible) attention is required in:

- Trauma.
- Newborns with bilateral HDN or a solitary kidney.
- Newborns with gross hematuria, urinary tract infections.
- Newborns with ambiguous genitalia, bladder or cloacal exstrophy, PUV, prune-belly syndrome, spina bifida.
- Children with acute abdominal or scrotal pain.
- Boys with priapism.

88. Patau's syndrome–trisomy 13-HSK, HDN, UDT.

- **Edwards' syndrome**–trisomy 18-HDN, micro penis.

- **Down syndrome**–trisomy 21- micro penis.
- **Tuner's syndrome**–anomalies of renal malrotation, cooarctation of aorta and lymphedema.

89. **Most common malignant abdominal tumor in infants**–neuroblastoma, followed by Wilms' tumor.
90. First-line test in suspected **occult spinal dysraphism**. Spinal ultrasound and optimal timing is before **6 months of age.**
91. Renal scintigraphy scans using **gallium-67** were more sensitive than DMSA scans in the diagnosis of acute pyelonephritis, especially in differentiating **new lesions** from old ones.
92. **Temperature**
    - Lower body temperatures in the early morning and temperatures approximately 1°C higher in the later afternoon or early evening.
    - Fever with temperatures <39°C (102.2°F) in healthy children do not require treatment.
93. A child with **acute scrotal pain must be presumed to have spermatic cord torsion** regardless of age until proven otherwise.

    It is associated with –scrotal wall swelling, erythema, or superior displacement of the testis.
94. **"Silk glove" sign** suggestive of a **thickened patent processus vaginalis** may be present if a hernia is intermittent.
95. **In the infant with a possible intersex condition:**
    - **Symmetrical gonadal examination** (gonads palpable on each side or impalpable on both sides) suggests a global disorder such as CAH or androgen insensitivity.
    - **Asymmetry in the gonadal examination** suggests a localized problem such as mixed gonadal dysgenesis or true hermaphroditism.
96. **Hydrocele in infant:**
    - In the absence of volume changes within the hydrocele, the processus vaginalis is usually not patent and the **newborn hydrocele resolves <1 year** without surgery.
    - Persistence of a hydrocele beyond >1 year even in the absence of volume changes usually indicates a **patent processus vaginalis and is an indication for surgical ligation** of the processus vaginalis.

97. In the absence of balanitis or UTI, the **prepuce should not be retracted** but allowed to separate naturally till 4 years of age.

98. **Micropenis**

- If the penis in a term infant is < 1.9 cm.
- Karyotype should be performed.
- Hypothalamic-pituitary-testicular axis should be assayed.

99. **An "atypical" presacral dimple may indicate spina bifida or cord tethering if:**

- Dimple is off center.
- >2.5 cm from the anal verge at birth.
- Deeper than 0.5 cm.
- **Skin markers** to suggest occult spinal abnormalities.
- Subcutaneous lipomas, dermal sinuses, tails and localized hypertrichosis.

100. **Pyuria** >5 WBC/ HPF for girls and > 3WBC/HPF for boys (adults >5 WBC/HPF in females and in males any WBC/HPF is significant).

101. **Microscopic hematuria**–5 RBC/HPF in at least two of three urine analysis over 2 to 3 weeks (adults >3 RBC/HPF is significant).

- **An absence of RBC in the urine with a positive dipstick**–hemoglobinuria or myoglobinuria.

102. **Normal urine protein excretion** in children–<4 mg/m^2/hr, or <100 mg/m^2/day.

- **Children > 2 years–normal protein (mg/dl)/creatinine (mg/dl)** ratio- <0.2.

103. **Hypercalciuria** urinary calcium excretion >4 mg/kg/day while the child is well and ingesting a normal diet.

104. **Hemolytic-uremic syndrome (HUS)**

- **Triad** (1) hemolytic microangiopathic anemia (2) thrombocytopenia (3) renal insufficiency.
- In children, HUS may be the **typical form**, associated with diarrhea, or an atypical form.
- Severity of renal involvement is not related to the severity of anemia, it does appear to be related to the **severity of the gastrointestinal prodrome.**

- **E. coli (O157:H7)** produce a verotoxin that binds to enterocytes and gains access to the microcirculation.
- E. coli O157:H7 should be isolated from stool of affected children, and recovery is better when samples are obtained within 6 days from onset of diarrhea.

105. Fanconi syndrome

- Interfere with energy production by the **proximal tubule** may result in generalized dysfunction.
- Polyuria and signs of dehydration.
- Rickets (hypophosphatemia, calcitriol deficiency), muscle weakness (hypokalemia), growth failure (acidosis), or constipation (dehydration).
- Hypouricemia.

106. Bartter's syndrome

- **Hypokalemia, metabolic alkalosis**, polyuria and growth failure.
- Hypokalemia is common to both Bartter's syndrome and RTA; however, Bartter's syndrome is characterized by alkalosis.
- Hypercalciuria, may result in nephrocalcinosis.

107. Gitelman's syndrome

- Results from mutations in the distal tubule and resembles effects of thiazide-like diuretics.
- Hypocalciuria (in contrast with Batter's syndrome which has hypercalciuria)

108. Nephrogenic diabetes insipidus

- Polyuria, excessive thirst and **hypernatremia**.
- **Inability to concentrate the urine** due to a defect in the renal tubular response to vasopressin.
- The most common form is **X-linked recessive** mutation of the vasopressin receptor.
- **Diagnosis**–insufficiently concentrated urine (UOsm < 300) in the presence of hypernatremic dehydration.
- **Treatment**–combination of hydrochlorothiazide and amiloride.

109. Estimation of the GFR using the **Schwartz Formula**

Age <18 mo	Height (cm) × 0.45/creatinine (mg/dl)
Age >18 mo and weight <70 kg	Height (cm) × 0.55/creatinine (mg/dl)
Male with weight >70 kg	Height (cm) × 0.70/creatinine (mg/dl)

110. Most common cause of renal insufficiency in children–obstructive uropathy.

111. Risk of UTI:

- **Only during the first year of life**–males > females.
- **Rest of life**–females > males
- Uncircumcised boys > circumcised boys.

112. Least to most reliable for UTI diagnosis–(1) "bagged specimen"; (2) midstream void; (3) catheterization; or (4) suprapubic bladder aspirate.

113. The most reliable urinary specimen for culture–obtained by suprapubic bladder aspiration.

114. Combination of positive leukocyte esterase and nitrite testing and microscopic confirmation of bacteria–100% sensitivity for detection of UTI.

- When all are negative the negative predictive value approaches 100%.

115. The ideal prophylactic agent:

- Low serum.
- High urinary concentrations.
- Have minimal effect on the normal fecal flora.
- Easily administered and tolerated.
- Cost-effective.

116. Main advantage of radionuclide VCUG

- Lower radiation exposure.
- More sensitive for reflux detection.
- Most useful for periodic reflux reevaluation or for screening siblings who have a low risk of reflux.

Limitations of radionuclide VCUG

- Should not be used to evaluate first infections in infants or young boys in whom risk of genitourinary abnormality is high and urethral visualization important.
- Poor spatial resolution.

117. The presence of a **"spinning top urethra"** in a school-aged girl may be an important indicator of dysfunctional voiding

118. **XGPN**–The "**bear paw" sign** with areas of low-attenuation nonenhancing dilated calyces and abscesses within areas of high-attenuation enhancing renal parenchyma may be present.

119. **Bilateral Renal Agenesis (BRA)**

- Male > Female.
- Structures of Wolffian duct origin (vas deferens, seminal vesicle, and epididymis) are normally formed.
- Injury occurred at the time when ureteral bud is formed (the 5th or 6th week of gestation).
- Most of the children who are born alive **do not survive beyond 48 hours.**
- Adrenal glands are usually normally positioned.
- Potter facies and the presence of oligohydramnios are pathognomonic.
- Fetus fails to produce proline, which is needed for collagen formation in the bronchiolar tree. The kidney is the primary source of proline. Thus, **pulmonary hypoplasia result from the absence of renal parenchyma** and not from diminished amniotic fluid.

120. **Unilateral Renal Agenesis (URA)**

- URA > BRA.
- Males >female.
- Left > right.
- The fault lies in ureteral bud.
- The ipsilateral ureter is completely absent in >50%.
- **Ipsilateral adrenal glandflattened or lying down.**
- Reproductive organ abnormalities–F> M occurs in 25% to 50%
- Males with absence of the vas deferens, 80% were found to have URA.

- Other systems involved–CVS (30%), GIT (25%), and musculoskeletal (14%) systems.
- URA patients are not increasingly susceptible to other diseases.

121. Supernumerary kidney

- Accessory organ with its own collecting system, blood supply and distinct encapsulated parenchymal mass.
- Ipsilateral and contralateral kidneys are normal.

122. Renal ectopia

- Left > right.
- Ectopic kidney is usually smaller, and it may not conform to the usual reniform shape.
- The renal pelvis is usually anterior (instead of medial) to the parenchyma because the kidney has incompletely rotated.
- 56% of ectopic kidneys have a HDN collecting system due to:
  - o **PUJO–35% (Most common).**
  - o VUJO–15%.
  - o Grade 3 reflux–25%.
  - o Malrotation–25%.
- The length of the ureter is according to the position of the kidney. **It is rarely redundant.**
- (In contrast ptotic kidney, in which the ureter has achieved its full length before the kidney drops so that ureter becomes redundant).
- **Rarely, the adrenal gland is absent or abnormally positioned.**
- Most ectopic kidneys are clinically asymptomatic.

123. Thoracic kidney

- The kidney usually lies in the posterolateral aspect of the diaphragm in the foramen of Bochdalek.
- The diaphragm at this point thin out and **kidney is not within the pleural space.**
- **The ureter is elongated** to accommodate the excessive distance to the bladder.
- **Ureter never enters ectopically into the bladder or other pelvic sites.**

124. Renal fusion

- **Most common form of renal fusion**–Horseshoe kidney (HSK).

- Crossed ectopia–kidney is located on the side opposite from which its ureter inserts into the bladder.
- Males > females.
- **Left-to-right ectopia** is seen three times more frequently than right-to-left ectopia.
- **Most common variety**–unilaterally fused kidney with inferior ectopia.
- Least common variety–fusion with superior ectopia.
- Normal trigone.

125. HSK

- Incidence 0.25%
- Abnormality occurs between the 4th and 6th week of gestation, after the ureteral bud has entered the renal blastema.
- Pelvis and ureters of HSK are anteriorly placed, crossing ventrally to the isthmus.
- **Inferior mesenteric artery** prevents full ascent by obstructing the movement of the isthmus.
- In 95% of patients, the **kidneys join at the lower pole**.
- It is located adjacent to the **L3 or L4 vertebra** just below the origin of the inferior mesenteric artery from the aorta.
- Isthmus is usually bulky with its own blood supply
- Calyces point posteriorly.
- UPJ obstruction causing significant hydronephrosis and occurs in 30%.

126. Anomalies of rotation

- It is frequently observed in patients with Turner's syndrome.
- The kidney and renal pelvis normally rotate 90 degrees ventromedially during ascent.

127. Multiple renal arteries–any kidney supplied by more than one vessel.

- **Anomalous vessels or aberrant vessels**–arteries that originate from vessels other than the aorta or main renal artery.
- **Accessory vessels**–two or more arterial branches supplying the same renal segment.

- **The lower renal segment, is often supplied by an accessory vessel**

128. **On the basis of vascular supply, the renal parenchyma is divided into five segments**–apical, upper, middle, lower and posterior.
    - The main renal artery divides initially into an anterior and posterior branch.
    - The anterior branch supplies the upper, middle and lower segments of the kidney.
    - The posterior branch invariably nourishes the posterior and lower segments.
    - The vessel to the **apical segment has the greatest variation** in origin.
129. **Endourologic incision of an obstructed UPJ** should be done laterally and posteriorly instead of anteriorly to avoid injury to this vessel.
130. **Calyceal diverticulum**
    - Is a cystic cavity within the kidney that is lined by transitional epithelium
    - Communicates with a calyx or less commonly with the renal pelvis through a narrow isthmus
    - Small diverticula are usually asymptomatic
    - The diagnosis is best made by CT or MR urography.
131. **Hydrocalycosis**–cystic dilation of a major calyx with a demonstrable connection to the renal pelvis; it is lined by transitional epithelium.
132. **Fraley syndrome**–dilation of the upper calyx due to obstruction of the upper infundibulum by vessels or stenosis.
133. **Megacalycosis**
    - Nonobstructive enlargement of calyces resulting from malformation of the renal papillae.
    - The calyces are dilated and malformed and may be increased in number.
    - The renal pelvis is not dilated, nor is its wall thickened, and the UPJ is normally funnelled without evidence of obstruction.
    - Congenital.

- M : F–6:1 and has been found only in white patients.
- Bilateral disease has been seen almost exclusively in males.
- Segmental unilateral involvement occurs only in females.

134. Pseudotumor (hypertrophied column of Bertin)

- Localized mass, usually situated between the infundibula of the upper and middle calyceal groups.
- The column may be sufficiently large to compress and deform the adjacent pelvis and calyces, suggesting like a mass on IVU.

135. TSC1, is located on chromosome 2 and **TSC2,** on chromosome 16.

PKD1 gene is located on chromosome 16, and **PKD2** gene is on chromosome 4.

136. Ask-Upmark kidney (segmental hypolplasia)

- Most patients are >10 years of age.
- Associated with severe hypertension, headaches, and hypertensive encephalopathy.
- Proteinuria and some degree of renal insufficiency may be present if bilateral.
- Kidney is smaller than normal.
- Partial or total nephrectomy may control the hypertension.

137. Most common site in the body for cysts–kidney.

Ducts dilated to four times their normal diameter (i.e., 200 μm) are called cysts.

138. Cysts with hyperplastic lining, sometimes with nodules of hyperplasia or polyps that project into the cyst lumen–ADPKD, tuberous sclerosis, VHL disease and ARCD.

139. Ectatic collecting ducts seen in–ARPKD and medullary sponge kidney.

140. Multicystic dysplasia and benign multilocular cyst, is an exception in that it arises before formation of the nephron.

141. Cystic disease of kidney

Genetical

- **ARPKD.**
- **ADPKD.**

- **Juvenile nephronophthisis/medullary cystic disease complex:**
  - o Juvenile nephronophthisis (autosomal recessive).
  - o Medullary cystic disease (autosomal dominant).
- **Congenital nephrosis** (familial nephrotic syndrome) (autosomal recessive).
- **Familial hypoplastic glomerulocystic disease** (autosomal dominant).
- **Tuberous sclerosis** (TS), **von Hippel-Lindau disease** (VHL).

142. Multicystic–dysplastic entity.

Polycystic–number of separate entities, mostly inherited, all without dysplasia and all with nephrons throughout the kidney.

143. Presentation of cysts

- **ARPKD**–utero to the age of 20 years.
- **ADPKD**–utero to autopsy.
- **Tuberous sclerosis**–utero to <30 years.
- **VHL**–almost always by the age of 30.
- **Bilateral simple cysts**–> 35 years.
- **ARCD** after ESRD develops.

144. Sonographic differential diagnosis of a newborn with bilateral, large, cystic kidneys.

Homogenous, hyperechogenic kidneys without macrocysts:

- ARPKD.
- Sporadic glomerulocystic kidney disease.
- Contrast nephropathy.
- Renal vein thrombosis.

With diffuse macrocysts:

- ADPKD.
- Sporadic glomerulocystic kidney disease.
- Tuberous sclerosis.

145. ARPKD

- Only mutations of a single gene, named PKHD1, located on chromosome 6 (6p12), are responsible for the disease. The gene produces a protein called fibrocystin

- 50% of affected newborns die in the first few hours or days of life.
- All patients are bilateral and have congenital hepatic fibrosis
- Younger the patient at presentation with ARPKD, the milder the liver disease.
- Younger the patient with congenital hepatic fibrosis, the milder the renal cystic disease.
- Very enlarged, homogeneously hyperechogenic kidneys.
- IVU with delayed films may show functioning kidneys with characteristic radial or medullary streaking **(sunburst pattern)** caused by dilated collecting tubules filled with contrast medium.

146. ADPKD

- 100% penetrance (AD)
- 50% of an affected individual's offspring will likewise be affected
- Genes involved are PKD1 (chromosome 16) PKD2 (chromosome 4) and PKD3
- Most cases are identified when the patients are between **30-50 years of age.**
- **Associated anomalies**–cysts of the liver, pancreas, spleen and lungs; aneurysms of the circle of Willis (berry aneurysms); colonic diverticula; aortic aneurysms and mitral valve prolapse.
- **Hepatic cysts,** usually appear later than renal cysts. These cysts are more likely to be found in adults than in children and more frequently in females.
- **Intracranial hemorrhages** in patients with ADPKD represent.
  - o Subarachnoid bleeding secondary to berry aneurysms.
  - o Rupture of intracerebral arteries.
- Usually have **bilateral cysts**. However, the disease can manifest asymmetrically, with cysts on only one side at first or with a unilateral renal mass.
- Incidence of **RCC in patients with ADPKD is no higher** than that in the general population.
- Pain (flank and/or abdominal) is the most common presenting symptom in adults.
  - o Mass effect (cysts impinging on abdominal wall or neighboring organs),

- o Bleeding into the cysts,
- o Urinary tract infection (including infected cysts)
- o Nephrolithiasis

147. Juvenile Nephronophthisis/Medullary Cystic Disease Complex

	Juvenile Nephronophthisis	**Medullary Cystic Disease**
Inheritance	AR	AD
ESRD	By age 13 years	20–40 years
Medullary cysts	Develop after renal failure	May develop before onset of renal failure
Tubular basement membrane	Thickened	May not be thickened
Symptoms	Polyuria, polydipsia, anemia, growth retardation (>2 years) Hematuria and usually appear after	Polyuria, polydipsia, anemia, proteinuria (symptoms patient is fully grown)

148. Congenital nephrosis (CNF)–enormously enlarged and edematous placenta, which accounts for >25% of the birth weight.

Diffuse mesangial stenosis (DMS)–associated with Drash syndrome (nephrotic syndrome, Wilms' tumor, and male pseudohermaphroditism).

- CNF and DMS–both characterized by normal-sized kidneys, initially with pronounced proximal tubular dilatation.
- DMS–glomeruli have an accumulation of PAS–positive and silver phosphate-staining mesangial fibrils.

149. Tuberous sclerosis complex

- **Triad**–epilepsy (80%), mental retardation (60%), and adenoma sebaceum (75%).
- Adenoma sebaceum are flesh-colored papules of angiofibroma and are prevalent in the malar area.
- An earlier skin lesion that is a white papule in the shape of an "ash leaf".
- The hallmark lesion of the CNS is a superficial cortical hamartoma of the cerebrum.
- **Contiguous gene syndrome (i.e., defects in both *TSC2* and *PKD1*).**

- The renal cysts are of a unique histologic type in that they have a lining of hypertrophic, **hyperplastic eosinophilic cells.**
- Renal cysts (20%), renal angiomyolipoma (40% to 80%), and **RCC (2%).**

150. VHL disease

Autosomal dominant

- Cerebellar and retinal hemangioblastomas; cysts of the pancreas, kidney, and epididymis; epididymal cystadenoma; pheochromocytoma; and clear cell RCC.
- The gene associated with the transmission of VHL is located on **chromosome 3.**
- Renal cysts and tumors often are multiple and bilateral.
- **Renal cysts, most common and often earliest manifestation,** are seen in 76% of patients.
- Pheochromocytoma occurs in 10% to 17% of affected individuals.
- **Most common cause of death**–RCC.

151. Multicystic dysplastic kidney (MCDK)

- The kidney does not have a reniform configuration, and no calyceal drainage system.
- Kidney has the appearance of "**a bunch of grapes**", with little stroma between the cysts.
- **Most common type of renal cystic disease,** and it is one of **the most common causes of an abdominal mass in infants.**
- No clear indication for removal of the kidney unless an increased amount of solid tissue is identified.
- **Haphazard distribution of cysts** of various sizes without a larger central or medial cyst and without visible communications between the cysts.
- Hydronephrotic kidneys show some function on a **DMSA scan,** whereas renal uptake is seldom seen in MCDK.

152. Benign multilocular cyst (cystic nephroma)

- Majority of patients present <4 years or >30 years.
- The patient is twice as likely to be **male if <4 years** and eight times as likely to be **female if >30 years.**

- In children, an asymptomatic flank mass is the most common finding.
- Adults present with either a flank mass, abdominal pain, or hematuria.
- Bleeding is secondary to herniation of the cyst through the transitional epithelium into the renal pelvis.
- The only way to determine the diagnosis of a multilocular cystic lesion, is by surgical excision.
- The treatment for multilocular cystic lesions in most children is nephrectomy.

153. **Diverticula** has linings of transitional epithelium, whereas **simple cysts** is lined by a single layer of flattened or cuboidal epithelium.

154. **Benign simple cyst on sonography**

- Sharply defined, thin distinct smooth wall.
- Spherical or oval with no internal echoes.
- Good transmission of sound waves with acoustic enhancement behind the cyst.

When these criteria are not met, CT with contrast medium enhancement needs to be made.

155. **Bosniak's Classification of Simple and Complex Cysts**

Category I Good through-transmission (i.e., acoustic enhancement) No echoes within the cyst

Sharply, marginated smooth wall

Requires no surgery.

Category II Benign with some radiologic concerns including septation, minimal calcification and high density

Requires no surgery.

Category II F Calcification in wall of cyst may even be thicker and more nodular than in category II

Septa have minimal enhancement, especially those with calcium

Requires no surgery.

Category III More complicated having more calcification, more prominent septation of a thicker wall than a category II lesion

More likely to be benign than malignant

Requires surgical exploration and/or removal.

Category IV Clearly a malignant lesion with large cystic components, irregular margins; solid vascular elements

Requires surgical removal.

155. The CT criteria for a simple cyst:

1. Sharp, thin, distinct, smooth walls and margins.
2. Spherical or ovoid shape.
3. Homogeneous content.
4. The density ranges from -10 to +20 HU, similar to the density of water, and no enhancement should occur after the intravenous injection of contrast medium.

156. Hyperdense cyst (i.e., between 20 and 90 HU) it still likely to be a simple cyst if no enhancement occurs and other criteria of CT and sonography are met.

157. Unilateral renal cystic disease

- Large renal cysts of varying size appearing side by side, often numerous at one pole.
- Absence of cyst development in the contralateral kidney.
- Family members should not be affected with cystic disease.
- Considered as a variation of the presentation of simple cysts.

158. Medullary sponge kidney

- Dilatation of the distal portion of the collecting ducts with numerous associated cysts and diverticula.
- On IVU have the appearance of the **bristles on a brush.**
- At times the collecting ducts are more ectatic and are filled with calcifications, giving an appearance suggestive of a **"bouquet of flowers".**
- **The most common presentation is renal colic,** followed by UTI and gross hematuria.
- The urographic features of the disorder are as follows:
  1. Enlarged kidneys, sometimes with calcification, particularly in the papillae.
  2. Elongated papillary tubules or cavities that fill with contrast medium.
  3. Papillary contrast blush and persistent medullary opacification.

- **Thiazides** are effective for lowering hypercalciuria and limiting stone formation.
- If thiazides cannot be used, **inorganic phosphates** may be appropriate.

159. When RCC develops in ESRD

- 80% of the time RCC in ESRD patients is associated with ARCD.
    1. Age at occurrence averages **5 years younger** in patients with ESRD.
    2. **M: F ratio is significantly greater** in ESRD patients with RCC than in the general population with RCC (7:1 and 2:1, respectively).
    3. **Incidence of RCC in ESRD is 3 to 6 times** that of the general population.
- ARCD is associated with CRF and most often seen in patients on long-term hemodialysis.
- It consists of hyperplastic renal cysts and frequently adenomas; either can progress to RCC.
- The cysts usually regress with transplantation.
- If RCC develops, it mostly does so <10 years of dialysis.

160. The terms **peripelvic and parapelvic generally describe cysts around the renal pelvis or renal sinus.**

161. The term **renal sinus cyst** is be reserved for all other cysts that are not derived from the renal parenchyma but rather from the other structures of the sinus, such as arteries, lymphatics, and fat.

- The predominant type of renal sinus cyst appears to be one derived from the **lymphatics**. Most often these cysts are **multiple, and often they are bilateral.**

162. The total requirements for maintenance fluids can be calculated using the Holliday-Segar formula

Children receive either 5% dextrose (D5) 1/ 4 normal saline (NS) + 20 mEq/L potassium chloride (KCl) or D5 1/2 NS + 20 mEq/L KCl.

163. The American Society of Anesthesiologists (ASA) has proposed practice guidelines that may be followed when determining NPO restrictions in children

- Fasting from clear fluids for 2 hours prior to anesthesia.

- Fasting from breast milk for 4 hours and formula feeds for 6 hours is recommended.
- Fasting period for solid food is 6 hours for regular meals and 8 hours for fat-containing meals.

164. Pediatric pain scale

Scale	Type	Age
PIPP	Behavioral and physiologic parameters Procedural pain	Preterm and term infants
CRIES	Behavioral and physiologic parameters Postoperative pain	32-60 weeks
FLACC	Behavioral parameters	<3 years
FACES	Self report	3-12 years
VAS	Self report	>7 years

165. Surgical antimicrobial prophylaxis is recommended for

- All surgery in neonates <72 hours of age because of possible exposure to maternal pathogens and, particularly, compromised immunologic capacity
- Major class II surgery
- All class III and IV surgical procedures

166. Most common cause of significant dilation of the collecting system in the fetal kidney–UPJ obstruction (far exceeding the incidence of MCKD).

167. "Ostling's folds" are now considered folds that are not obstructive and disappear with a person's linear growth.

168. Most common cause of extrinsic UPJ obstruction–an aberrant, accessory, or early-branching lower pole vessel.

- These vessels pass anteriorly to the UPJ and contribute to mechanical obstruction.

169. UPJ obstruction may also be seen with severe VUR

- These conditions coexist in 10% of cases.
- The ureter elongates and develops a tortuous course.
- A kink may develop in the UPJ area, a point of relative fixation, and may cause obstruction secondarily.

- **Obstructive lesion needs to be corrected initially,** even though the VUR contributed to the initial problem.

170. In UPJ obstruction most common anomaly encountered in the opposite kidney–UPJ obstruction. (Renal dysplasia and MCDK is the next most common observed contralateral lesions).

171. To improve diagnostic accuracy of ultrasonography in UPJO.

- **Renal parenchyma-pelvicaliceal**–A ratio of <1.6 correlates well with an obstructive process and need for pyeloplasty, whereas patients with a ratio >1.6 can be safely observed.
- **Resistive index (RI) values**–were much higher in the kidneys that had an obstructive pattern on diuretic renography ($RI \geq 0.75$).

172. Parenchymal maturation, occurs at 3 months of age.

173. There is no correct time to give a diuretic.

- Some prefer the diuretic prior to tracer (usually 15 minutes, F -15), some with the tracer (times 0 or 2 to 3 minutes, F 0), and other give the diuretic when the renal pelvis is full of tracer (15 to 20 minutes, F +20).

174. Role of MRI urography is in defining urinary tract anatomy, calculate differential renal function, and assess urinary tract obstruction.

- In comparison with USG and nuclear renography, dynamic contrast enhanced MRI is superior to assess urinary tract obstruction.

175. The Davis intubated ureterotomy

- Depends on secondary epithelialization from the incised ureter.
- Indication–when multiple or extensive strictures of the proximal ureter are present but cannot be bridged by a pelvic flap.
- Its use requires maintenance of ureteral continuity on at least one side and the presence of an indwelling ureteral stent for **6 weeks (time needed for full circumferential regeneration of all layers of the ureter).**

176. Ureterocalicostomy is performed when there is:

- Extensive proximal ureteral strictures.
- Intrarenal pelvis.
- Diminished pelvis that prevented the performance of a tension-free anastomosis.

177. Ureterocalicostomy, key points include:

- Amputating the lower pole of the kidney.
- Preserving all periureteral tissue and blood supply.
- Creating a widely spatulated tension-free, mucosa-to-mucosa anastomosis.
- Adequate internal stenting.
- Perioperative fat can be placed around the anastomosis, but closing the lower pole capsule over the renal parenchyma should be avoided.

178. The **retroperitoneal lateral approach** provides the advantage of dealing with most situations requiring a **pyeloplasty**.

- **Only indications for performing pyeloplasty through transperitoneal approach are in the HSK and the ectopic kidney.**

179. Acucise balloon is inflated across the UPJ narrowing for treatment of PUJO.

180. Antegrade endopyelotomy requires access to the kidney by a midpole posterior calix.

181. A duplex kidney–two separate pelvicalyceal systems.

- **Bifid system**–if ureters join at the level of the UPJ.
- **Bifid ureters**–if the ureters join more distally but are still proximal to the bladder level.
- **Double ureters**–if ureters that drain their respective poles and empty separately into the genitourinary tract.

182. A "simple ureterocele" lies completely within the bladder.

- **A "ectopic" ureterocele**–those that extended to the bladder neck or distally to the urethra.
- **A stenotic ureterocele**–narrowed or pinpoint opening and is found inside the bladder.
- **Sphincteric**–if ureterocele has an orifice distal to the bladder neck.
- **A cecoureterocele**–intravesical orifice and a submucosal extension that dips into the urethra.

183. In the male, the embryologic equivalents of the mesonephric duct are the epididymis, vas deferens, seminal vesicles and prostate.

In the female, the mesonephric duct proximal to the ureteric bud becomes the epoöphoron, paroöphoron and Gartner's duct.

184. **An ectopic ureter can drain into any of these female structures**–fallopian tube, uterus, upper vagina or vestibule.

185. **In males, the posterior urethra is the most common site** of termination of an ectopic ureter. Drainage into seminal vesicle is three times more often than the ejaculatory duct and vas deferens combined.

   In the female, the urethra and vestibule are the most common sites.

186. **Of all ectopic orifices,** 80% are associated with a duplicated collecting system.

   In females, more than 80% are duplicated, but in males, most ectopic ureters drain single systems.

187. Continuous incontinence in a girl with an otherwise normal voiding pattern after toilet training is the **classic symptom of an ectopic ureteral orifice.**

188. **Ureterocele**

   - Occur most frequently in females (4:1 ratio) and almost exclusively in whites.
   - 10% are bilateral.
   - 80% of all ureteroceles arise from the upper poles of duplicated systems.

189. **Ureterocele**–IVU often demonstrates the **characteristic cobra-head (or spring-onion)** deformity, an area of increased density similar to the head of a cobra with a halo or less dense shadow around it.

190. **Ureterocele incision is recommended in** all neonates as well as in older children with either an.

   - Intravesical ureterocele.
   - Ureterocele associated with a functioning upper pole.
   - Single-system ureterocele.

191. **Preferred method of incising the ureterocele**–a transverse incision through the full thickness of the ureterocele wall using the cutting current.

Making the incision as distally on the ureterocele and as close to the bladder floor as possible lessens the chance of postoperative reflux into the ureterocele.

192. Three areas of the ureter are particularly liable to ureteral stenosis:

- In order of decreasing frequency, UPJO, the distal ureter just above the extravesical junction, and rarely, the mid ureter at the pelvic brim.

193. Trifid ureter–most commonly all three ureters unite and drain through a single orifice.

194. Paquin's dissections of the UVJ in children suggest.

- 5:1 ratio of tunnel length to ureteral diameter in nonrefluxing junctions.
- 1.4:1 ratio in refluxing UVJs.

195. International Classification of VUR

Grade	Description
I	Into a nondilated ureter
II	Into the pelvis and calyces without dilatation
III	Mild to moderate dilatation of the ureter, renal pelvis, and calyces with minimal blunting of the fornices
IV	Moderate ureteral tortuosity and dilatation of the pelvis and calyces
V	Gross dilatation of the ureter, pelvis and calyces; loss of papillary impressions; and ureteral tortuosity

196. Radiographic investigation for VUR has generally been directed to:

- Children younger than 5 years.
- Children with a febrile UTI.
- Male with a UTI regardless of age or fever, unless sexually active.

197. DMSA scanning provided 98% sensitivity and 92% specificity for **scar detection.**

198. Natural history

1. Spontaneous resolution of reflux is very common.
2. High-grade reflux is less likely to resolve spontaneously.
3. Sterile reflux is benign.

4. Extended use of prophylactic antibiotics is benign.
5. The success rate with surgical correction is very high.

199. Surgical approach for reflux management

- **Intravesical**
  - o **Suprahiatal**
    - – Politano-Leadbetter Technique.
  - o **Infrahiatal**
    - – Cohen Cross-Trigonal Technique

      (Suited for small bladders or thick-walled bladders (PUV or neuropathic). **Procedure of choice** in conjunction with bladder neck reconstructive–procedures because the superior displacement of the ureters provides room for adequate elongation of the bladder neck).
    - – Glenn Anderson.
- **Extravesical**
  - o Lich and Gregoir.
- **STING technique (subureteric Teflon injection)**
  - o For endoscopic correction of reflux.
- **Deflux** is currently the preferred agent for endoscopic correction.

200. Agents used for Endoscopic Correction of Vesicoureteral Reflux

Nonautologous Materials
Polytetrafluoroethylene (PTFE) Cross-linked bovine collagen Polydimethylsiloxane Dextranomer hyaluronic copolymer (Deflux)
Autologous Materials
Chondrocytes Fat Collagen Muscle

201. Recommendations for the management of vesicoureteric reflux in childhood: (EAU Guidelines 2012)

- Regardless of the grade of reflux or presence of renal scars, all patients diagnosed within the first year of life should be treated initially with antibiotic prophylaxis.

- Parenteral antibiotic treatment should be initiated for febrile infections.
- Definitive surgical or endoscopic correction is preferred treatment in patients with frequent infections.
- Surgical correction should be considered in patients with persistent high-grade reflux (grades IV/V).
- The outcome of open surgical correction is better than endoscopic correction for higher grades of reflux, whereas satisfactory results can be achieved by endoscopic injection for lower grades.

202. Megaureter management

- **Plication or infolding (Kalicinski and Starr)** is useful for a moderately dilated ureter. However, tissue bulk poses a problem with an extremely large ureter.
- Plication of ureters >**1.75 cm in diameter** has been associated with more complications.
- **Excisional tapering** is preferred for a more severely dilated ureter or a ureter that is markedly thickenened (Hendren).

203. Prune belly syndrome (PBS)

- 95% occurring in males (5% in females).
- Renal dysplasia.
- The ureters are typically dilated, tortuous and redundant.
- VUR present in 75% of children.
- The bladder appears massively enlarged with a pseudodiverticulum at the urachus.
- On voiding, the bladder neck opens widely into a dilated prostatic urethra.
- 50% void spontaneously with normal voiding pressures, normal flow rates and low PVR.
- The vas and seminal vesicles are often atretic, although either may be dilated or thickened.
- **Bilateral intra-abdominal testes** lying over the iliac vessels are the most typical findings.
- **Transabdominal bilateral orchidopexy at about 6 months** of age is currently considered the approach of choice.
- Uneven involvement with the medial and inferior **abdominal muscle typically most deficient.**

204. **Megacystis-megaureter syndrome**

It is a nonobstructive condition in contrast to PUV which is an obstructive lesion

Voiding studies will demonstrate an open posterior urethra and differentiates megacystis-megaureter from PUV or PBS.

205. **The single most important determinant of survival** in PBS is usually the severity of the urinary tract anomaly, in particular, the degree of renal dysplasia.

206. **Other names that have been applied to PBS include**–triad syndrome, Eagle-Barrett syndrome, and abdominal musculation syndrome.

207. **Accurate diagnosis of PBS** can be made as early as 11 to 14 weeks of gestation.

208. **Incomplete forms of the syndrome**–lack the typical abdominal wall features but have the common uropathy and cryptorchidism.

209. **5% of PBS patients are female**, most of them have abdominal wall deficiency and the abnormal urinary tract.

210. Risk of bladder exstrophy in the offspring of individuals with bladder exstrophy and epispadias is 1 in 70 live births, **a 500-fold greater incidence than in the general population.**

211. **Reflux in the closed exstrophy bladder occurs in 100% of cases,** and subsequent surgery is usually required at the time of bladder neck reconstruction.

212. The initial staged approach to functional bladder closure included three separate stages:

- **Bladder, abdominal wall closure, and urethral closure** onto the penis in the newborn period with bilateral innominate and vertical iliac osteotomy.
- **Epispadias** repair at 6 months to 1 year of age.
- **Bladder neck reconstruction** along with antireflux procedure at age 4 to 5 years.

213. **Modern staged reconstruction of bladder**

- **Early bladder, posterior urethral and abdominal wall closure,** usually with osteotomy.

- Reconstruction of a **continent bladder neck and reimplantation of the ureters.**
- **Early Epispadias repair between 6 months and 12 months of age**, after testosterone stimulation.
- **Bladder neck repair usually occurs when the child is 4 to 5 years of age**, has an adequate bladder capacity, and, most important, is ready to participate in a postoperative voiding program.

214. Urethroplasty and penile reconstruction, if the urethral groove has adequate length, in the exstrophy patients is the **modified Cantwell-Ransley repair.**

215. **Bladder capacity is measured** with the child under anesthesia with a gravity cystogram at the 1-year of the initial closure.

Bladder capacity at the time of bladder neck reconstruction is an important determinant of eventual success

Bladder neck reconstruction can be planned if, median bladder capacity is **85 mL.**

216. **Exstrophy variant**

- **Pseudoexstrophy**–characteristic musculoskeletal defect of the exstrophy anomaly with no major defect in the urinary tract has been named.
- **Superior vesical fissure variant**–membrane ruptures only at the uppermost portion, and a superior vesical fistula results that actually resembles a vesicostomy. Bladder extrusion is minimal and is present only over the normal umbilicus.
- **Duplicate exstrophy**–occurs when a superior vesical fissure opens but there is later fusion of the abdominal wall and a portion of the bladder elements (mucosa) remains outside.
- **Covered exstrophy**–this has also been referred to as split symphysis variant. A common factor in these patients is the presence of musculoskeletal defect associated with classic exstrophy but no significant defect of the urinary tract.

217. **Complete penile disassembly technique**–this approach allows the tissue deformation in exstrophy to return more closely to an anatomically oriented position.

- Disassembly technique with complete primary repair of exstrophy (CPRE) or Mitchell technique is used exclusively for the surgical treatment of newborns with exstrophy.

- CPRE technique appears to be the most widely used single-stage anatomic approach to exstrophy.

218. **The obliterated urachus** becomes the median umbilical ligament and connects the apex of the bladder with the umbilicus.
219. Four different urachal anomalies have been described:
    1. **Patent urachus (50%).**
    2. Umbilical-urachus sinus (15%).
    3. Urachal cyst (30%).
    4. Vesicourachal diverticulum (3% to 5%).
220. **Primary paraureteral diverticula** are seen in smooth-walled bladders, occur isolated, are intermittent, and occur in children with no infravesical obstruction.

    Secondary paraureteral diverticula are found in trabeculated bladders as one of many diverticula in the bladder, are always present, and are caused by infravesical obstruction.
221. **Primary diverticula** arise as a localized herniation of bladder mucosa at the ureteral hiatus and are most likely caused by a **congenitally deficient bladder wall.**
222. **Young's classification is used for PUV.**
223. **Type I PUV:**
    - **Most common type**
    - There is a ridge lying on the floor of the urethra, continuous with the verumontanum, which takes an anterior course and divides into two fork-like processes in the region of the bulbomembranous junction.
    - The valve is made of a fibrous stroma covered on each side by transitional epithelium.
    - There is **no muscle** within the valve.
    - **Lack plicae colliculi.**
224. **Type II PUV**
    - Arises from the verumontanum and extending along the posterior urethral wall toward the bladder neck.
    - **Type II folds are not obstructive** and probably result from **hypertrophy of muscles.**

- They can be seen in response to many **obstructive conditions,** such as urethral strictures, PUV, anterior urethral valves and DESD.
- These type II folds are **no longer referred to as valves.**

225. **Type III PUV**
    - Type III valve is a membrane lying transversely across the urethra with a small perforation near its center.
    - The membrane is distal to the verumontanum and sometimes is elongated, like a windsock, reaching the bulbous urethra.
    - Only 5% of the total.
    - Attributed to incomplete dissolution of the urogenital portion of the cloacal membrane.
    - Type III valves have a **worse prognosis.**
226. Pulmonary hypoplasia is the **most common cause of mortality** in valve patients.
227. **The differential diagnosis of bilateral hydronephrosis includes**
    - posterior urethral valves
    - prune-belly syndrome
    - bilateral ureteropelvic junction obstruction
    - bilateral high-grade vesicoureteral reflux
    - bilateral ureterovesical junction obstruction
    - congenital urethral atresia
    - anterior urethral obstruction
228. **The classic USG findings in patients with valves:**
    - Bilateral hydroureteronephrosis.
    - Distended bladder
    - Thickened bladder wall.
    - **"Keyhole" sign** of a dilated bladder above a dilated prostatic urethra is also helpful.
    - Valves may be missed if the screening ultrasound is done before 24 weeks' gestation
229. **Voiding cystourethrography (VCUG)**–most important study in diagnosis of PUV because it defines the anatomy and gross function of the bladder, bladder neck, and urethra.

MAG3 is the most useful agent for this imaging because it provides functional data and adequate imaging of both the parenchyma and collecting system.

230. **Initial management in PUV**–immediate establishment of urinary catheter drainage from the bladder.

 This should be performed **even if the diagnosis has not been confirmed** by VCUG.

231. **Primary ablation is the preferred surgical procedure** to treat PUV and vesicostomy is reserved for very small or very ill infants.

232. If the **creatinine concentration remains >2.0** after 10 days of adequate bladder decompression and if hydronephrosis is unimproved, upper tract diversion may be considered.

 (**Vesicostomy** remains an excellent alternative treatment in these difficult situations).

 If the **creatinine concentration drops <2.0**, it is safe to rely on improved bladder drainage for additional kidney improvement.

233. **VUR in PUV**

 - Between 50% and 70% of patients with PUV will have VUR at the time of diagnosis.
 - Reflux resolves after valve ablation in 20%- 32% of refluxing ureters.
 - Children with initial bilateral reflux are more likely to have reflux resolve than are those with unilateral reflux.

234. **Hydronephrosis and PUV**

 - Almost all patients with PUV have severe hydroureteronephrosis at diagnosis.
 - Nonrefluxing hydronephrosis resolves in 49% of patients after valve ablation.

235. **Full valve bladder**

 - Coined by Mitchell.
 - Despite successful valve ablation, intrinsic bladder dysfunction leads to deterioration of the upper urinary tracts and incontinence.
 - The combination of poor sensation, high bladder volumes, and poor compliance produces storage pressures high enough to prevent adequate drainage of the upper tracts.

236. Indicator that fetal intervention would not be helpful to improve renal function

Aspirated fetal bladder urine with high sodium content and isosthenuria (similar specific gravity compared with serum values)

237. Valves is the only urologic anomaly to be considered for antenatal intervention

238. There are four basic predictors of renal function in patients with PUV:

- **Ultrasound appearance**–amount of dysplasia.
- **Serum chemistries**–Initial creatinine concentration of 3.6 mg/dL, post-drainage creatinine concentration of 2.4 and 1-year nadir of 1.7 are associated with worse long term function..
- **Age at diagnosis**–infants who presented <1 year of age had a worse prognosis than those who presented later in life.
- **Presence of reflux**–carries a poor prognosis.

239. Anterior urethral valves

- Obstruction is rare compared with PUV.
- Although these obstructive structures may be called valves, they often occur in the form of a diverticulum of the urethra, with one wall acting as an obstructive "valve".

240. Koff's formula–Bladder capacity (mL) = [Age (yr) + 2] × 30.

241. Uroflowmetry

- **Normal pattern**–smooth bell shape.
- **Overactive bladders**–tower shape.
- **Outlet obstruction**–low plateau-shape.
- **Sphincteric overactivity**–staccato pattern.
- **Acontractile or underactive bladders**–interrupted flow.

242. Nocturnal enuresis: (EAU Guidelines 2012)

- Alarm treatment is the best form for arousal disorder.
- Success rates of 70% can be obtained with desmopressin (DDAVP), 200-400 μg.
- A nasal spray is no longer recommended due to an increased risk of overdose.
- Imipramine, achieves only a moderate response rate of 50% and has a high relapse rate.

243. **Myelomeningocele accounts for >90% of all open spinal dysraphic states** and most spinal defects occur at the lumbosacral level.

244. **Sacral agenesis**

- **Absence of part or all of two or more lower vertebral bodies.**
- **IDDM mothers** have a 1% chance of giving birth to a child with this disorder.
- **The presentation is bimodal**–with more than three fourths of the disorders being detected in early infancy and the remainder discovered between 4 and 5 years of age.
- High index of suspicion in patients with–**flattened buttocks** and a low, short gluteal cleft.
- The diagnosis is most easily confirmed with a **lateral film of the lower spine.**
- **On urodynamic evaluation,** equal number of individuals manifest either an upper or a lower motor neuron lesion (35% vs 40%, respectively); 25% have no sign of denervation at all.
- The number of **affected vertebrae does not seem to correlate** with the type of motor neuron lesion present.

245. **Transureteroureterostomy**

- **Better ureter should be implanted into bladder,** draining the other across into it.
- The crossing ureter should be carefully mobilized with all of its adventitia and as much periureteral tissue as possible to preserve blood supply.
- Care must be taken not to angulate the crossing ureter immediately beneath the **inferior mesenteric artery.**
- The crossing ureter is widely anastomosed to the **posteromedial** aspect of the recipient ureter.
- The **recipient is not mobilized** or brought medially to meet the end of the other ureter.

246. **Psoas hitch**

- The bladder should be secured to the psoas muscle and fascia with **nonabsorbable sutures.**
- Broad, shallow sutures on the psoas muscle and fascia should be under taken **without trapping the sciatic nerve.**

- **The contralateral bladder pedicle may be divided** to increase bladder mobility and the length of the hitch.
- **Ureteral reimplantation** should be performed before the bladder psoas hitch.

247. Bladder neck reconstruction

- **Young's technique**–excising a portion of the bladder neck and significantly tightening the bladder neck over a silver probe.
- **Dees**–extended the length of excised tissue through the trigone.

Leadbetter

- Elevated the ureters off the trigone, placing them in a more cephalad position on the bladder floor.
- This allowed tubularization of the trigone and further enhanced lengthening of the urethra.
- This technique has **minimal success in individuals with neurogenic dysfunction.**

Fascial sling

- Coaptation and elevation of the bladder neck causes approximation of opposing epithelial surfaces and increased outlet resistance.
- Patients who undergo a sling procedure must be prepared for CIC.
- Used more extensively and with **better results in girls with neurogenic sphincter incompetence**.
- Success of the sling, appears to be improved with augmentation cystoplasty.

Bulking agents

- Limited role for increasing outlet resistance and should be reserved for a select group of patients.
- Patients with marginal native outflow resistance are probably better candidates.

Artificial urinary sphincter

- Placement of the cuff should be at the level of the **bladder neck** in all female patients and prepubertal boys.
- **Bladder neck** is also the most desirable and effective location in pubertal boys and adult men with neurogenic sphincter incompetence.
- The **bulbar urethra** can be used as an alternative site in adult men with mature spongiosum.

- It is the continence mechanisms that **does not negatively affect spontaneous voiding.**
- **CIC** is an important adjunct in 75% of children with neurogenic sphincter incompetence and can be performed successfully through the cuff.

248. Urethral lengthening

Tanagho technique

- Cephalad-based anterior detrusor wall tube.
- Closure of the tubularized bladder neck forms circularly oriented muscle fibers that work as a sphincter mechanism.
- **Poor success rate in the neurogenic population.**

Kropp technique

- Based on an anterior detrusor wall tube that is kept in continuity with the urethra, tubularized, and implanted into a submucosal tunnel within the trigone.
- Urethral lengthening and construction of a flap valve for **neurogenic bladder neck** and sphincter dysfunction.
- **Effective** technique; however, **difficulty with catheterization** is a common problem and significant concern.

Pippi Salle procedure

- Maximize the benefits of the Kropp technique.
- Anterior bladder onlay flap.
- Posterior wall of the neourethra is intact, providing less problem during catheterization.

249. Gastrocystoplasty

- Gastric mucosa is a barrier to chloride and acid resorption and secretes HCl.
- **Serum chloride decreases and serum bicarbonate increases.**
- Hypokalemic, hypochloremic metabolic alkalosis.
- Hematuria-dysuria syndrome.

250. All intestinal segments has **increase in serum chloride and decrease in serum bicarbonate level.**

- The majority of bladder stones are **struvite.**

- **Sigmoid colon** followed by stomach and then ileum were more likely to require reaugmentation.
- **Ileum** seems the least likely to demonstrate remarkable urodynamic abnormalities and **stomach** the most.

251. **The main disadvantage to ureterocystoplasty** is the limited population of patients with a nonfunctioning kidney draining into a megaureter.

252. **The main disadvantage of autoaugmentation** is a limited increase in bladder capacity such that adequate preoperative volume may be the most important predictor of success.

253. **Hypospadias**–ectopic urethral meatus on the ventral aspect of the penis, scrotum, or perineum with or without ventral penile curvature.

254. **Hypospadias classification:**
    - **Anterior/distal**–glanular, coronal, and subcoronal–**(50% to 70%).**
    - **Middle**–distal penile, midshaft and proximal penile.
    - **Posterior / proximal**–penoscrotal, scrotal and perineal.

255. Urethral folds fuse ventrally in the midline in the **11th week of gestation**, forming the urethra.

256. **A high index of suspicion for an intersex state** should accompany presumed males with any degree of hypospadias and cryptorchidism.

257. **Prepubertal exogenous testosterone** administration does not adversely affect ultimate penile growth.

    Hormonal stimulation has been used in <1% of distal repairs versus 25% of proximal to perineal cases and is recommended when the glans appears small

258. **Gittes and McLaughlin**–first to describe artificial erection.

259. **Best time for surgery for hypospadias is**–6 and 12 months of age.

260. Fourfold increase in urethral stricture rate after hypospadias repair with PDS compared with **chromic or polyglycolic acid suture.**

261. **Ventral curvature (VC)**
    - It may resolve with ventral degloving and dartos dissection.
    - VC <30 degrees remaining after ventral dissection can be corrected by midline dorsal plication.

- VC >30 degrees after ventral dissection can be straightened by either single ventral corporeal incision with grafting or multiple ventral corporeal incisions without grafting.
- During these maneuvers the urethral plate and adjacent corpus spongiosum often can be maintained intact by elevating them from the corpora.
- Persistent VC after these maneuvers requires urethral plate transection

262. Repair techniques

- **Distal hypospadias**–advancement, tubularization or flap techniques.
- **Middle hypospadias**–tubularization or vascularized flap techniques.
- **Proximal defects**–tubularization, vascularized flap, two-stage techniques, or the incorporation of extragenital skin for repair.

263. Distal hypospadias

- **Advancement techniques**–meatoplasty and glanuloplasty (MAGPI) technique, with excellent functional and cosmetic results provided there is adequate urethral mobility and no penile curvature.
- **Tubularization techniques**–Thiersch-Duplay urethroplasty.
- A modification of the Thiersch-Duplay technique described **by Snodgrass**. The tubularized incised plate (TIP) urethroplasty combines modifications of the previously described techniques of urethral plate incision and tubularization.
- **Flap techniques**–local tissue flap techniques for coronal and subcoronal defects is the **Mathieu, perimeatal-based flap** technique.
- **Barcat balanic groove.**
- **Pyramid procedure**–for megameatus intact prepuce (MIP) variant of hypospadias.

264. Middle hypospadias

- Onlay island flap (OIF) technique.
- Split prepuce in-situ onlay.
- TIP urethroplasty.

265. Posterior hypospadias

One stage repair

- Double-onlay preputial flap.
- Transverse preputial island flap (TPIF) employs preputial skin for formation of a tubularized neourethra transferred to the ventrum.

Two stage repair

- At the first stage, **orthoplasty** is performed and the prepuce is repositioned ventrally.
- **The second stage is performed >6 months** after completion of the first stage.
- **The primary goal of the second stage of the** procedure is to create a neourethra that bridges the defect between the hypospadiac meatus and the tip of the penis.
- **Preferred technique**–tubularization of local skin in Thiersch-Duplay fashion.

266. Most common complication of hypospadias and circumcision repair–bleeding.

267. Reoperative hypospadias surgery should be undertaken >6 months after the previous failure.

- No attempt at repair should be entertained until all edema, infection, and/or inflammation has resolved and healing is complete.

268. Indication of circumcision

- In uncircumcised boys >7 years with phimosis that is resistant to topical corticosteroids.
- Boys with phimosis that causes ballooning of the foreskin or recurrent balanitis.

269. Circumcision prevention:

- Penile cancer.
- Urinary tract infection (UTI).
- Sexually transmitted disease including HIV infection.
- Phimosis as well as lessers the risk of balanitis.

270. Newborn circumcision has potential medical benefits and advantages as well as disadvantages and risks. When circumcision is being considered, the benefits and risks should be explained to the parents and informed consent obtained.

271. **Eutectic mixture of local anesthetic (EMLA;** lidocaine and prilocaine).

- EMLA cream poses a risk for methemoglobinemia.

272. **The most common late complication of newborn circumcision–** meatal stenosis.

273. **The normal urethral meatus** is

- 10 French before 4 years of age
- 12 French from 4 to 10 years of age
- 14 French after 10 years of age

274. **In cases of partial glans removal**

- Excised tissue should be preserved and immediately sutured back to the penis.
- When repair is performed <8 hours after the injury, the penis heals well.

275. **Micropenis**

- **Normally formed penis that is at least 2.5 SD below mean in size.**
- **When penis of a full-term newborn < 1.9 cm long.**

276. **Buried penis can be differentiated from a micropenis,** with the latter not having a normal penile stretched length

277. **Micropenis**

- Ratio of the length of the penile shaft to its circumference is normal.
- Corpora cavernosa are severely hypoplastic.
- Scrotum is usually fused but often diminutive.
- Testes are usually small and frequently undescended.
- **The most common causes of micropenis are** hypogonadotropic hypogonadism, hypergonadotropic hypogonadism (primary testicular failure) and idiopathic.
- Results from a hormonal abnormality that occurs after 14 weeks of gestation.
- **Investigation**
    - o **A karyotype should be performed.**
    - o **Testicular function** by measuring T levels before and after hCG stimulation.

- o **Anterior pituitary screening tests** include serial measurements of serum glucose, sodium, potassium, and serum cortisol concentrations and thyroid function tests.
- o **MRI of the head** to determine the anatomic integrity of the hypothalamus and the anterior pituitary gland as well as the **midline structures of the midbrain**.

278. Penile torsion

- Rotational defect of the penile shaft.
- Shaft is rotated in a **counterclockwise direction (i.e., to left side).**
- Penile size is normal and the condition is unrecognized.
- Correction is unnecessary if the rotation is <60 to 90 degrees from the midline.

279. The most commonly used classification of urethral duplication is that of Effman

Type I is partial urethral duplication

Type II is complete urethral duplication

Type III describes urethral duplication as part of bladder duplication.

280. Most common cause of priapism in children is sickle cell disease.

281. Child with stuttering priapism

- 1st line therapy–Oral α-adrenergic agent (pseudoephedrine).
- 2nd line therapy–Oral β agonist (terbutaline).
- 3rd line therapy–GnRH analog plus flutamide.

282. During gestation

- **4th to 6th weeks**–genital ridges organize, followed by migration of primordial germ cells.
- **7th week**–testicular differentiation is initiated by the *SRY* gene.
  - o Primitive Sertoli cells have developed.
  - o MIS expression is detectable and is limited to Sertoli cells only.
  - o Gubernaculum appears.
- **8th week**–fetal testis begins to secrete testosterone and MIS
  - o MIS is secreted by Sertoli cells and causes degeneration of the müllerian structures.

- **12th to 14th weeks**–testosterone synthesis is regulated by maternal hCG.
- **15th weeks**–germ cells differentiate into gonocytes on entering the testicular cords to become fetal spermatogonia.
- **23rd weeks**–testes lie dormant within the abdomen, during this time the processus vaginalis continues its elongation into the scrotum.
- **24th and 28th weeks**–75% of testes passes through the inguinal canal.
- **30th and 32nd weeks**–testicular descent is normally complete.

283. **Cryptorchidism**–affects **3%** of full-term male newborns.
    - **70% to 77% of cryptorchid testes will spontaneously descend, usually by 3 months of age.**
    - **By 1 year of age**, the incidence of cryptorchidism declines to **1%.**

284. **Factors that predict complete spontaneous descent by 3 months of age include:**
    - Low birth weight **(principal determinant).**
    - Bilateral cryptorchidism.
    - Normal scrotal anatomy.
    - Testis that are positioned lower along the normal path of descent.
    - (Boys with a small or poorly rugated scrotum and those with hypospadias are more likely to be cryptorchid at 3 months).

285. **Most common ectopic location of testis is**–superficial pouch between the external oblique fascia and Scarpa's fascia, a structure that has been termed the Denis-Browne pouch.

286. 80% of undescended testes are clinically palpable and 20% are nonpalpable.

    "Nonpalpable testis" implies-intra-abdominal, absent (vanishing), atrophic, or missed on physical examination.

287. **A vanishing or absent testis**–the anatomic hallmark is blind-ending spermatic vessels that are found just proximal to the internal inguinal ring (IIR).

288. A "retractile testis":

- Withdraws spontaneously out of the scrotum toward the inguinal canal by an active cremasteric reflex but can easily be brought down into a dependent position within the scrotum and remains there after traction has been released.
- Most common encountered between the ages of 3 and 7 years.
- The retractability of the testes is caused by an overactive cremasteric reflex.
- Children with retractile testes should be monitored yearly, at least upto puberty, until the testes are no longer retractile and remain intrascrotal.

289. Transabdominal descent–hormonal control by MIS.

Inguinoscrotal phase of descent–mediated by androgen (Testosterone and DHT).

290. Probable factors required for normal descent of testis:

- Endocrine factors
  - o Androgens
  - o MIS
  - o Estrogen
  - o Descendin
- Gubernaculum.
- Genitofemoral Nerve and Calcitonin Gene-Related Peptide (CGRP)
- Epididymis.
- Intra-abdominal pressure.

291. The relative risk of malignant transformation in an undescended testis is 2.5 to 8 overall and 2 to 3 in boys undergoing prepubertal orchidopexy

292. Earliest postnatal histologic abnormality in cryptorchid testes

- Hypoplasia of the Leydig cells, observed in first month of life.

The histopathologic hallmarks associated with cryptorchidism

- Evident between 1 and 2 years of age.
- Decreased numbers of Leydig cells.
- Degeneration of Sertoli cells.

- Delayed **disappearance** of gonocytes.
- Delayed **appearance** of adult dark (Ad) spermatogonia.
- Failure of primary spermatocytes to develop.
- Reduced total germ cell counts.

293. Two critical prepubertal steps in germ cell maturation and proliferation are:

1. Transformation of the fetal stem cell pool (gonocytes) into the adult stem cell pool (Ad spermatogonia) at 2 to 3 months of age.
2. Transformation of Ad spermatogonia into primary spermatocytes (meiosis) at 4 to 5 years.

294. Orchidopexy performed at an early age will protect against the development of malignancy is inconclusive.

An indication for orchiopexy is to permit a more thorough examination of the testis, which would theoretically allow for earlier detection of malignant degeneration.

295. A patent processus vaginalis is found in >90% of patients with an UDT. Cryptorchidism associated with **epididymal anomalies–90%.**

296. Approximately **10% of testicular tumors** arise from an UDT.

297. Torsion of a UDT should be considered in any child with abdominal or groin pain and an empty ipsilateral hemiscrotum.

298. Endocrine factors:

- The diagnosis of bilateral anorchia should be considered if a male karyotype is confirmed.
- MIS and inhibin B are specific testicular markers.
- If gonadotropin levels, FSH in particular, are increased in a prepubescent boy, further endocrine workup is unnecessary because it represents bilateral anorchia.
- If gonadotropin levels are normal in a boy with bilateral nonpalpable testes, an hCG stimulation test can be performed to further establish the diagnosis.

299. Definitive treatment of UDT–between 6 and 12 months of age.

300. Every effort should be made to preserve any testicular tissue at an early age, especially in children with unilateral or bilateral intra-abdominal testes.

- **Orchiectomy**–reserved for postpubescent males with a contralateral normally descended testis when the cryptorchid testis is abnormal or too far from the scrotum to allow for tension-free placement without compromising the vascular integrity of the testis.

301. Role of hormonal therapy

- Two types of medical treatment of a UDT–exogenous hCG and exogenous GnRH or LHRH.
- **Successful results reported in:**
  - o Older groups of children.
  - o Testes that were retractile or below the external inguinal ring.
- **Not indicated in:**
  - o Previously operated testes.
  - o Prior surgery that would result in inguinal scar tissue formation.
  - o Ectopic testes.
  - o Associated with inguinal hernia.
- **Overall efficacy of hormonal treatment is <20% for cryptorchid testes.**

302. Prentiss maneuver is performed by passing the testis under the floor of the inguinal canal to an exit site just above the pubic tubercle.

303. Arterial blood supply of testis:

- Primary testicular artery (branch from aorta).
- Deferential artery of the vas deferens(branch of inferior vesical artery).
- Cremasteric arteries(branch of inferior epigastric artery).

304. Most important requirement for successful Fowler-Stephens orchiopexy–long, looping vas (present in less than a third of boys with true intra-abdominal testes).

305. The Fowler-Stephens test

- Method of testing the collateral blood supply to the testis.
- Can also performed by temporarily occluding the testicular artery with a vascular clamp for 5 minutes and inspecting the testis for color.
- Performed by making a small incision in the tunica albuginea of the testis.

- **If the blood supply at this point considered tenuous, a two-stage repair** should be performed to allow for development of the collateral circulation.

306. Advantage of two-stage orchiopexy with spermatic vessel ligation:

1. Allows for development of collateral blood supply to compensate for division of the main blood supply to the testis.
2. Allows for greater mobility of the testis to place it within the scrotum.

307. Most accurate means of determining whether a testis is intra-abdominal–diagnostic laparoscopy.

308. There are three distinct possible findings–when laparoscopy is used to assess a nonpalpable testis.

1. Blind-ending vessels above the internal ring (vanishing testis).
2. Cord structures entering the internal ring (viable intracanalicular testis versus an intracanalicular or scrotal atrophic testis).
3. Intra-abdominal testis.

309. Intra-abdominal testis:

Normal

- <2 cm from IIR–orchidopexy.
- > 3 cm from IIR–divide spermatic vessels-staged Fowler Stephens orchidopexy.
- Very high–autotrasplantation.

Abnormal/atrophic–orchidectomy.

310. Absent testis

Vessels exiting internal ring–

- Normal vessels-explore.
- Atretic vessels–remove remnant with contralateral fixation.

Blind ending vessels–no further exploration.

311. Success rate in management of UDT

- **84% for microvascular orchiopexy.**
- 81% for standard abdominal orchiopexy.
- 77% for staged Fowler-Stephens orchiopexy.
- 67% for standard Fowler-Stephens orchiopexy.

312. Torsion of spermatic cord (intravaginal)

- Injury to the testicular parenchyma may begin as soon as **4 hours** after occlusion of the cord.
- Torsion of the cord within the space of the tunica vaginalis, result from lack of normal fixation.
- **Absence of a cremasteric reflex** is a good indicator of torsion of the cord.
- High resolution US visualization has 100% sensitivity for the combination of cord twist and/or reduced blood flow in diagnosing–torsion
- Radionuclide imaging, originally the investigation of choice for assessment of an acute scrotum, is more limited because it allows evaluation of only testicular blood flow.
- **Exploration of the contralateral hemiscrotum** must be carried out.
- The contralateral testis must be fixed to prevent subsequent torsion.

313. Torsion of testicular and epididymal appendages

- Most common cause of acute scrotum in prepubertal children
- Localized tenderness of the **upper pole** of the testis or epididymis.
  - At **upper pole** tender nodule may be palpated.
  - Infarcted appendage is visible through the skin as a **"blue dot sign".**
  - In cases in which the inflammatory changes are more significant, scrotal wall edema and erythema may be severe.
  - The **cremasteric reflex should be present**, and the testis should be mobile.
  - Radionuclide scans or CDUS may show **normal or increased flow.**
  - **Nonoperative management** allows most cases to resolve spontaneously.

314. Men with vasal agenesis should be screened with renal USG.

- In men with bilateral vas agenesis, the incidence of renal anomalies is 14% to 21%.
- In men with unilateral agenesis, it is 26% to 79%.

- The most common renal anomaly found is **unilateral renal agenesis.**

315. **Presence of a Y chromosome**, independent of the number of X chromosomes, resulted in the development of a male embryo.

    In the **absence of a Y chromosome** the embryo developed as a female.

316. **In human, the hypothetical Y chromosomal gene is termed** the testis-determining factor (TDF).

317. ***SRY* is localized to** the smallest region of the Y chromosome

318. **Secretion of MIS by the Sertoli cells at 7 to 8 weeks' gestation.** It is a member of TGF-β family, and the human gene has been cloned and mapped to chromosome 19.

    - **Testosterone secretion by**–the fetal testes is detectable shortly after the formation of Leydig cells in the interstitium at **9 weeks' gestation.**
    - **Estrogen synthesis is** detectable just after **8 weeks** of gestation.

319. **First sign of male phenotypic differentiation is**–degeneration of the müllerian ducts adjacent to the testes as a result of MIS secretion by the Sertoli cells.

320. **Genitalia of the male fetus is completed with closure of the elongated urogenital cleft by**–12 to 13 weeks' gestation.

321. **A. Disorders of Gonadal Differentiation**

    - **Seminiferous tubule dysgenesis.**
    - **Klinefelter's syndrome.**
    - **Syndromes of gonadal dysgenesis**
        - o Turner's syndrome.
        - o Pure gonadal dysgenesis.
        - o Mixed gonadal dysgenesis.
        - o Partial gonadal dysgenesis
        - o Bilateral vanishing testis/testicular regression syndromes.

    B. True hermaphroditism

    C. Masculinized Female (Female Pseudohermaphroditism)

    - o CAH(21-hydroxylase, 11β-hydroxylase, 3β-hydroxysteroid dehydrogenase deficiencies).

    D. Undermasculinized Male (Male Pseudohermaphroditism)

- **Variants of CAH affecting corticosteroid and testosterone synthesis:**
  - o StAR deficiency.
  - o 3βpHydroxysteroid dehydrogenase deficiency.
  - o 17α-Hydroxylase deficiency.
- **Disorders of testosterone biosynthesis.**
  - o 17, 20–Lyase deficiency.
  - o 17β-Hydroxysteroid oxidoreductase deficiency.
- **Disorders of androgen-dependent target tissue:**
  - o Androgen receptor and postreceptor defects.
  - o Syndrome of complete testicular feminization.
  - o Syndrome of partial androgen resistance.
- **Disorders of testosterone metabolism by peripheral tissues**
  - o 5α-Reductase deficiency
- **Persistent müllerian duct syndrome.**

322. Klinefelter's syndrome (XXY)

- **Presence of an extra X chromosome is the genetic hallmark.**
- **Most common major abnormality of sexual differentiation.**
- **Males with at least one Y chromosome and at least two X chromosomes.**
- Eunuchoidism.
- Gynecomastia (Plasma estradiol levels tend to be high).
- Azoospermia.
- Small, firm testes.
- Serum levels of testosterone are low-normal and those of gonadotropins are elevated.
- Patients tend to be taller.
- Absolute volume of Leydig cells is not increased.
- Fertility, with the benefit of ICSI, has been reported.

323. Turner syndrome (XO)

- Presence of only one normally functioning X chromosome with female phenotype.
- Lymphedema with short stature or primary amenorrhea.

- Broad chest, widespread nipples and webbing of the neck.
- Renal anomalies :
  - o Horseshoe kidney–10%.
  - o Duplication or renal agenesis–20%.
  - o Malrotation–15%.
  - o Multiple renal arteries–90%.
- Risk of gonadoblastoma, an in-situ germ cell cancer, is 7% to 30%.

324. 46, XX "pure" gonadal dysgenesis

- Closely related to those with Turner's syndrome.
- Normal female external genitalia, normal müllerian ducts with absence of wolffian duct structures.
- Normal height, bilateral streak gonads, sexual infantilism, and a normal 46,XX karyotype.

325. Mixed gonadal dysgenesis

- **Second most common cause of ambiguous genitalia after CAH.**
- Unilateral testis, which is often intra-abdominal.
- Contralateral streak gonad.
- Persistent müllerian structures associated with varying degrees of inadequate masculinization.
- Most patients have a 45,XO/46,XY karyotype.

326. Embryonic testicular regression and bilateral vanishing testes

- Patients with a 46,XY karyotype.
- Absent testes with clear evidence of testicular function at some point during embryogenesis.
- Diagnosis can be made on the basis of a 46,XY karyotype and castrate levels of testosterone despite persistently elevated serum LH and FSH.

327. True hermaphrodites

- Have both testicular tissue with well-developed seminiferous tubules and ovarian tissue with primordial follicles.
- It may take the form of one ovary and one testis or, more commonly, one or two ovotestes.

- External genitalia are ambiguous but masculinized to variable degrees and 75% are raised as male.

328. Masculinized female (female pseudohermaphroditism)

- Disorder of phenotypic sexual development in which 46,XX individuals with ovaries have a partially masculinized phenotype and ambiguous genitalia.
- Most common cause of the masculinized female–CAH.
- Most common cause of ambiguous genitalia in the newborn–CAH.

329. CAH (21-hydroxylase)

- Deficiency of steroid 21-hydroxylase is responsible for **95% of cases of CAH.**
- Exhibit one of the two classic forms of the disease: **75% present with salt wasting and 25% with simple virilisation.**
- Formation of hydrocortisone is ↓ →compensatory ↑ ACTH→↑ adrenal steroids proximal to the enzymatic defect→↑ **testosterone, the active androgen in CAH.**
- **Plasma levels of progesterone and 17-hydroxyprogesterone ↑.**
- Urinary levels of **17-ketosteroids and pregnanetriol ↑.**
- **A pelvic USG demonstrating the presence of müllerian tissues is confirmatory.**

330. Undermasculinized male (male pseudohermaphroditism)

- 46,XY individuals with differentiated testes who exhibit varying degrees of feminization phenotypically.

331. Complete androgen insensitivity (testicular feminization) is characterized :

- **46,XY karyotype,** bilateral testes, female-appearing external genitalia, and absence of müllerian derivatives.
- Postpubertal patient with findings of amenorrhea, absence of pubic hair, or inguinal hernias containing testes.
- It is confirmed by a 46,XY karyotype and a normal male androgen and gonadotropin profile.
- USG confirms the absence of müllerian tissue, and a vaginal examination confirms a blind-ending vagina without a cervix.

332. Syndrome of partial androgen resistance (Reifenstein's)

- Male with perineoscrotal hypospadias, cryptorchidism, rudimentary Wolffian duct structures, gynecomastia and infertility.

333. 5α-reductase deficiency is secondary to mutations in the type II gene.

- Newborns with a **46,XY karyotype** and a phenotype that may vary from penoscrotal hypospadias to, more commonly, markedly ambiguous genitalia.
- **Phallus is quite small,** appearing as a normal or enlarged clitoris.
- A urogenital sinus is present, with **separate vaginal and urethral openings** and labioscrotal fusion.
- The vaginal pouch is short and blind-ending.
- Testes and epididymides are located in the labia, inguinal canals, or abdomen; and the vasa terminate in the blind-ending vaginal pouch.
- At puberty, partial masculinization occurs with an increase in muscle mass, development of male body habitus, increase in phallic size and onset of erections.
- **Sperm production and fertility** is reported.
- **Enlargement of the prostate and hairline recession do not develop.**

334. Persistent müllerian duct syndrome (PMDS) or hernia uteri inguinale

- 46,XY karyotype and normal male external genitalia.
- Unilateral or bilateral UDT, bilateral fallopian tubes, a uterus, and an upper vagina draining into a prostatic utricle.
- Diagnosed after müllerian tissue is encountered during inguinal herniorrhaphy or orchidopexy.

335. The Mayer-Rokitansky-Küster-Hauser (MRKH) syndrome

- Associated with variable absence or hypoplasia of the **cervix, uterus and fallopian tubes.**
- **Ovaries** are almost always present and functional.
- This syndrome is **second only to gonadal dysgenesis** as a cause of primary amenorrhea.
- **46, XX karyotype** and are normal-appearing females with

normal secondary sex characteristics.

- The external genitalia appear normal, but only a shallow vaginal pouch is present.
- The most common clinical presentation is **primary amenorrhea.**
- **Congenital abnormalities of the skeletal system** have been described in 10% to 20% of cases.
- **Upper urinary tract anomalies** occur in approximately one third of patients and include renal agenesis, pelvic kidney, and horseshoe kidney.
- **Based on the morphology** of the retained müllerian structures, divided into typical and atypical forms.
- **In the typical form (type A)**, the patient has symmetrical uterine remnants and normal fallopian tubes not associated with upper tract abnormalities.
- **The (10%) atypical form (type B)** is characterized by asymmetric uterine buds or abnormally developed fallopian tubes. Urinary tract anomalies occur more commonly.
- Treatment entails **creation of a neovagina,** surgically or by means of dilation, to allow for sexual function and drainage of menstrual fluid if necessary.

336. Large intestine is the bowel segment of choice for vaginoplasty.

Ileum

- Two specific indications for use of an ileal segment for bowel vaginoplasty are previous irradiation of the deep pelvis and the absence of large intestine (i.e., cloacal exstrophy).
- Stenosis has been reported more frequently after the use of ileum.

Bowel vagina vs McIndoe procedure (dissecting a canal between the rectum and urethra and lining this area with split-thickness skin grafts)

Advantages

- Lubricating properties of mucus (which may help facilitate intercourse).
- Decreased incidence of postoperative contracture (and hence the reduced need for postoperative dilatation).

Disadvantages

- Frequent need to wear pads because of the chronic vaginal discharge.

- Daily douching may be necessary to evacuate the mucus.
- Potential transmission of blood-borne pathogens such as hepatitis and HIV.

337. A persistent urogenital sinus most commonly occurs in genital ambiguity states (Most commonly due to CAH).

338. With urogenital sinus abnormalities and cloacal anomaly– genitography and endoscopy are mandatory to define the anatomy.

339. Definitive repair of a cloaca is carried out at 6 to 12 months of age

340. Vaginoplasty

Cut-back vaginoplasty

- Rarely used and is appropriate for only simple labial fusion.

Flap vaginoplasty

- Applicable to a low (distal) vaginal confluence.
- Should never be used for patients with a very high vaginal confluence because it may result in a short hypospadiac urethra, vaginal voiding, many infections, and even incontinence.

Pull-through vaginoplasty

- Used for a very high confluence.

Complete vaginal replacement

- Used only for a rudimentary or absent vagina.

341. Diagnoses based on karyotype and anatomic symmetry

Karyotype- 46XY-	Symmetric anatomy-	Undervirilized male
	Asymmetric anatomy-	Mixed gonadal dysgenesis
Karyotype- 46XX-	Symmetric anatomy-	Overvirilized female
	Asymmetric anatomy-	Ovotesticular disorder of sex differentiation.

342. Imaging in pediatric urolithiasis

- Unenhanced helical computed tomography (CT) has become the most accurate and efficient first choice in initial imaging
- Ultrasonography should be considered as a screening tool in the workup for nonemergent abdominal or flank pain

343. In managing stone disease in the pediatric population,

- Renal calculi <3 mm are likely to spontaneously pass
- Stones >4 mm in the distal ureter are likely to require endourologic treatment

344. **Indication for ESWL** in pediatric population- uncomplicated renal and proximal calculi <15 mm

Indications for PCNL in the pediatric population-

- Large upper tract stone burden (>1.5 cm)
- Lower pole calculi >1 cm
- Concurrent anatomic abnormality impairing urinary drainage and stone clearance
- Cystine or struvite composition

345. **Most common bladder abnormality associated with ESRD**–low-capacity, hypertonic bladder with poor compliance.

346. **Indications for augmentation prior to transplantation include**

- Capacity <75% of that expected for age
- Pressures >30 cm H_2O
- Being catheterized every 3 hours
- Maximal anticholinergic medications.

347. **Native nephrectomy before transplant is indicated for**

- Malignant hypertension,
- Profound nephrotic syndrome with malnutrition,
- Recurrent upper tract infection
- Massive reflux.

348. **Neuroblastoma**

- **Most common extracranial solid tumor of childhood.**
- **Most common malignant tumor of infancy.**
- >95% of cases are diagnosed in children by 10 years of age.
- **70% children have metastatic disease at diagnosis.**
- Neuroblastoma is known to arise from cells of the neural crest that forms the adrenal medulla and sympathetic ganglia.
- Tumors may occur anywhere along the sympathetic chain within the neck, thorax, retroperitoneum, pelvis or adrenal gland.
- **75% arise in the retroperitoneum**, 50% in the adrenal and 25% in the paravertebral ganglia.
- These tumors can undergo **spontaneous regression.**

349. Neuroblastoma–prognostic factors

Adverse prognostic factors:

- Deletion of the short arm of chromosome 1.
- Amplification of the N-myc oncogenes.
- Higher stage.

Good prognostic factors:

- Aneuploidy of tumor DNA.
- Young age at presentation.
- Nonadrenal primary tumors.
- DNA index greater than 1.0.

350. Increased levels of urinary metabolites of catecholamines, VMA and HVA, are found in 90% to 95% of patients.

351. International Neuroblastoma Staging System

Stage		Definition
1	–	Localized tumor with complete gross excision, with or without microscopic residual disease.
2A	–	Localized tumor with incomplete gross excision.
2B	–	Localized tumor with or without complete gross excision, with ipsilateral nonadherent LN positive for tumor.
3	–	Unresectable unilateral tumor infiltrating across the midline, with or without regional LN involvement; localized unilateral tumor with contralateral regional LN involvement; or midline tumor with bilateral extension by infiltration (unresectable) or by LN involvement.
4	–	Any primary tumor with dissemination to distant LN, bone, bone marrow, liver, skin and/or other organs.
4S	–	Localized primary tumor (as defined for stage 1, 2A or 2B), with dissemination limited to the skin, liver and/or bone marrow (less than 10% tumor) in infants <1 year.

352. Treatment

- **Children with stage I have a DFS rate of >90% with surgical excision alone.**
- Chemotherapy was required in only 10% of stage I and 20% of stage II patients and achieved excellent overall survival in the stage II patients.

- N-myc amplification, unfavorable histology, age older than 2 years, and positive lymph nodes predicted **lower overall survival.**
- **Stage III and stage IV**–surgery is usually performed 13 to 18 weeks after initiation of chemotherapy so that three to four courses of treatment can be completed.

353. Ganglioneuromas

- In older children
- Usually located in the posterior mediastinum and retroperitoneum, with only a small number arising in the adrenal glands.
- Often grow to very large size before they cause symptoms as a result of compression of adjacent structures or extension into the spinal canal.

354. Rhabdomyosarcoma (RMS)

- **Most common soft tissue sarcoma in infants and children.**
- **Third most common solid tumor** in children after neuroblastoma and Wilms' tumor.
- **Vagina and paratesticular region having a better prognosis than** bladder/prostate primaries.
- **Embryonal RMS is the most common subtype.**
- **Botryoid and spindle cell variants of embryonal RMS are associated with excellent survival.**
- Sixty to eighty percent of paratesticular RMS is **stage I** at diagnosis.
- Patients > 10 years have a higher risk for retroperitoneal relapse and should undergo staging with ipsilateral RPLND before chemotherapy.

355. Wilms tumor

- Wilms' tumor, or nephroblastoma, is the most common primary malignant renal tumor of childhood.
- 80% of cases occurring in those <5 years.
- **Genitourinary abnormalities** (renal fusion anomalies, cryptorchidism, hypospadias)–4.5% of patients with Wilms' tumor.
- **Denys-Drash syndrome**–male pseudohermaphroditism, renal mesangial sclerosis and nephroblastoma.
- **WAGR syndrome**–Wilms' tumor, aniridia, genital anomalies, mental retardation.

- **BWS–macroglossia, nephromegaly, hepatomegaly and hemihypertrophy.**

356. **WT1**–11p13 resulted from chromosomal deletions in patients with the WAGR syndrome. Mutations of WT1 occur in DDS.

WT2–11p15 locus associated with BWS.

Loss of the long arm of chromosome 16 (detected in approximately 20%).

Loss of the short arm of chromosome 1p (detected in approximately 10%).

357. Staging System of the Children's Oncology Group

Stage

I – Tumor limited to the kidney and completely excised.

II – Tumor beyond the kidney, but is completely resected. Extrarenal vessels may contain tumor thrombus or be infiltrated by tumor.

III – Residual nonhematogenous tumor confined to the abdomen: LN involvement, any tumor spillage, rupture or biopsy, peritoneal implants, tumor beyond surgical margin either grossly or microscopically, or tumor not completely removed.

IV – Hematogenous metastases to lung, liver, bone, brain, etc.

V – Bilateral renal involvement at diagnosis.

358. Treatment Protocol Used in the National Wilms' Tumor Study-5

Stage/Histology	**Radiotherapy**	**Chemotherapy**
Stage I, II FH Stage I anaplasia	None	AMD plus VCR (18 weeks)
Stage III, IV FH Stage II-IV focal anaplasia	1080 cGy	AMD, VCR and DOX (24 weeks)
Stage II-IV diffuse anaplasia	Yes	AMD, VCR, DOX, CPM and etoposide
Stage I-IV CCSK Stage I-IV RTK	Yes	Carboplatin, etoposide and CPM

AMD, dactinomycin; CCSK, clear cell sarcoma of the kidney; CPM, cyclophosphamide; DOX, doxorubicin; FH, favorable histology, VCR, vincristine; RTK, Rhabdoid tumor of kidney.

359. **Situations in which preoperative chemotherapy is routinely recommended:**

- Bilateral Wilms' tumors.
- Tumors inoperable at surgical exploration.
- Tumor extension into inferior vena cava above the hepatic veins.

360. **Rhabdoid tumor of the kidney (RTK) is the most aggressive and lethal childhood renal tumor**

361. **Congenital mesoblastic nephroma (CMN) is the most common renal tumor in infants.**

362. **RCC is the most common renal malignancy in the second decade of life.**

363. **i(12p) is** found in intratubular germ cell neoplasia.

364. **Most common nongerminal testicular tumors in children–** Gonadal sex cord stromal tumors.

   Most common of the sex cord tumors–Leydig cell tumor.

365. **Most common tumors found in association with intersex disorders**–Gonadoblastomas.

366. **Most common malignancies that spread to the testis in children–** Leukemia and lymphoma. Children with ALL who have bulky disease at diagnosis have been reported to have upto a 20% incidence of testicular relapse.

367. **Radiographic assessment of the genitourinary tract for a possible injury in :**

- All patients with penetrating trauma.
- Blunt trauma patients with:
  1. A significant deceleration or high-velocity injury.
  2. Significant trauma that has resulted in fractures of thoracic rib cage, spine, pelvis, or femur, or bruising of the torso/perineum, or signs of peritonitis.
  3. Gross hematuria.

4. Microscopic hematuria (<50 RBC/HPF) associated with shock (SBP<90 mm Hg).

368. Repeat CT with delayed images should be obtained 3 days and 3 months after the trauma and also DMSA, at 1 week after trauma in patients with :

- Grade 3 renal lacerations associated with devitalized fragments.
- Grade 4.
- Grade 5.

369. Most sensitive method for the diagnosis and classification of pediatric genitourinary trauma–triphasic abdominal and pelvic CT.

370. The two most likely genitourinary injuries to be missed by single-phase CT or single-shot IVP–urinomas and isolated ureteral injuries.

371. Consensus Recommendations for Management of Renal Trauma

Non-operative

Grade 1 or 2 renal injury irrespective of traumatic etiology.

Isolated grade 3, 4 and hemodynamically stable grade 5 renal injuries.

Absolute requirement for surgical intervention

Uncontrollable renal hemorrhage (usually grade 4 vascular or grade 5 injuries).

Persistent or delayed hemorrhage not responding to angiographic embolization.

Expanding pulsatile retroperitoneal mass found on surgical exploration for coexisting intra-abdominal injuries.

Retroperitoneal (renal) exploration recommended (verify contralateral renal function)

Blunt/penetrating trauma, inadequate preoperative radiographic staging due to vascular instability of patient, retroperitoneal hemorrhage found on exploration.

Blunt/penetrating trauma, radiographic screening studies reveal grade 3 with devitalized renal fragments, grade 4 or 5 renal injury, coexisting intra-abdominal injuries.

372. Findings on triphasic CT associated with UPJ disruption are :

- Good renal contrast agent excretion with medial extravasation of contrast agent in the perirenal and upper ureteral area.
- Absence of parenchymal lacerations.
- No visualization of the ipsilateral distal ureter.

373. In a clinically stable patient in whom the diagnosis of **UPJ disruption is made within 5 days after the traumatic insult,** immediate surgical repair is the preferred treatment.

374. Absolute indications for bladder imaging after blunt abdominal trauma are:

- Presence of gross hematuria coexisting with a pelvic fracture.
- Inability to void.

Relative indications for bladder imaging after blunt abdominal trauma:

- Urinary clot retention.
- Perineal hematoma.
- History of prior bladder augmentation.

375. Traumatic bladder lacerations in children are two times more likely to extend through the bladder neck compared with the same injury in an adult.

376. Differences between pediatric and adult urethral injuries:

- Pelvic fracture is more likely to be unstable and associated with a severely and permanently displaced prostatic urethra.
- Displacement of the prostate off the pelvic floor makes a complete posterior urethral disruption more common in boys than men.
- In children, concurrent bladder and urethral injuries may occur in upto 20% of the patients, with coexisting anterior longitudinal tears through the bladder neck and sphincteric complex.
- In prepubertal girls, pelvic fractures more likely to be associated with a urethral injury than in adult women.

377. Investigation of choice to rule out the presence of a urethral injury–RGU.

378. **Endoscopic urethrotomy** for short, <1-cm nonobliterative bulbar and penile urethral strictures is commonly performed for pediatric urethral stricture disease.

379. **An anastomotic urethroplasty** through either the perineal, transpubic, trans-symphyseal, or combined approach is the procedure of choice for distraction urethral injuries in both children and adults.

380. **Repair of traumatic urethral strictures of the bulbar, proximal and penile urethra of >4 cm in length** in children.

- Pursued using a one-stage flap procedure from the prepuce or penile shaft skin or a dorsal graft urethroplasty using a free skin graft or buccal mucosa.
- If the defect is great enough that the flap or graft must be used in a circumferential manner two or multiple-stage approach is preferred.
- The use of a staged reconstruction is based on–recurrent strictures are more likely to occur when any flap or graft is used in a circumferential manner (tube) as a single-stage procedure.
- Staging the operation by performing a classic two-stage Johannson urethroplasty or preferentially a multiple-staged preputial flap or buccal graft urethroplasty.

Chapter 18
UROIMAGING

3.1

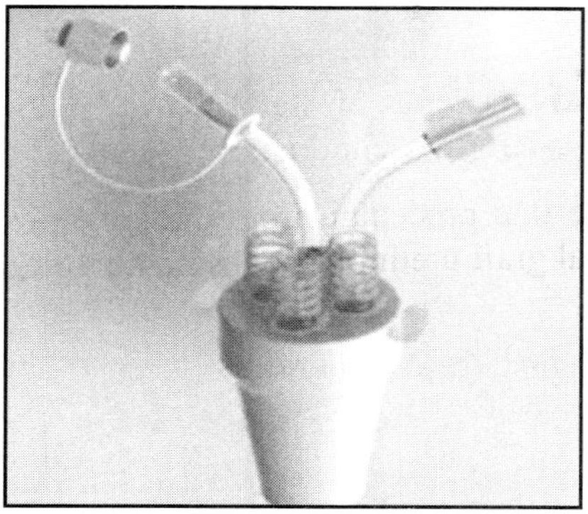

a) Name the equipment?

b) What is the purpose of this equipment?

Answer:

a) Port for single port surgery

b) Most commonly used for laparoscopic simple and donor nephrectomy

3.2

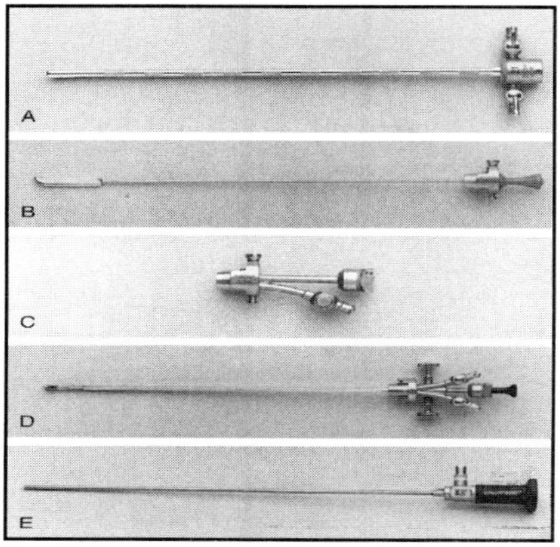

a) What does this image suggest?

b) All the above equipment compiles to form?

Answer:

a) A, metal sheath; B, obturator; C, bridge; D, deflector system; and E, lens

b) Rigid cystoscope

3.3

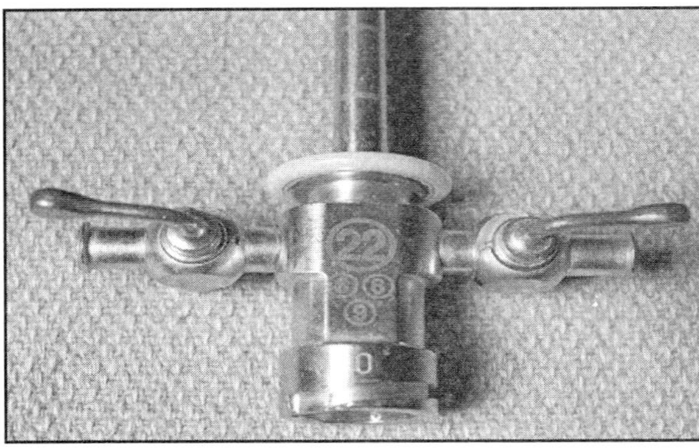

a) Describe the markings on the scope?

Answer:

a) The largest number indicates the outer diameter (22 Fr).

The smaller numbers below indicate the size of the two largest simultaneous instruments (6 Fr) or single largest instrument (9 Fr) that may be passed through the sheath.

3.4

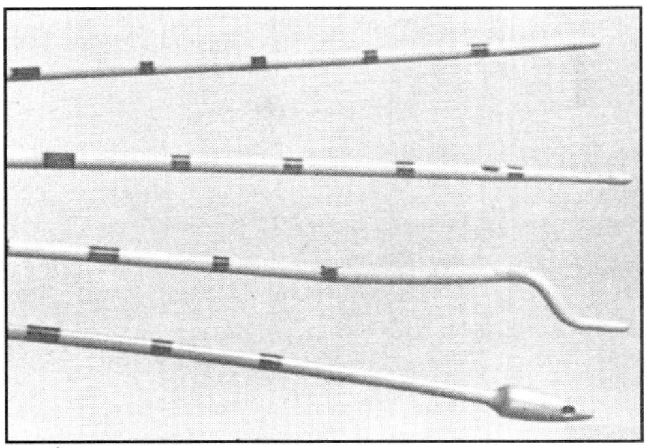

a) What does this figure suggest?

b) Best option for RGP?

Answer:

a) From top to bottom -Round, olive, spiral, and conical or "bulb" tips

b) Bulb or cone tip is most preferred

4.1

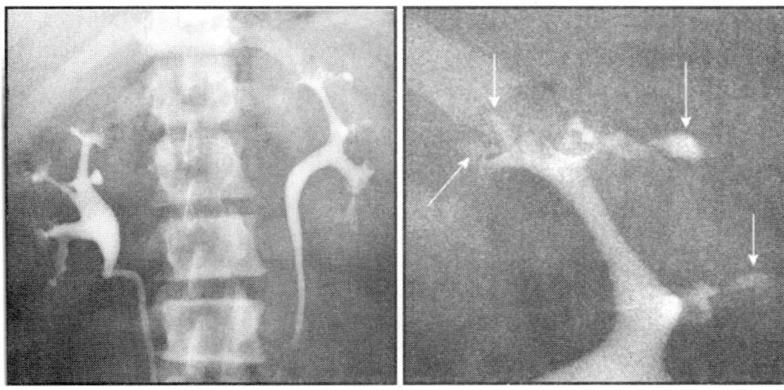

1. **What is this study? What does it show in this man with a long history of ankylosing spondylitis and recurrent bilateral loin pain?**
2. **What are the causes of this condition?**

Answer

1-IVU showing irregular calyces with contrast tracking out from the fornices into the papillae, producing an 'egg in cup' appearance.

Appearances are consistent with papillary necrosis, and in this case it was secondary to analgesic use.

2-Of all these, sickle cell disease and diabetes mellitus are the most common causes others being pyelonephritis, obstruction, TB and cirrhosis.

4.2

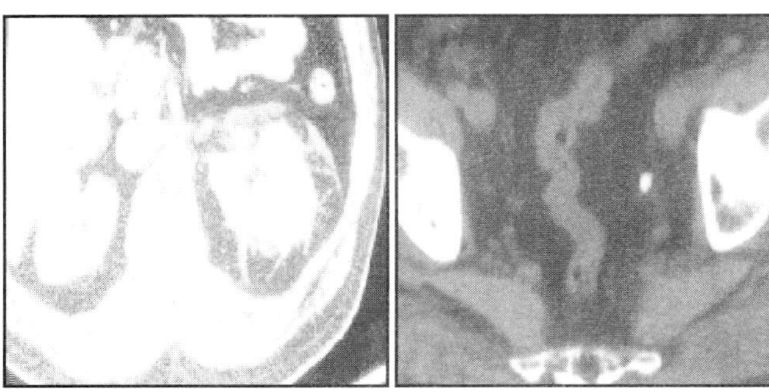

25 years old male with acute flank pain

a) **What are the findings in the above 2 slides?**

Answer:

a) Left perinephric stranding

Hydroureter

Left ureteric stone

Finding suggestive of ureteric stone with pyelonephritis

4.3

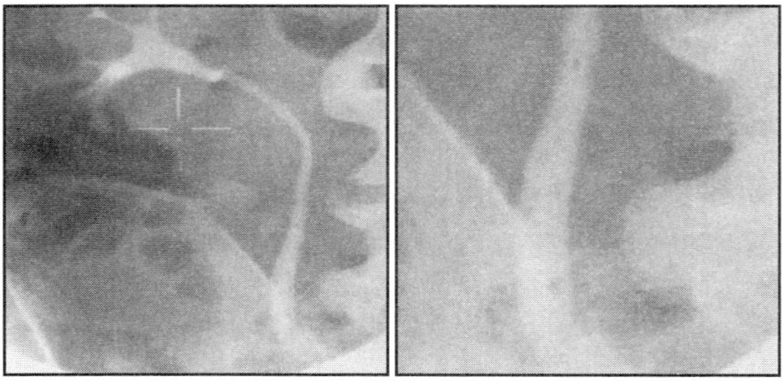

40 years old female with recurrent UTI

a) What are the findings in the above 2 slides?

Answer:

a) Submucosal haemorrhage has a cobblestone appearance

Sharply defined filling defects

Findings suggestive of ureteritis cystica

4.4

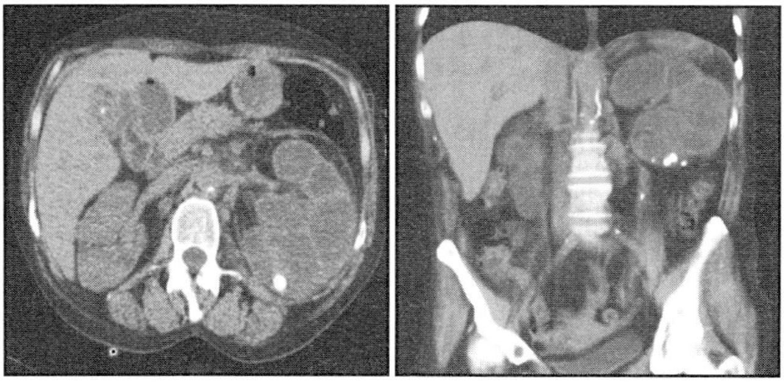

1. What do these images show and what is the diagnosis in this middle aged female with recurrent loin pain resistant to antibiotics?

2. **What is the treatment for this condition.**

Answer :

1. Left kidney is enlarged and contains multiple large, round, low attenuation (10–30 HU) lesions, but maintains a normal shape. The low attenuation lesions represent enlarged calyces, abscesses or granulomas (bear paw sign). A few calculi are seen within the kidney, perinephric stranding and thickening of Gerota's fascia.

   Appearances are of Xanthogranulomatous pyelonephritis (XGP).

2. Antibiotics and conservative therapy do not tend to be successful. Nephrectomy is the treatment of choice

4.5

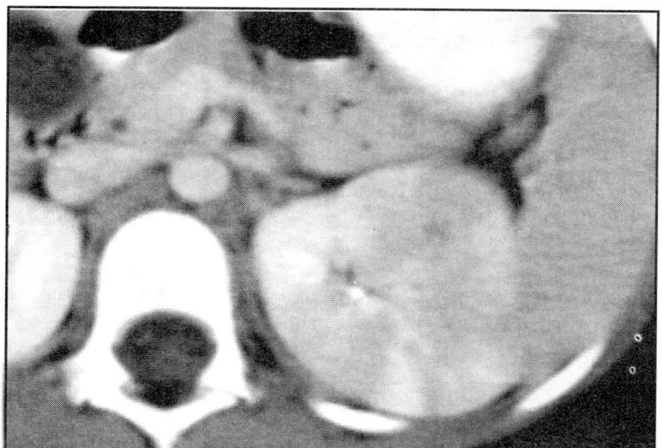

a) **What does this CT suggest?**

b) **What is the best treatment option?**

Answer:

a) CECT Scan showing acute left pyelonephritis.

b) Ambulatory patients should be treated with a fluoroquinolone for 7 days. Patients with complicated pyelonephritis and blood culture positive should be treated for 7 days with IV therapy. If blood cultures are negative 3-day IV therapy is sufficient. In either case, an appropriate oral antimicrobial drug should be continued in full dosage for an additional 10 to 14 days.

4.6

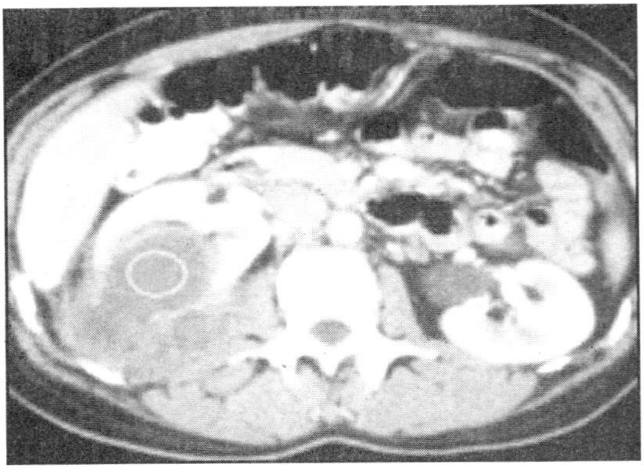

a) **What does this CT suggest?**

b) **Best treatment options?**

Answer:

a) Right renal abscess with perirenal extension

b) Less than 3 cm abscesses in diameter -IV antibiotics and careful observation

Abscesses 3 to 5 cm in diameter and smaller abscesses in immunocompromised hosts or those that do not respond to antimicrobial therapy percutaneous drainage

Abscesses greater than 5 cm in diameter -Surgical drainage

4.7

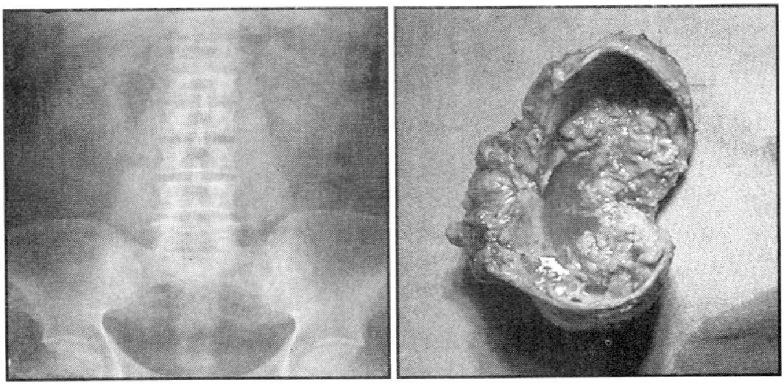

a) **What is the finding?**

b) **Which is the most common organism involved with the disease?**

Answer :

a) Specimen shows Xanthogranulomatous pyelonephritis (Stone, obstruction and infection)

b) Proteus

4.8

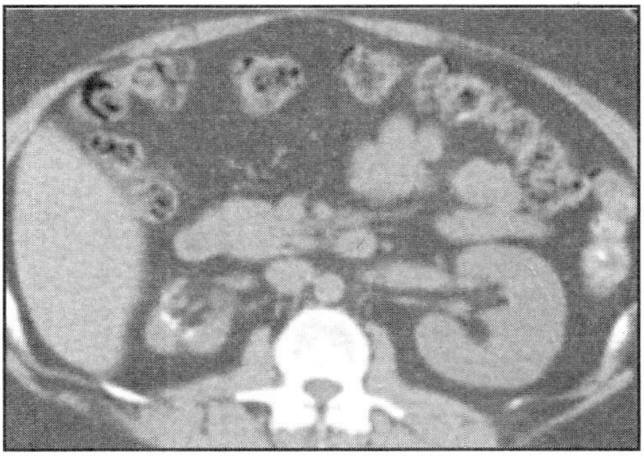

a) What does this CT suggest?

b) When leukocyte and hyaline casts are present in tubules it can be termed as?

Answer:

a) Small, deformed right kidney with multiple deep scars and dystrophic calcifications -Chronic pyelonephritis

b) Leukocyte and hyaline casts are sometimes present in the tubules; the latter may cause resemblance to the thyroid colloid, hence the description renal thyroidisation

4.9

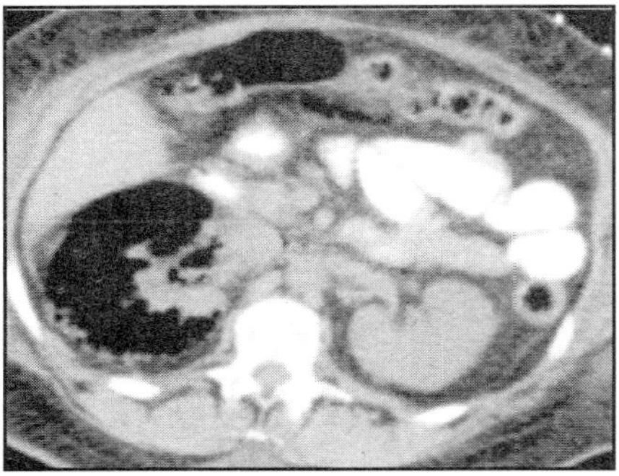

a) What does this CT suggest?

b) What is the classic triad and most common organism associated with it ?

Answer:

a) Type1 emphysematous pyelonephritis

b) Classic triad of fever, vomiting, and flank pain and most common organism associated with it is E Coli

4.10

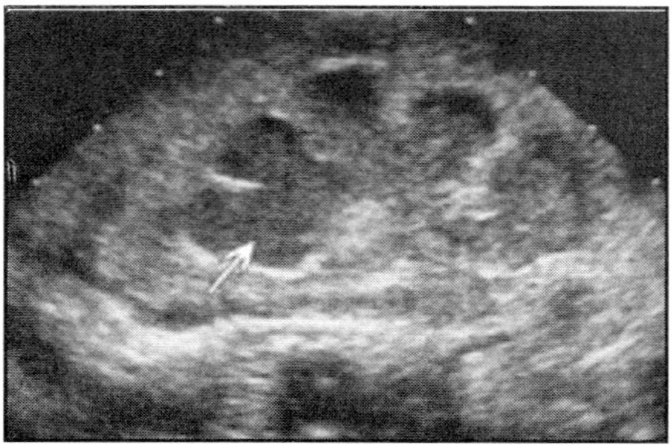

a) What does this USG suggest?

b) Best treatment option?

Answer:

a) USG image shows a dilated collecting system that is nearly completely filled with echogenic debris (arrow) secondary to pyonephrosis.

b) Appropriate antimicrobial drugs and drainage of the infected pelvis. A ureteral catheter can be passed to drain the kidney, but if the obstruction prevents this, a percutaneous nephrostomy tube should be placed

4.11

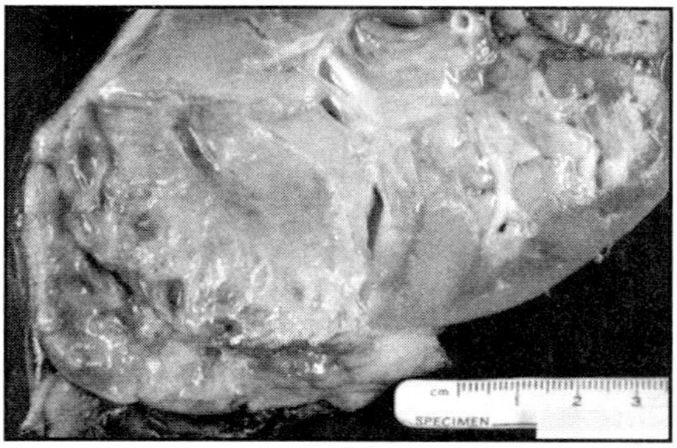

a) What does this specimen suggest?

b) Best treatment option?

Answer:

a) Specimen shows the thick-walled, yellowish capsule of the focal lesion-Xanthogranulomatous pyelonephritis

b) Antimicrobial therapy may be necessary to stabilize the patient preoperatively, and, occasionally, long-term antimicrobial therapy will eradicate the infection and restore renal function. If localized xanthogranulomatous pyelonephritis is diagnosed preoperatively or at exploration, it is amenable to partial nephrectomy

4.12

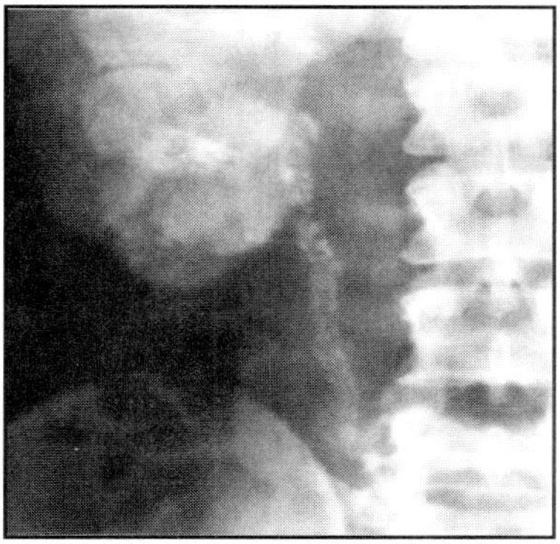

a) What does this specimen suggest?

Answer:

a) Calcifications of renal parenchyma due to tuberculosis. Abdominal radiograph demonstrates extensive calcifications forming a cast of the kidney and ureter.

4.13

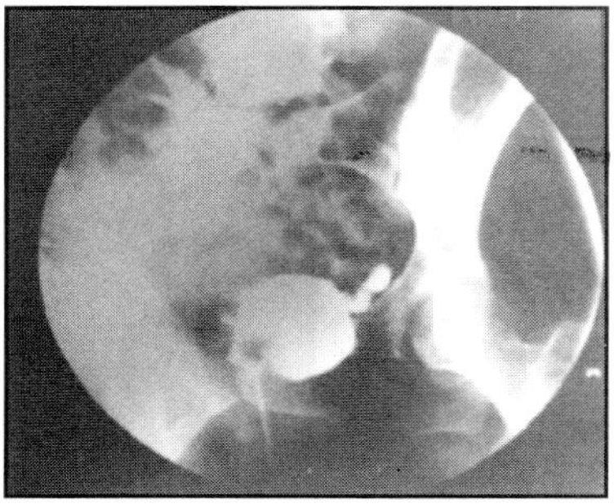

20 years old lady with extreme frequency

a) Name the study

b) Finding

Answer:

a) MCU

b) Thimble bladder with left VUR

4.14

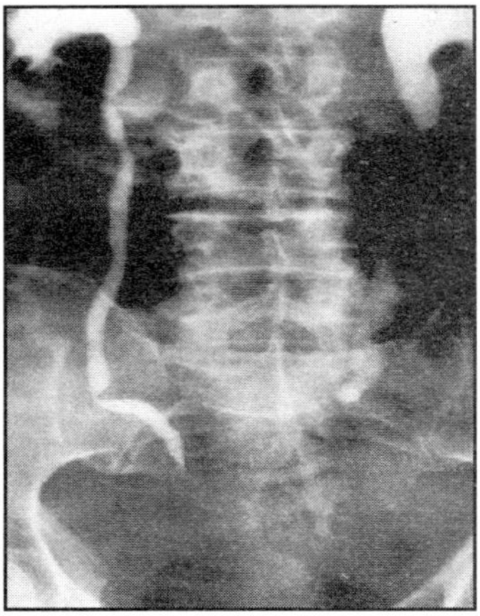

a) What is shown in the above figure?

b) What can be the condition associated with it?

Answer:

a) Bilateral lower ureteric stricture

b) Tuberculosis

4.15

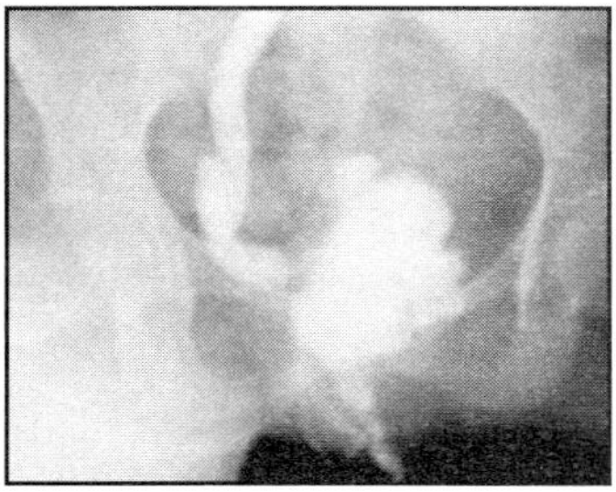

a) What is shown in the above figure?

b) What can be the condition associated with it?

Answer:

a) Thimble shaped irregular bladder with low capacity and UV junction stricture

b) Tuberculosis

4.16

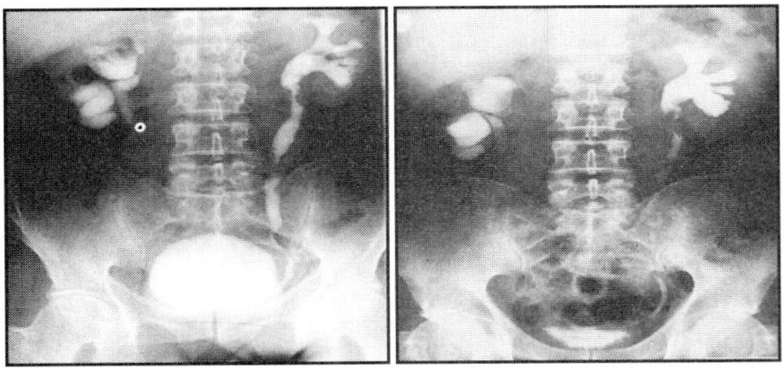

A 45-year-old man presents with dysuria and urinary frequency. Initial urinary tests reveal microscopic haematuria and sterile pyuria. A second 84-year-old man presents with night sweats and a swelling in his loin.

1. Describe the images shown and the likely diagnosis.

Answer :

1.IVU films shows left kidney with blunted, dilated calyces and the left ureter demonstrates an irregular 'jagged' contour with alternating strictures and dilatations.

The right kidney shows dilated calyces secondary to infundibular strictures, and cephalic retraction of an atrophic renal pelvis.

The appearances are highly suspicious for renal and ureteric tuberculosis

4.17

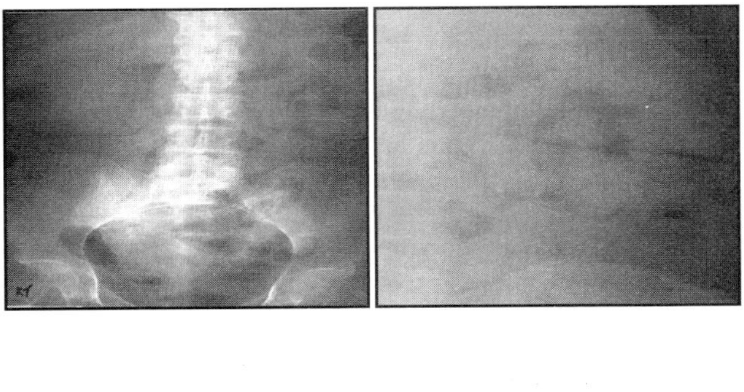

A 75-year-old diabetic woman presented with fever and flank pain.

1. **Describe the images and the most likely diagnosis?**
2. **What is the aetiology?**

Answer :

1. Plain film of the abdomen showing abnormal gas shadow outlining the left pelvicalyceal system and a further gas shadow centrally in the pelvis which outlines the bladder. Appearances are highly suggestive of emphysematous pyelonephritis.
2. This is an acute, life-threatening infection of the kidney with gas formation. It is associated with diabetes most commonly, but also immunocompromise or ureteric obstruction. The usual organisms are *E. coli, Klebsiella or Proteus* .

4.18

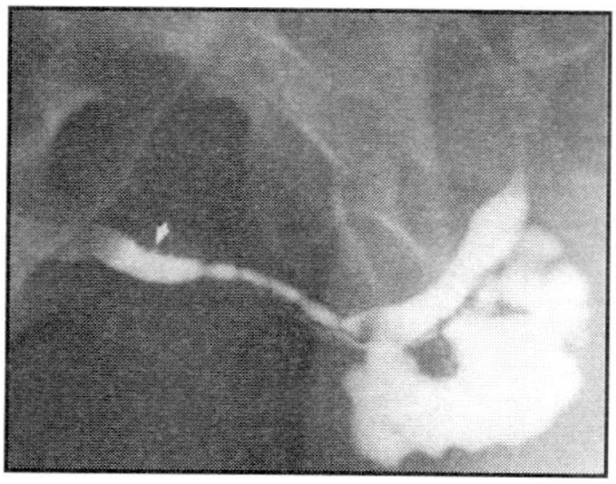

a) Name the investigation?

b) Mention initial management of the problem?

Answer:

a) RGU showing anterior urethral stricture with extravasation of contrast in patient with periurethal abscess secondary to stricture

b) Suprapubic catheterisation

4.19

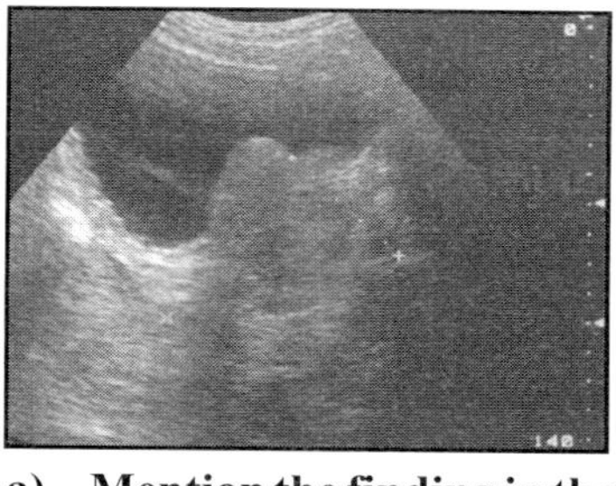

a) Mention the finding in the figure?

b) What is the most important differential diagnosis?

Answer:

a) It is the sagittal view of the prostate, figure shows the middle lobe of prostate extending into the bladder

b) Middle lobe of prostate can be confused with bladder mass

4.20

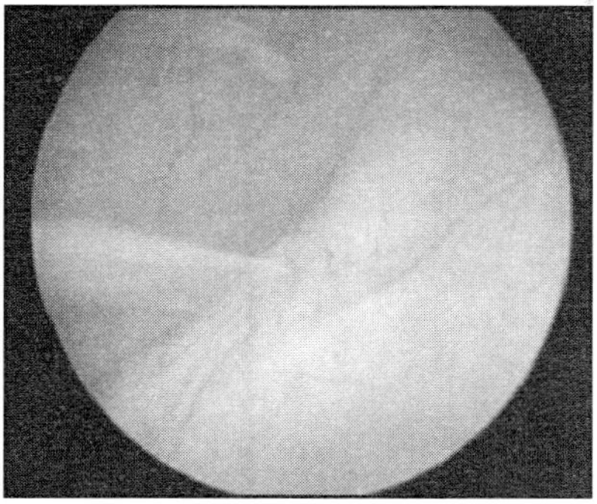

a) Mention the finding in the figure?

b) What is the treatment?

Answer:

a) Chyluria

b) DEC, 6 mg/kg/day in three divided doses for 2 weeks

Sclerosing therapy with0.2% betadine or silver nitrate

If above therapy fails then consider pyelolymphatic discconection

6.1

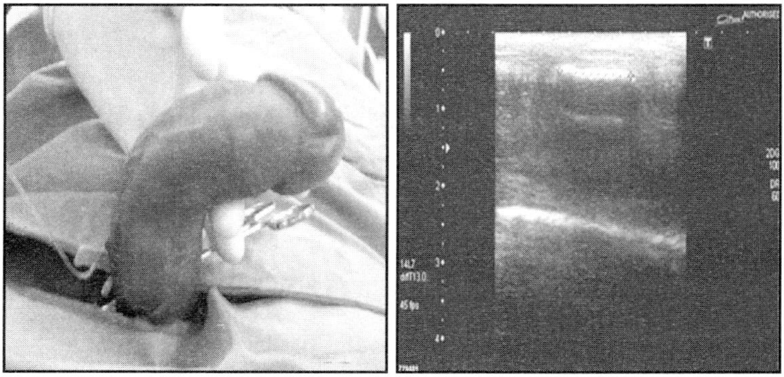

1. What is shown in the artificial erection test below, what is the diagnosis and what are the features of this condition?

2. How is this condition assessed?

Answer

1. 90° lateral curvature of the midshaft of the penis. The diagnosis is Peyronie's disease. The features include penile pain, curvature and fl accidity distal to the curve.

2. Palpation for a plaque in the fl accid state and photography or injection of the penis with a vasoactive agent may be required to formally document curvature.

   Figure (b) is a longitudinal grey-scale ultrasound image showing a long calcified tunical plaque along the dorsal surface of the cavernosa.

6.2

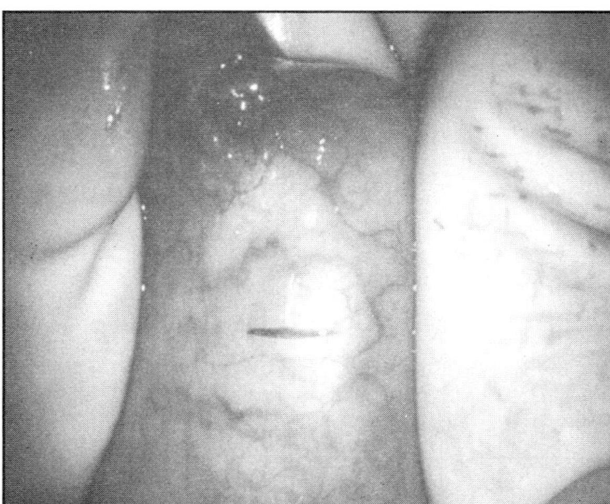

a) Mention the procedure done in the figure?

b) Indication of procedure?

Answer:

a) Testicular biopsy

b) Azoospermic patients with normal testicular size, palpable vas deferens, and normal serum FSH levels require a diagnostic testicular biopsy

7.1

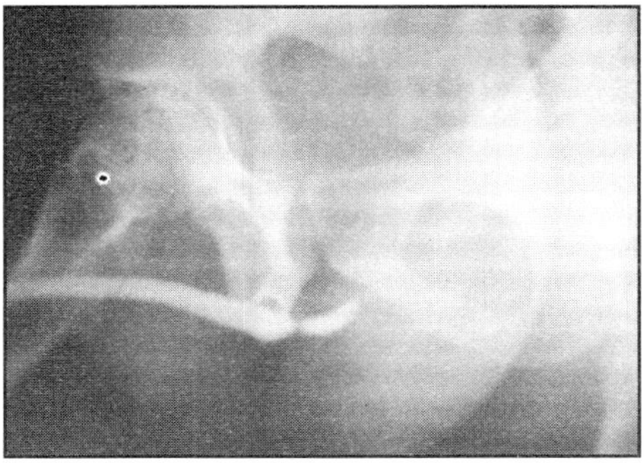

a) Name the study

b) Identify the diagnosis

Answer:

a) RGU

b) Bulbomembranous stricture

7.2

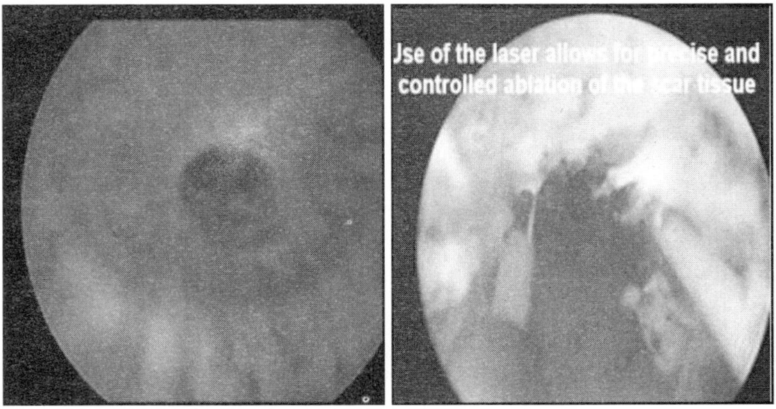

a) What is the finding?

b) Mention the procedure performed?

Answer:

a) Urethral stricture at urethroscopy

b) Laser Optic internal urethrotomy

7.3

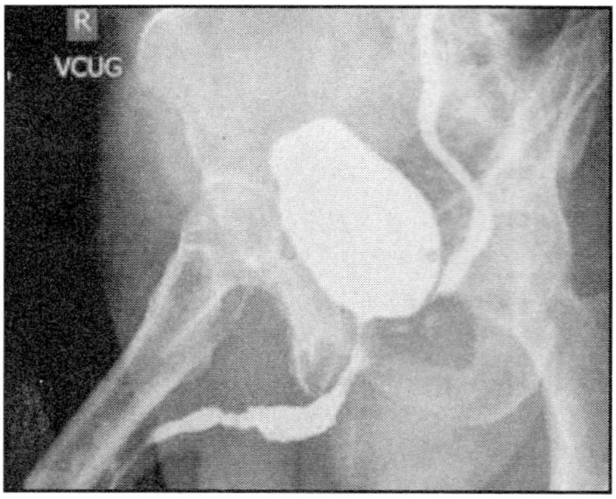

a) Name the investigation?

b) Mention the diagnosis?

Answer:

a) MCUG / VCUG

b) Stricture urethra with left sided VUR

7.4

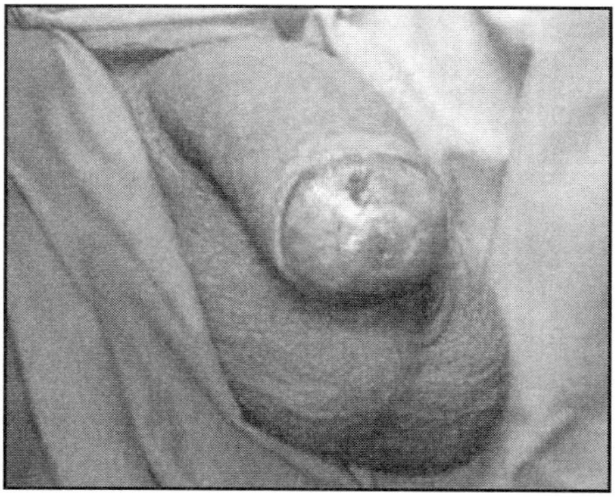

a) What is the finding and is it premalignant?

b) Mention the investigation require to evaluate the disease?

Answer:

a) BXO changes at glans and meatus. It is premalignant condition (9%)

b) RGU/MCU

7.5

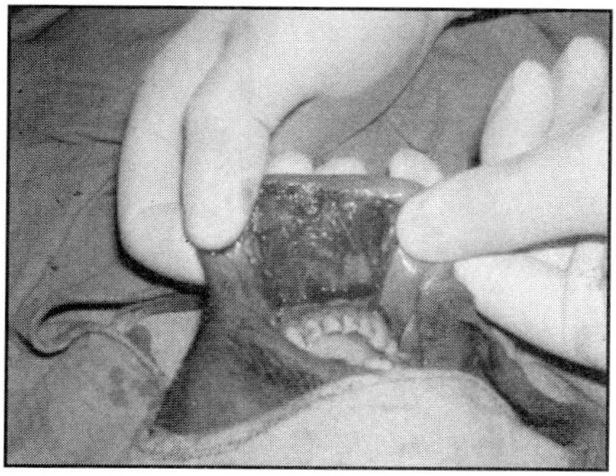

a) What is shown in the above figure?

b) What are its advantages over other grafts?

Answer:

a) Harvesting of buccal mucosa from cheek

b) Panlaminar plexus.

Graft can be thinned and still preserves its physical characteristics.

Graft is thought to have optimal vascular characteristics

7.6

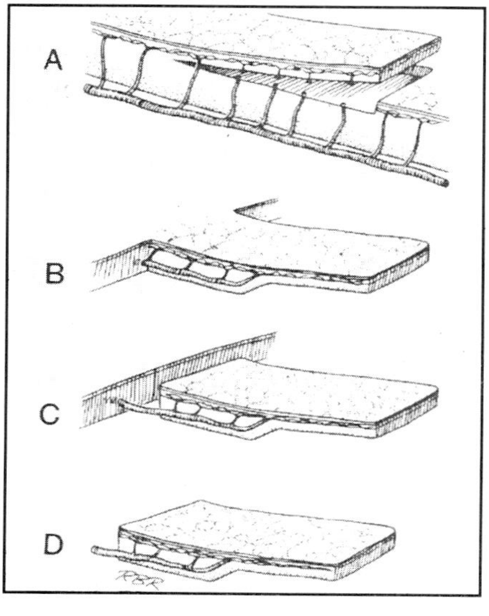

a) **Name the types of flap raised?**

Answer:

a) A-Random flap

B-Peninsular

C-Island flap

D-Free flap

7.7

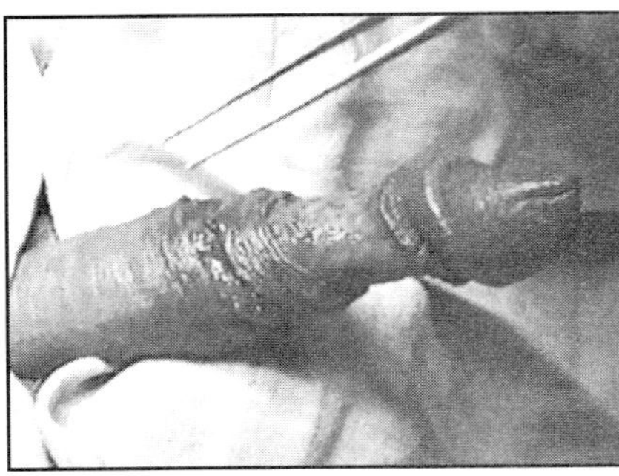

a) **Name the types of flap raised?**

b) **What are the advantages of this flap?**

Answer:

a) Circumferential penile flap

b) Advantages are

- Robust blood supply
- Upto 15 cm length can be acheived and does not rely on graft bed condition

7.8

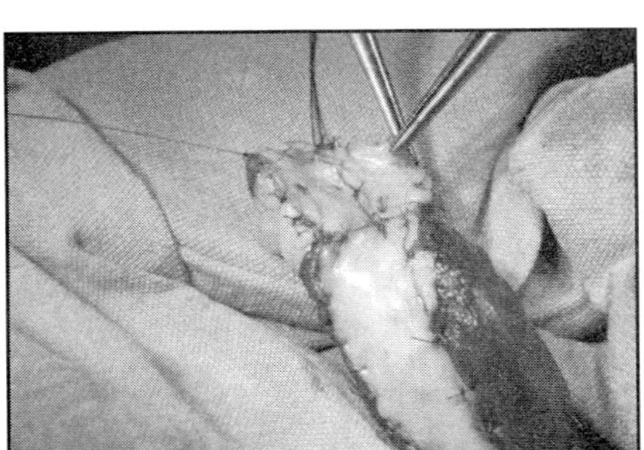

a) **Name the procedure being done?**

Answer:

a) Stage 1 Johansons urethroplasty with buccal mucosa implantation (Lay open with perineal urethroplasty)

7.9

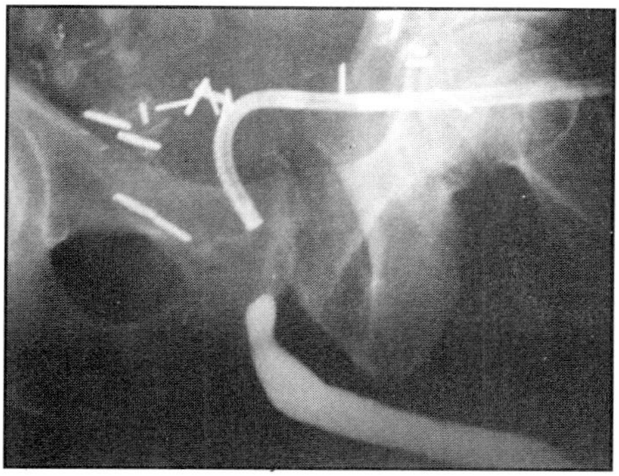

a) **What is the diagnosis?**

b) **What is the management?**

Answer:

a) RGU being done with bougie placed through SPC to determine the length of defect

b) Anastomotic urethroplasty is the procedure of choice in the totally obliterated bulbar urethra after a straddle injury

7.10

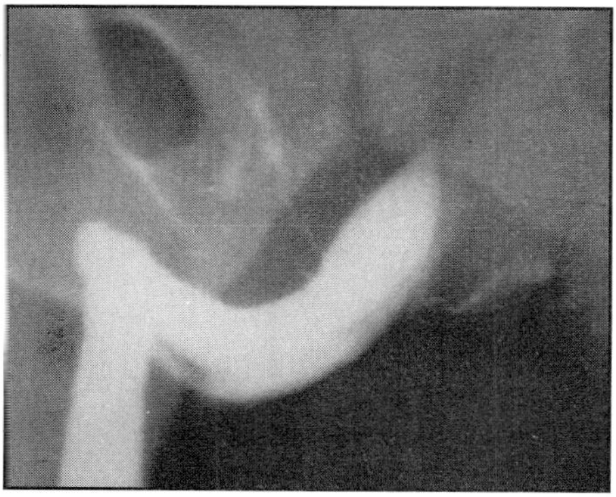

30 year old with history of pelvic trauma

a) **What are the findings in the above slide?**

Answer:

a) Local contrast extravasation confined to buck fascia

MCU is suggestive of straddle injury

7.11

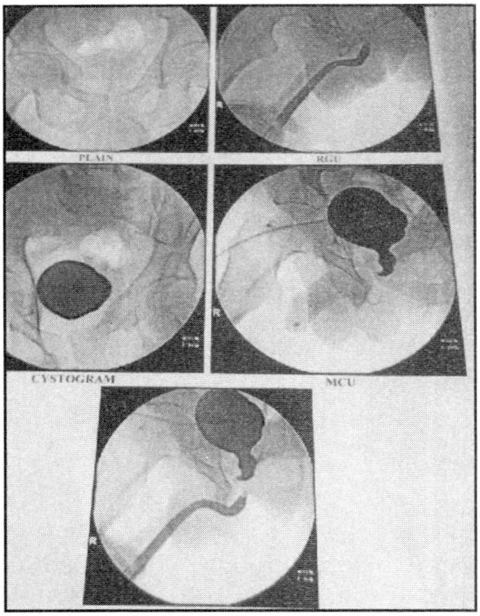

a) What is the finding?

b) Mention the investigation required to evaluate the disease?

Answer:

a) Pelvic fracture with urethral distraction injury

b) Open perineal anastamotic urethroplasty

7.12

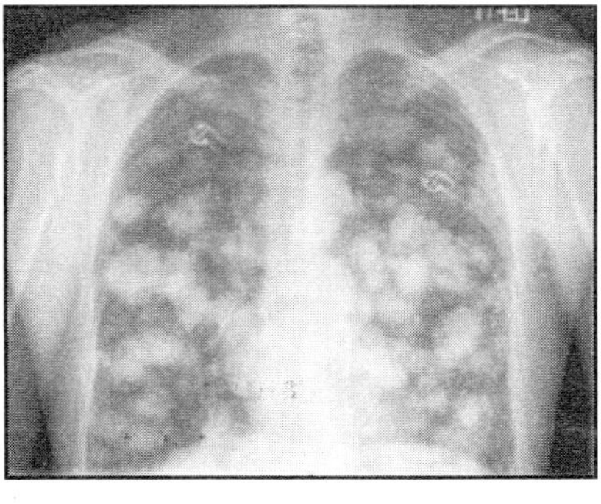

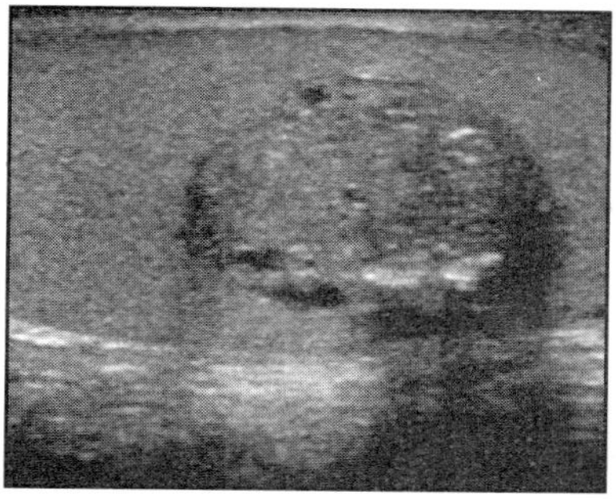

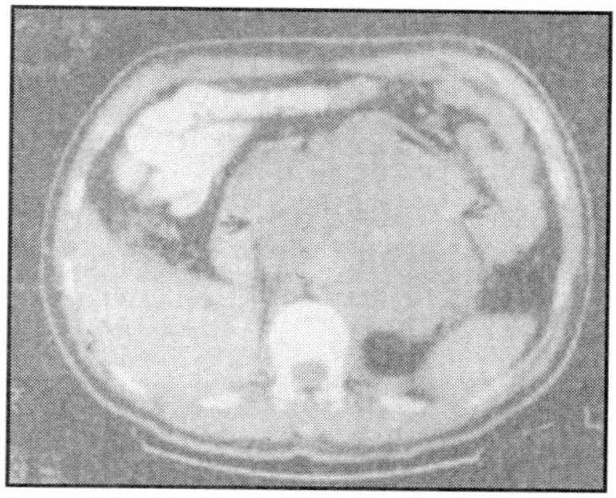

a) **What does this CXR, USG and CECT suggest?**

b) **Which is the most common histological type between 30-40 years of age ?**

Answer:

a) X ray chest of a patient with metastatic tumour (Cotton ball appearance)

USG showing heterogeneous testicular mass

CECT scan showing large para-aortic retro-peritoneal mass (patient of testicular tumour)

b) Seminoma is rare before age 10 years and after age 60 years, but it is the most common histologic type overall, with a peak incidence between 35 and 39 years

7.13

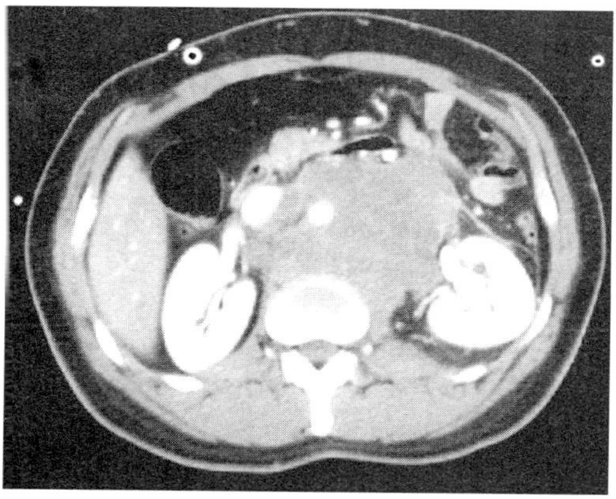

a) **What does this CT suggest?**

b) **What is the treatment of stage 2c seminoma testis?**

Answer :

a) CT abdomen showing extensive retroperitoneal lymphadenopathy in patient with seminoma of testis

b) Start cisplatin based chemotherapy, if residual mass is discrete and >3cm-surgical resection

7.14

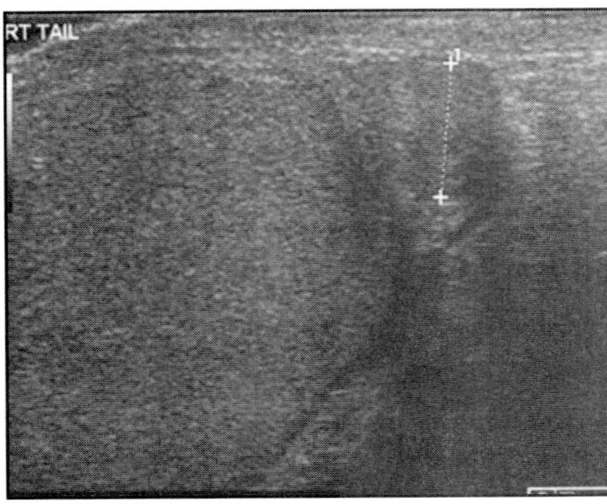

A 38-year-old man presents with a self-palpated, painless, small firm swelling in his right scrotum. He thinks it has been present for several years. The only abnormality found was within the right epididymal tail.

1. **Describe the abnormality.**
2. **What is the differential diagnosis for this lesion?**

Answer

1. These longitudinal sonographic images reveal a focal, oval, well-circumscribed solid epididymal tail mass (between callipers) of lower echo refl ectivity compared to the adjacent testis. There is increased vascularity within the lesion and the tail of the epididymis as a whole.
2. The age, presentation and location of the mass suggest a diagnosis of adenomatoid tumour of the epididymis. Adenomatoid tumours are the commonest tumour associated with the epididymis but arise from mesothelial cells.

   Other benign epididymal lesions include papillary cystadenomas, which are found with von Hippel-Lindau disease

9.1

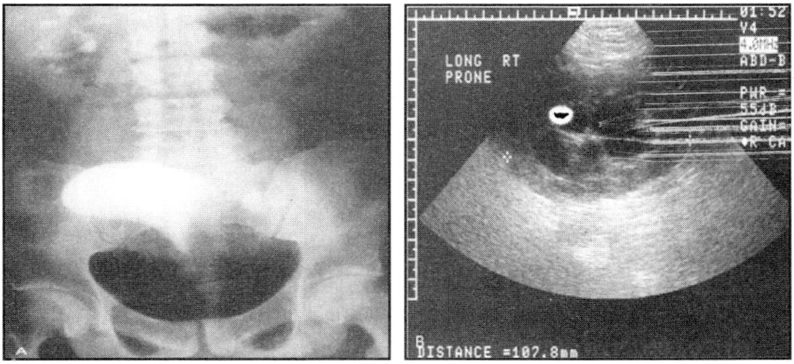

a) What are the findings?

b) What is the diagnosis?

Answer:

a) IVU demonstrates severe right hydronephrosis and the classic vertical elongation of the bladder (pear or gourd shape bladder). USG demonstrates characteristic findings of hydronephrosis with hypoechoic areas indicating dilated calyces.

b) Pelvic lipomatosis

9.2

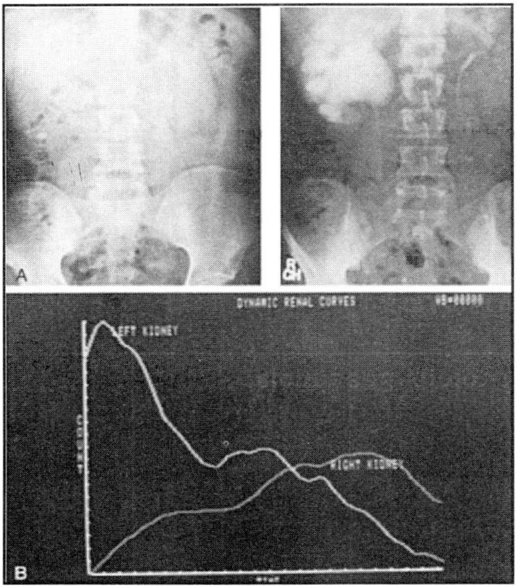

24 Years old male with history of right pyeloplasty 6 months back, now presented with following investigations on follow up:

a) What are the findings?

b) What is the diagnosis?

Answer :

a) X-ray KUB- Right lower pole stone of 1 cm.

IVU-After contrast medium is injected, there is obvious dilatation of the collecting system with a normal caliber ureter.

Diuretic renogram reveals a shift to the right in uptake by the right kidney, followed by a rapid fall-off of the radionuclide after injection of furosemide. This is consistent with dilatation without obstruction.

b) Right residual HDN following previous PUJO

9.3

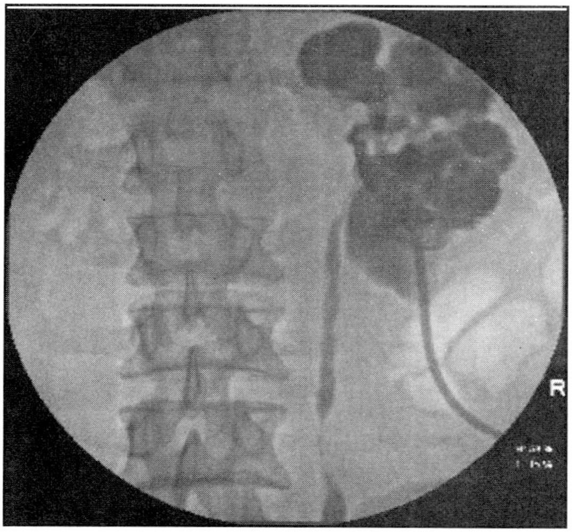

a) What is this investigation?

b) Best treatment option?

Answer:

a) Nephrostogram showing hydronephrotic kidney with long proximal ureteric stricture.

b) Ileal conduit

9.4

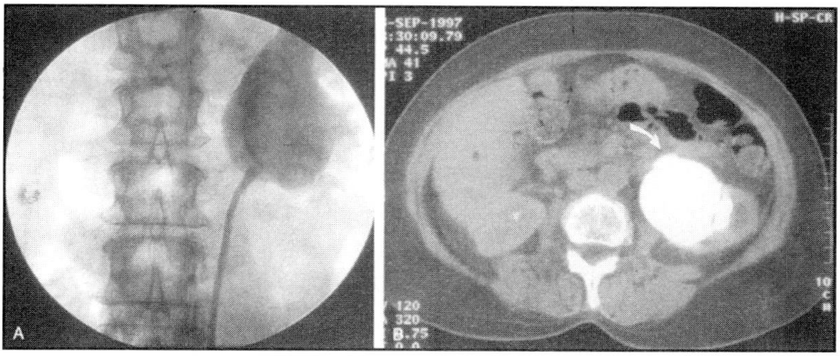

a) What is the diagnosis?

b) What is the management?

Answer:

a) RGU with left UPJ obstruction reveals a "high insertion" of the left ureter.

CT scan reveals the ureter inserting on the anatomically anterior aspect of the renal pelvis.

b) Dismembered pyeloplasty

9.5

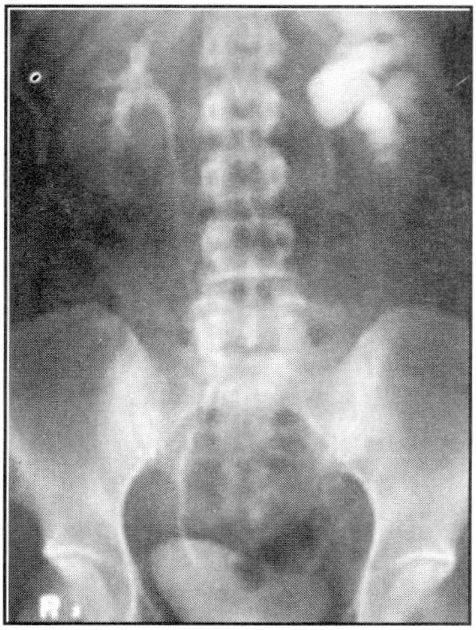

a) What does this IVU suggest?

b) Best treatment option?

Answer:

a) Left HDN with PUJO

b) Confirm diagnosis with DTPA followed by laparoscopic pyeloplasty

9.6

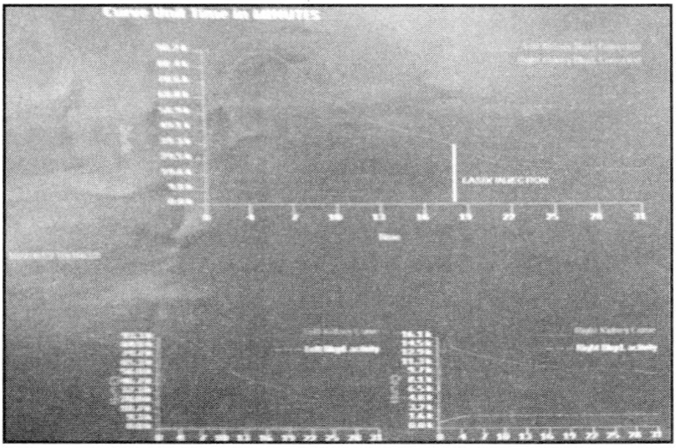

a) Identify the scan

b) Diagnosis

Answer:

a) DTPA

b) Right PUJ obstruction

9.7

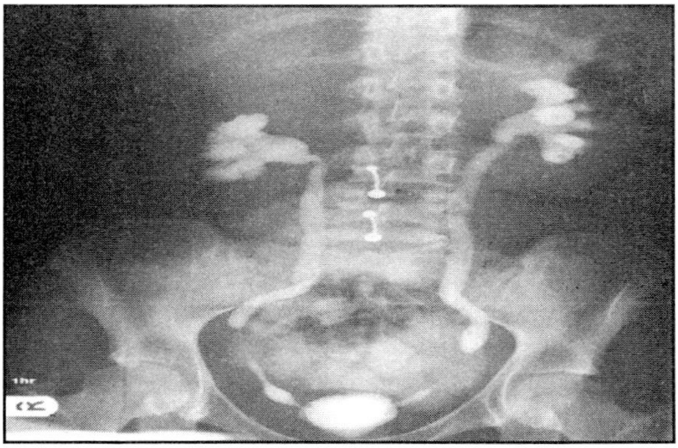

This woman presented with chronic pelvic and bilateral loin pain, which had cyclical variability. Microscopic haematuria was also noted.

1. **Describe the findings on this image taken as part of an intravenous urogram.**
2. **Suggest a differential diagnosis and further investigations.**

Answer

1. Postcontrast image from an IVU series showing smooth and dilated upper tracts but otherwise normal. This patient proved to have bilateral endometriosis.
2. The smoothness of the mucosal outline of the strictures would suggest an extra luminal mass of benign aetiology. Possible causes are endometriosis, post radiation, retroperitoneal fi brosis, extra-luminal compression by pelvic masses (e.g. ovarian cysts) pelvic infl ammatory disease, lymphadenopathy, collections or ischaemic strictures following pelvic surgery.

Further investigations that may help are CT/MRI +/− biopsy. Ureteroscopy is unlikely to contribute other than to confirm the strictures, but occasionally the nodules of endometriosis may be seen in the wall. The diagnosis is often made at diagnostic laparoscopy.

9.8

(a)

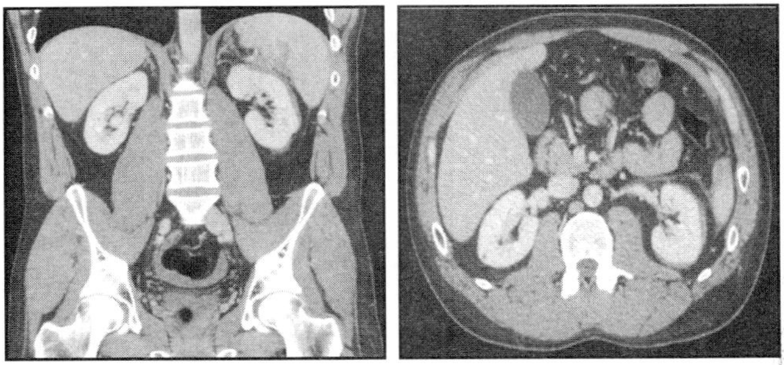

(b)

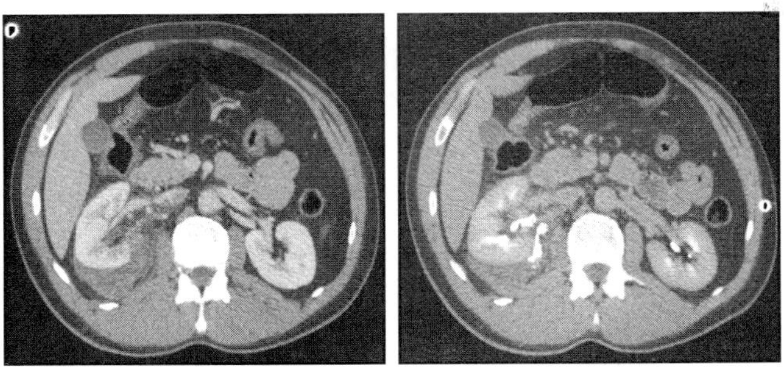

CT scans of a 25-year-old male who was involved in road traffic accident (RTA).

Describe the findings in figure (a) and (b).

Answer

(a) There is a crescentic low attenuation region following the convexity of the left renal cortex, compatible with subcapsular haematoma.

This is a Grade I renal injury

(b) Laceration extends outside the kidney resulting in a perinephric haematoma or collection.

On the delayed phase image contrast excreted into the collecting system has also leaked into the collection confirming damage to the collecting system i.e. grade IV injury.

9.9

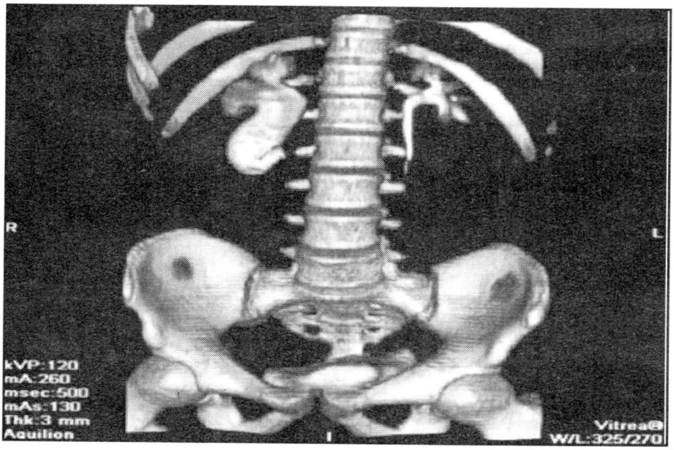

CT scan of a 16-year-old who presented with right loin pain and hamaturia, what is the diagnosis in this case and what operation was performed to rectify this congenital abnormality?

Answer.

The CT reconstruction shows appearances in keeping with a retrocaval ureter.

There is a classic S shaped bend in the upper ureter centred around the L3 vertebra

10.1

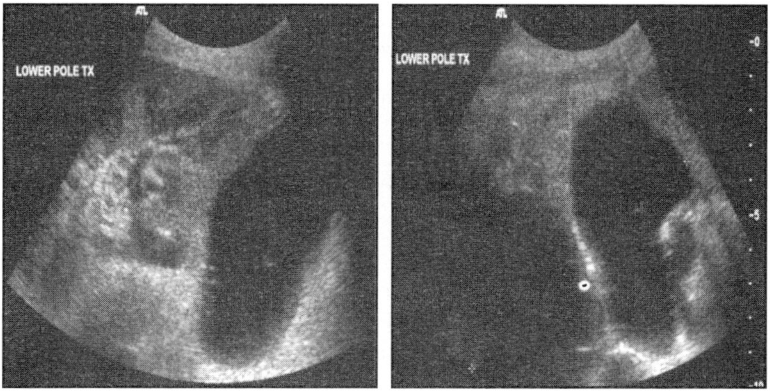

A routine post transplant US was performed on this patient 2 weeks following his surgery. The transplant is functioning normally, and the patient is well.

1. **Describe the findings.**
2. **What is the differential diagnosis?**
3. **How should this be managed?**

Answer :

1. These ultrasound images through the lower pole of the renal transplant show a fluid collection below the renal hilum.
2. This may represent:

   Urinary bladder (may lie adjacent to a transplant kidney)

   Urinoma

   Lymphocoele (5-15% of patients)

   Abscess

   Haematoma (tends to be more echogenic)
3. Drainage can usually be performed percutaneously under ultrasound guidance, but simple drainage is not always curative and surgical exclusion may be required. Regarding surgery, if this proves to be a lymphocoele then surgical marsupialisation is required.

11.1

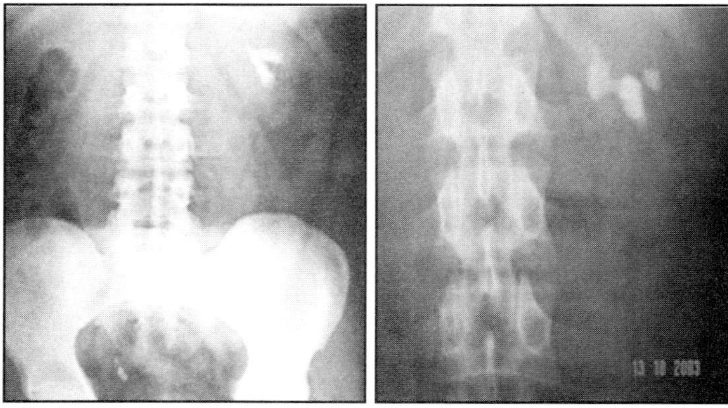

a) Identify the abnormality in both x ray

b) Treatment of choice and most common complication following the procedure

Answer:

a) Renal stone

b) Renal stone more than 2 cm treatment of choice is PCNL and most common complication following it is haemorrhage

11.2

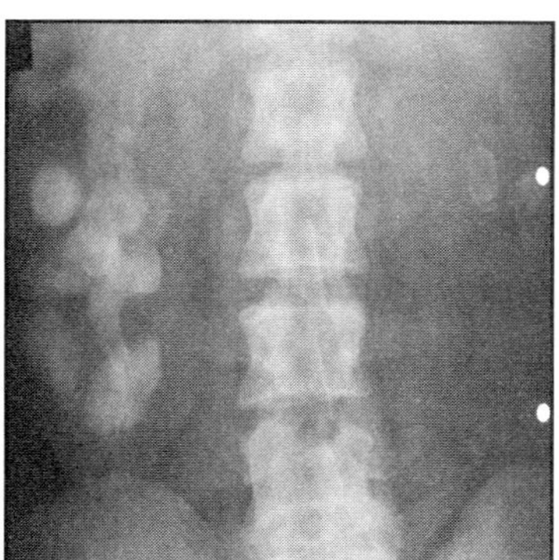

a) Identify the abnormality in x-ray

b) Most likely composition of this abnormality

c) Write five indications for metabolic work up

d) Incidence of stone in HSK and PUJO

Answer:

a) Staghorn stone

b) Struvite

c) Indications for a Metabolic Stone Evaluation

Recurrent stone formers

Strong family history of stones

Pathologic skeletal fractures

Osteoporosis

History of urinary tract infections with calculi

d) The incidence of renal calculi in patients with ureteropelvic junction obstruction and horse shoe kidney is 20% each

11.3

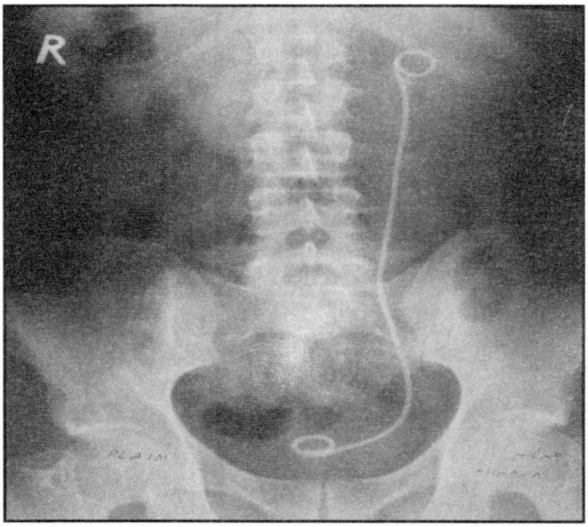

a) Identify the x-ray

b) Write indications for pre-ESWL DJ- stenting

c) What does 6/26 size stands for?

Answer:

a) Left DJ Stent in situ

b) Renal stone >20mm and in patients with solitary functioning kidney, DJS should be placed before ESWL

c) 6 Fr is the diameter of stent and 26 cm is the length of stent

11.4

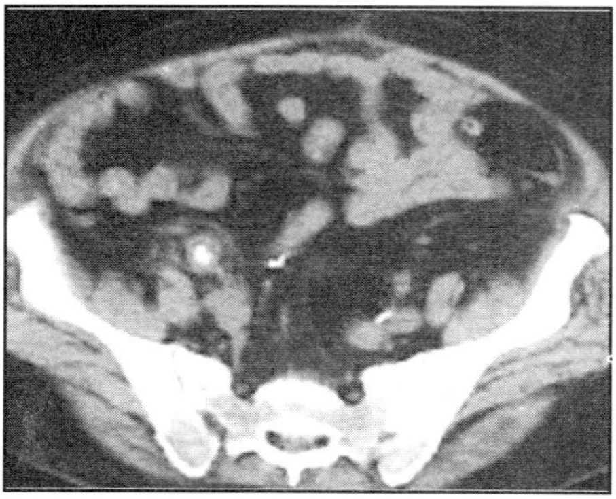

a) What are the findings in the above slide?

b) What can be the differential diagnosis of above finding?

Answer:

a) Right ureteral stone with hydroureteronephrosis

b) Ureteral clot or ureteral tumor

11.5

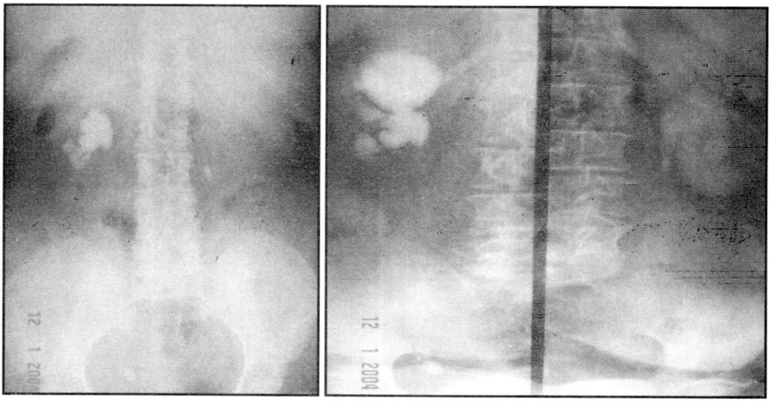

a) What is the diagnosis considering both X ray- KUB and IVU

b) Appropriate treatment options for Right & left side

Answer:

a) Right renal and lower ureteric stone and left upper ureteric stone

b) Right URSL followed by right PCNL. Push back and left ESWL

11.6

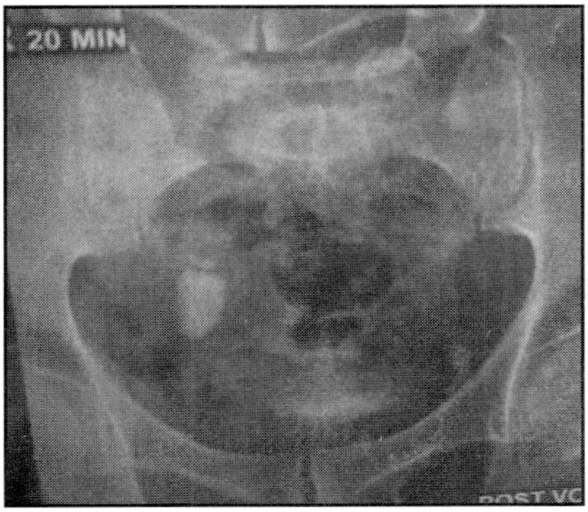

a) **What is the diagnosis in the above IVU**

b) **Appropriate treatment options**

Answer:

a) Right lower ureteric stone

b) Open or laparoscopic ureterolithotomy is the most appropriate option

11.7

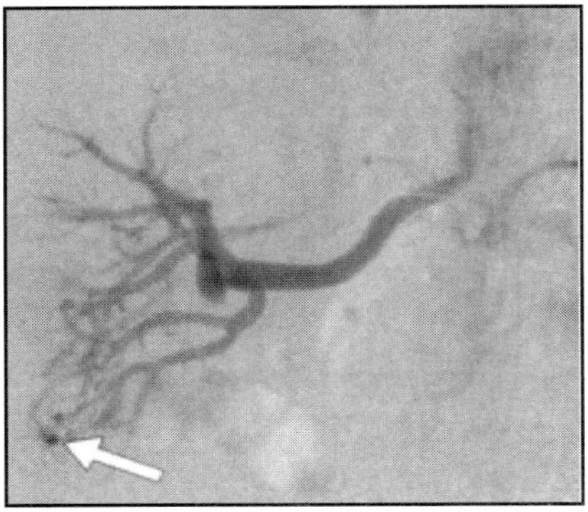

a) **What is the investigation**

b) **Name the findings seen in this investigation and condition associated with it.**

Answer:

a) Renal angiography

b) Psedoaneurysm and it can be following PCNL

11.8

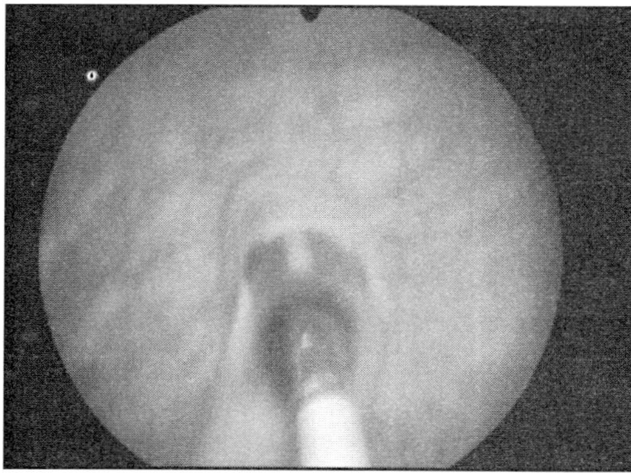

a) What is being done in the above image?

b) Indication

Answer:

a) Balloon dilatation of ureteric orifice.

b) Generally done when ureteroscope cannot be introduced through ureteric orifice.

11.9

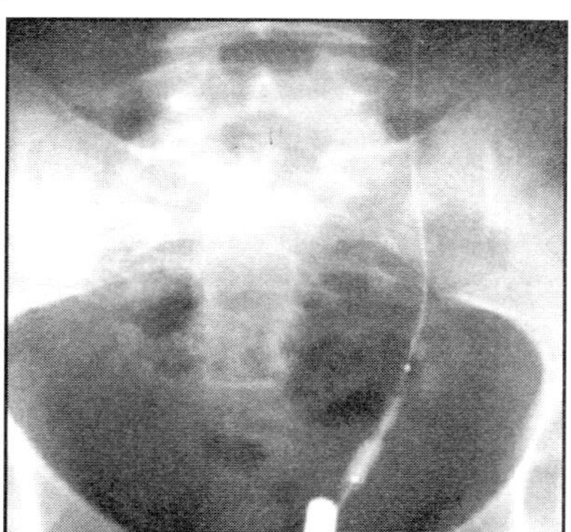

a) What is being done in this study?

b) How much is the pressure generated by this equipment?

Answer:

a) Balloon dilatation of ureteric orifice

b) 15 atm

11.10

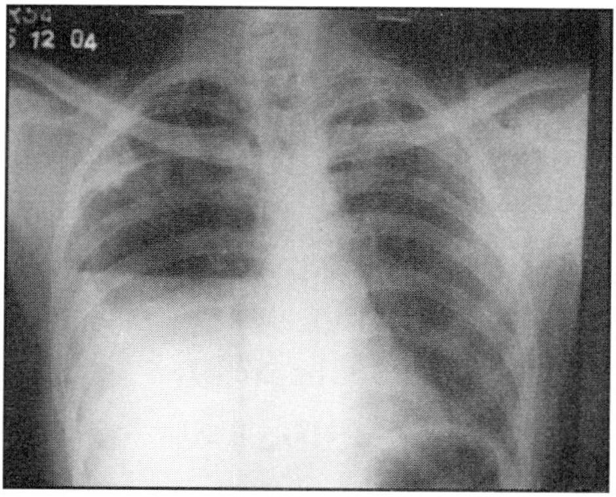

Chest X ray following PCNL

a) Finding

b) Treatment

Answer

a) Right hydropneumothorax

b) Intercostal drainage by chest tube

11.11

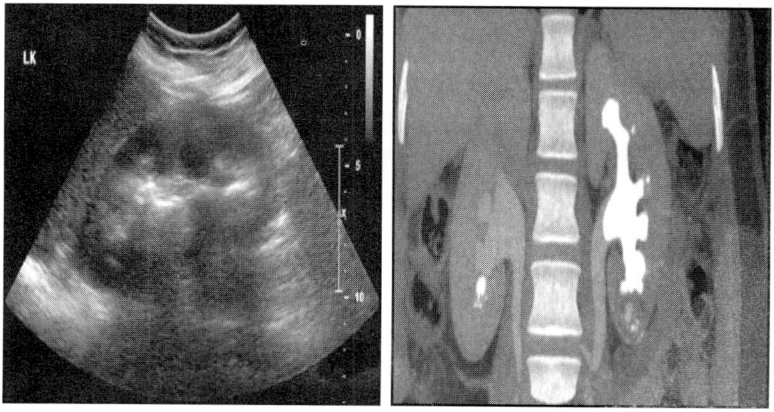

A 35-year-old lady presents with recurrent urinary tract infections.

1. Describe the US and CT findings.

2. Describe the management of this condition

Answer

1. The ultrasound scan demonstrates a large echogenic lesion occupying the central portion of the left kidney which casts an acoustic shadow.

CT image shows a large calcified stone which completely opacifi es the left renal pelvicalyceal system. A small stone is also seen in the infundibulum to a lower pole calyx of the right kidney. The appearance on the left is of a staghorn calculus which is composed of calcium magnesium ammonium phosphate (struvite).

2. Firstly the presence of infection should be excluded

The residual renal function should be measured (by a DMSA or MAG3 nuclear medicine test).

Then depending on the patient's co-morbidities and the likelihood of recovery of renal function either percutaneous nephrolithotomy, open pyelolithotomy or nephrectomy are the main treatment options.

11.12

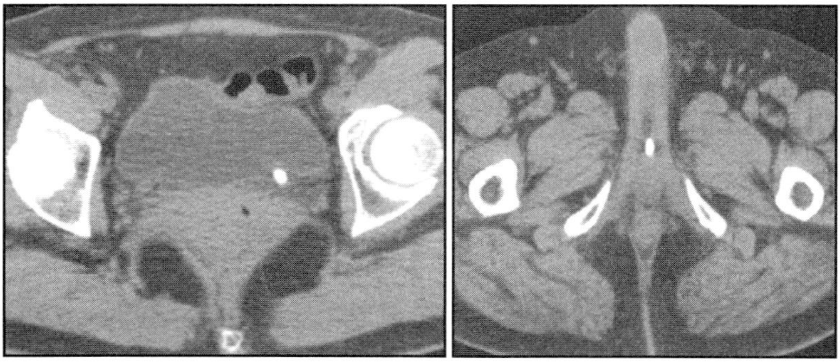

1. **What are the findings in figure at (a) and (b)**
2. **Management**

Answer

a) Stone at ureterovesical stone.

b) Stone in prostatic urethra

2. Management for ureterovesical stone is medical expulsion therapy for 7-10 days if stone is not expelled out, ureteroscopy is the treatment of choice

For prostatic urethra stone it is pushed back into bladder, than broken by lithotripsy and then removed by cystoscope

11.13

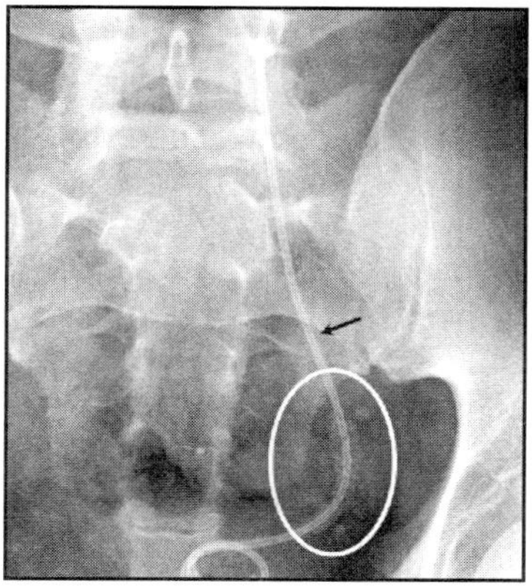

a) **Name the finding?**

b) **What is the best treatment for this?**

Answer:

a) Steinstrasse

b) Ureteroscopic intervention is definitive and predictable with an immediate success

11.14

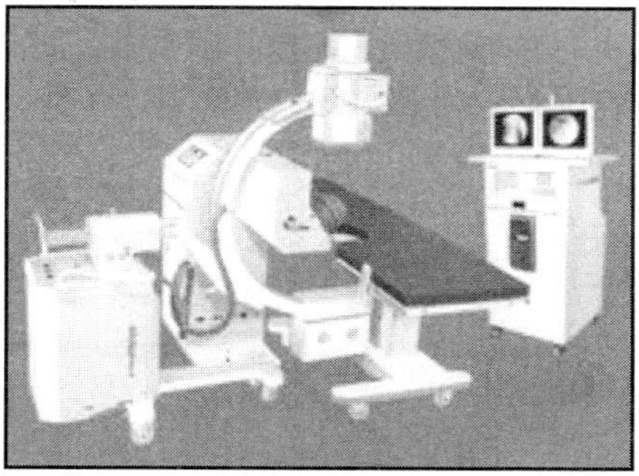

a) **Name the machine?**

b) **Name three primary types of generators?**

Answer:

a) ESWL machine

b) There are three primary types of shockwave generators: electrohydraulic (spark gap), electromagnetic, and piezoelectric.

11.15

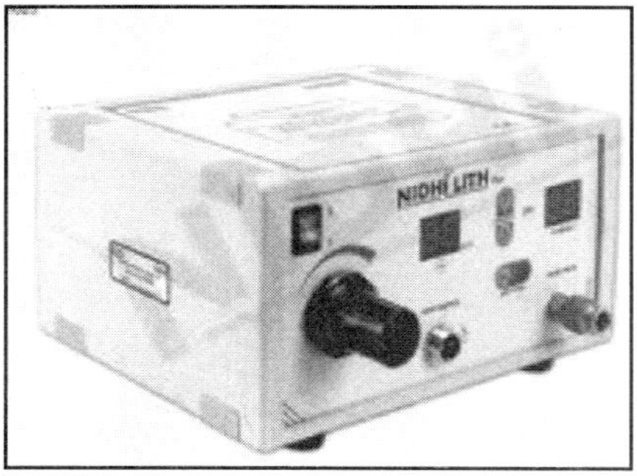

a) Name the equipment?

b) What is the main use, advantages and disadvantages of this equipment?

Answer:

a) Pneumatic lithotripter machine

b) This is mainly used for fragmentation of stones (Renal, ureteric or bladder)

Advantages-Low cost and low maintenance significantly least risk of ureteral perforation

Disadvantages-Relatively high rate of stone retropulsion

11.16

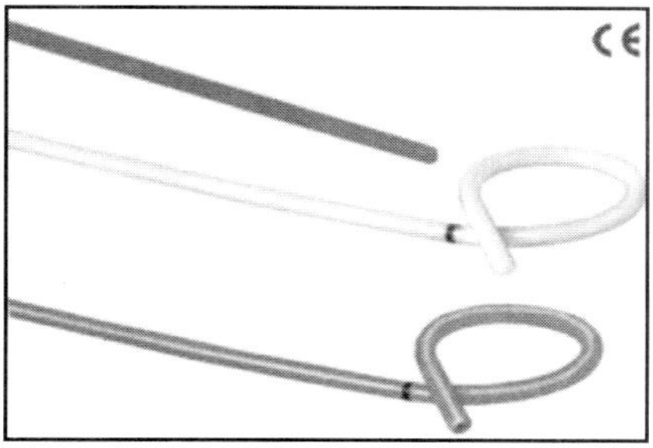

a) Name the above image?

b) What is the commonest polymer used for this?

Answer:

a) DJ stent

b) Polyurethane is the commonest polymer used in today's stents

11.17

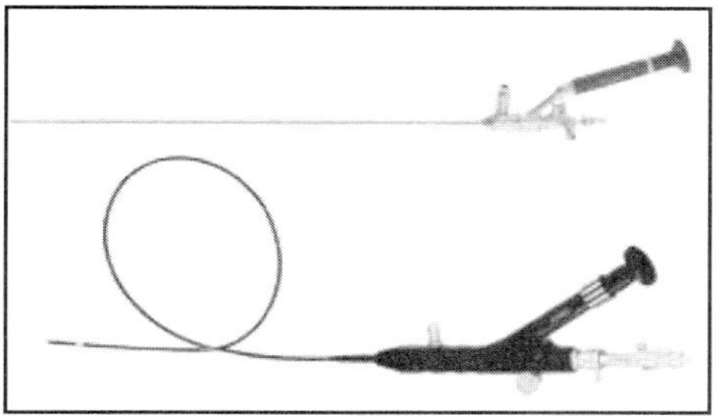

a) **Name the instruments**

b) **Name the advantage of one over another**

Answer:

a) Rigid and flexible ureteroscope

b)

Ureteroscope (semirigid)	**Advantages**: more durable, larger working channel for larger instruments , better visibility related to increased irrigating ability
	Disadvantages: may be more traumatic to the urethra/ureter, limited access within the ureter
Ureteroscope (flexible)	**Advantages**-Typically used for stones above the iliac vessels and in the kidney
	Disadvantages: flexible fiberoptics require frequent repairs, which are costly; smaller working channels have lower flow rates; the image is not as sharp as with semirigid endoscopes

12.1

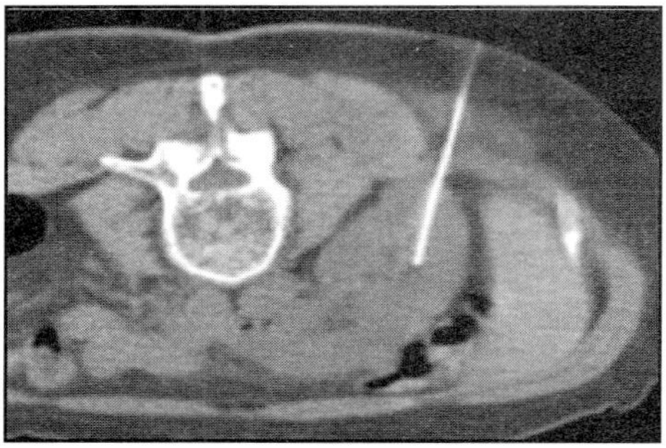

a) **What does this CT suggest**

b) Name the indication for carrying out this procedure

Answer:

a) CT guided biopsy of left renal mass

b) Patients suspected of having metastatic disease, renal abscess, or lymphoma can undergo CT guided biopsy

12.2

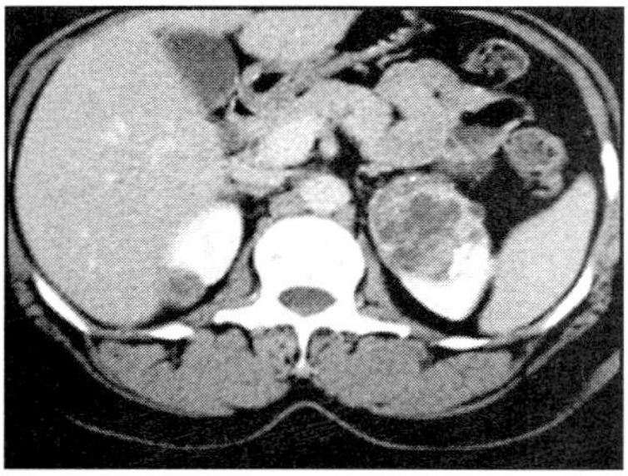

a) What is the diagnosis

b) Best treatment option

Answer:

a) CECT Scan- Left renal cell carcinoma (Heterogeneously enhancing lesion)

b) Best treatment option- Laparoscopic radical nephrectomy

12.3

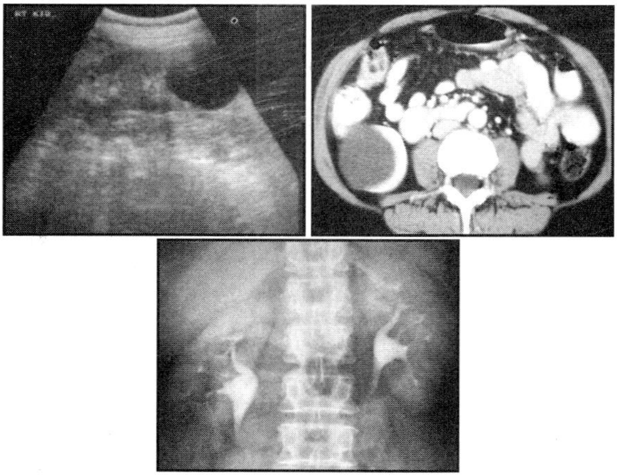

a) What are the findings?

b) What is the diagnosis?

Answer:

a) Anechoic mass on USG, water density mass on CT, mass on upper pole of right kidney on IVU

b) Suggestive of simple cyst

12.4

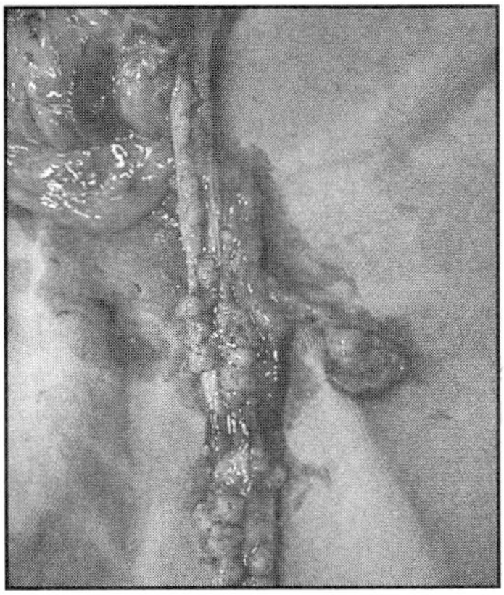

a) What is this specimen

b) Indication

Answer:

a) Radical nephroureterectomy

b) Invasive high grade lesion of ureter or renal pelvis

12.5

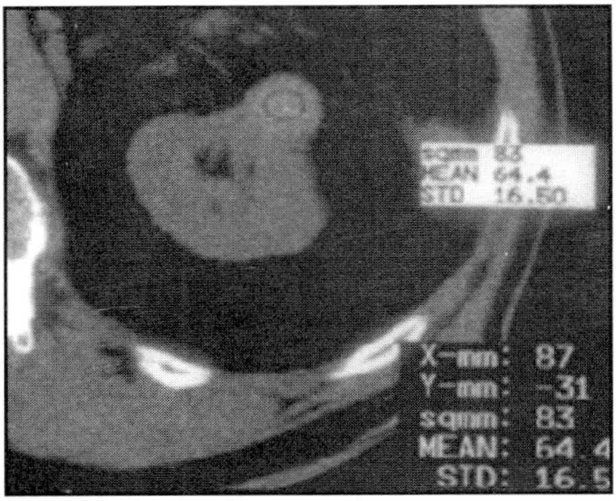

CECT-KUB

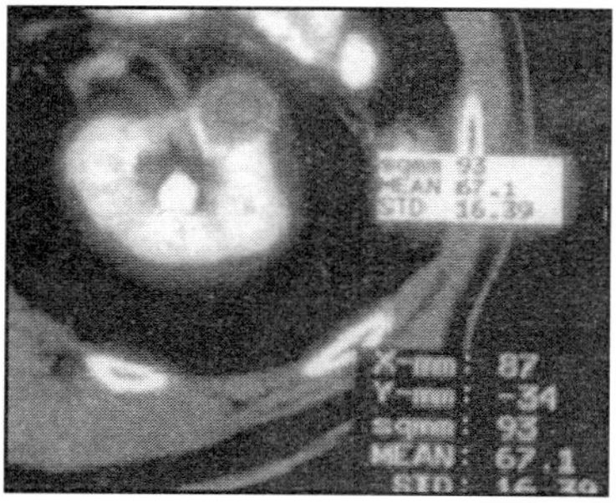

On 2 year follow up

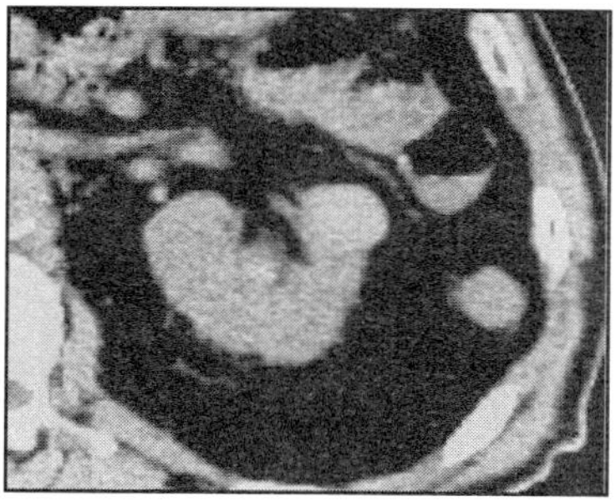

a) **What are the findings?**

b) **What is the diagnosis?**

Answer:

a) High density cyst. Homogenous with no enhancement. No change on 2 year follow up

b) Findings suggestive of Bosniak grade 2

12.6

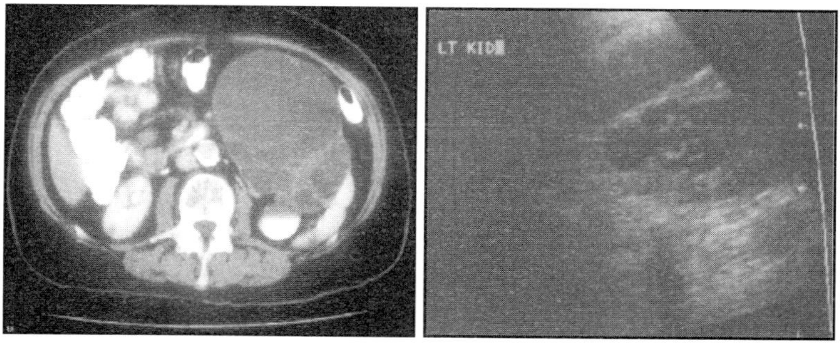

a) What are the findings?

b) What is the diagnosis?

Answer:

a) Multiple thick septation on USG, multilocular lesion and thickened septa with mild septal enhancement on CT

b) Suggestive of Bosniak grade 3

12.7

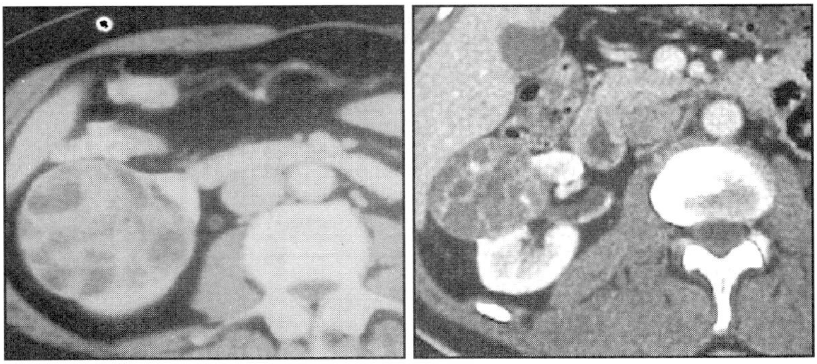

a) What are the findings?

b) What is the diagnosis?

Answer:

a) Multiple thick enhancing septa and nodular tissue on CT

b) Suggestive of Bosniak grade 4

12.8

(a)

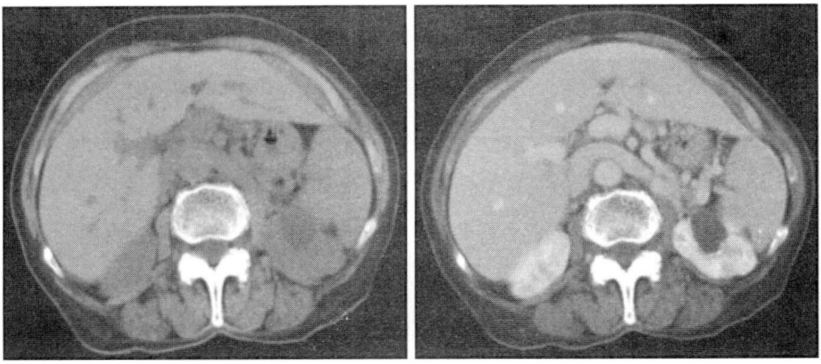

(b)

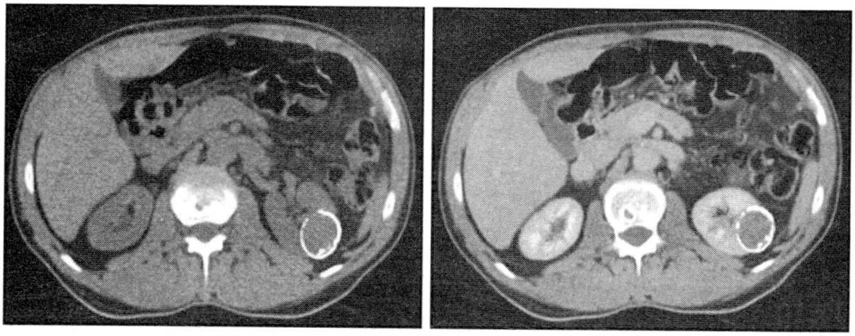

1. Describe the CT findings in Figs (a) and (b)
2. What is meant by a renal protocol CT?

Answers

1. Figure (a) are pre- and post-contrast axial CT images through the upper abdomen showing a simple cyst in the upper pole of the left kidney. There is no evidence of wall-thickening, septations, enhancement or calcifi cation. It is suggestive of Bosniak type I cyst

   Figure (b) are pre- and postcontrast axial CT images through the upper abdomen showing a cystic left renal lesion with thick peripheral calcifi cation. There is no evidence of septation, enhancement or solid elements. The cyst is classified as Bosniak IIF (Follow-up).

2. The renal mass protocol CT includes a pre and post contrast fine cut CT focused on the kidneys. The timings of the post contrast study is 60–90 s. With the benefit of a pre and post contrast study enhancement can be objectively evaluated a >20 unit density change after contrast implies vascularised tissue, and this is a key evaluation when searching for neo-vascularity.

12.9

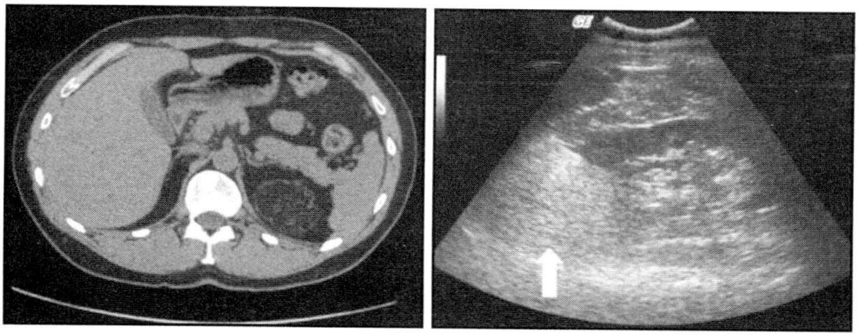

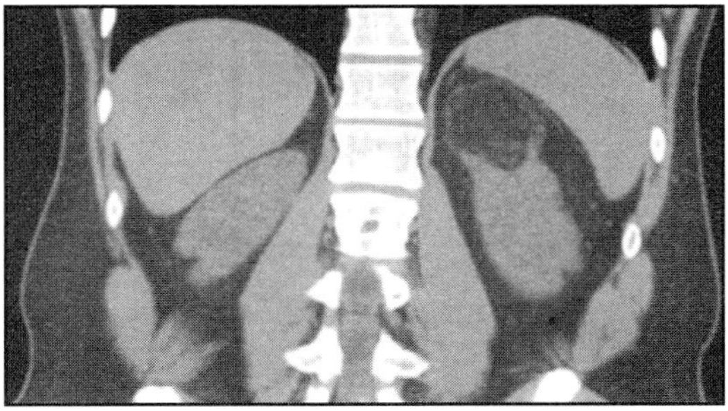

A 30-year-old women presents with non-specific chronic back pain.

1. **Describe images. What is the diagnosis?**
2. **What is the aetiology of the mass?**

Answer

1. Left kidney showing an exophytic mass in the upper pole of the left kidney. This mass has similar density to the subcutaneous and retroperitoneal fat on both CT and USS. The diagnosis is angiomyolipoma (AML).
2. AML is a hamartoma including various proportions of adipose tissue, spindle and epithelioid smooth muscle and abnormal blood vessels.

12.10

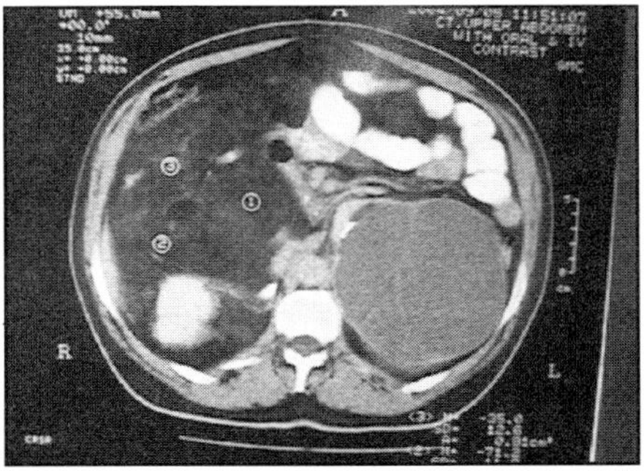

a) **What is the finding in the CT?**

b) **How much is the HU of marked area?**

Answer:

a) AML

b) -20 HU or lower

12.11

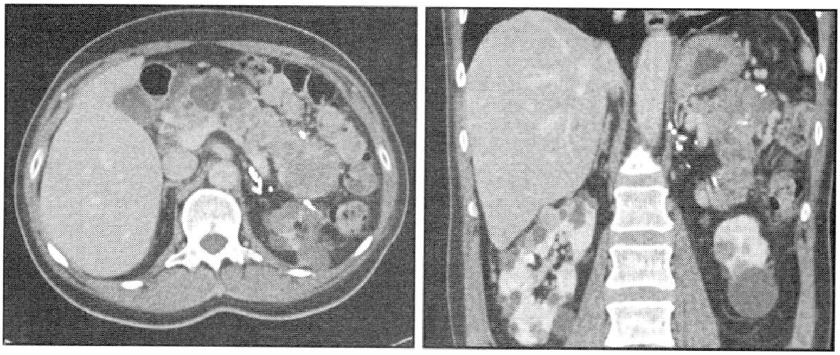

A 28-year-old female patient with pancreatic insufficiency was found to have multiple renal cysts on routine imaging.

1. **Describe the findings on her CT scan.**
2. **What is the likely unifying diagnosis?**

Answer

1. Post-contrast CT images of upper abdomen. There are multiple cysts within the pancreas and kidneys.

   Multiple pancreatic and renal cysts of a variety of types are characteristic of von Hippel Lindau (VHL) disease.

2. Von-Hippel Lindau disease is an autosomal dominant condition. The von Hippel- Lindau gene is located on the short arm of chromosome 3 (3p26p25), only 20% are familial, the rest are sporadic mutations.

12.12

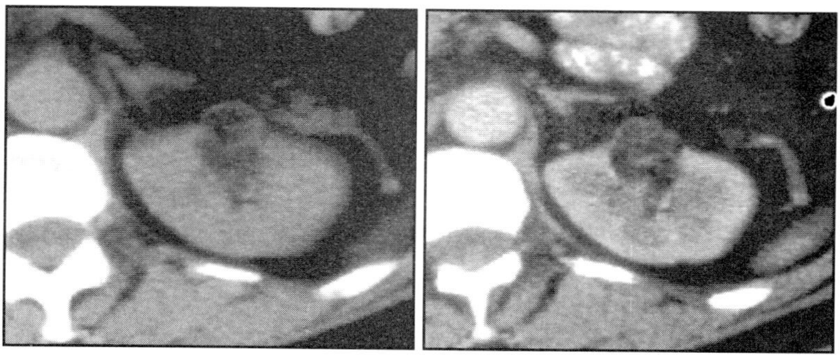

45 years old female with echogenic mass

a) **What are the findings in the above 2 slides?**

Answer :

a) Intrarenal lesion with low density

Above CT and MRI is suggestive of AML

12.13

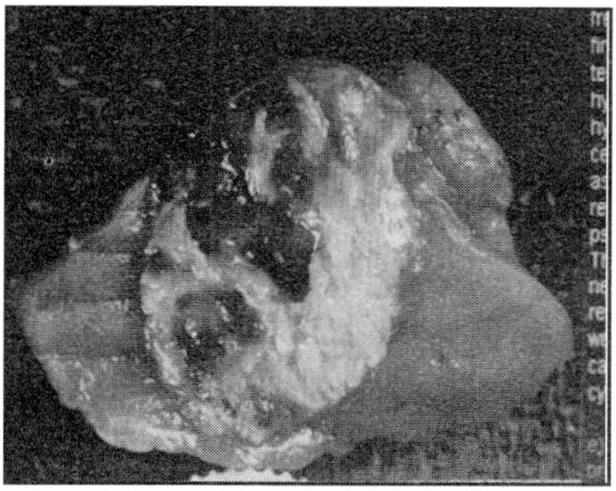

a) What is this specimen?

b) Name two familial syndrome associated with it?

Answer:

a) Radical nephrectomy specimen showing Renal cell carcinoma

b) Von HippelLindau and Birt-Hogg-Dubé

12.14

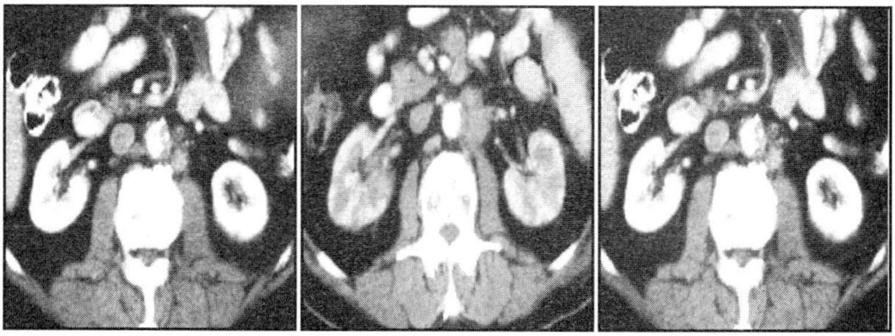

72 years old male with recent development of back pain

a) What are the findings in the above 3 slides?

Answer :

a) Poorly defined hypodense areas with normal contour of kidney

Increased periortic lymphadenopathy, suggestive of renal lymphoma

12.15

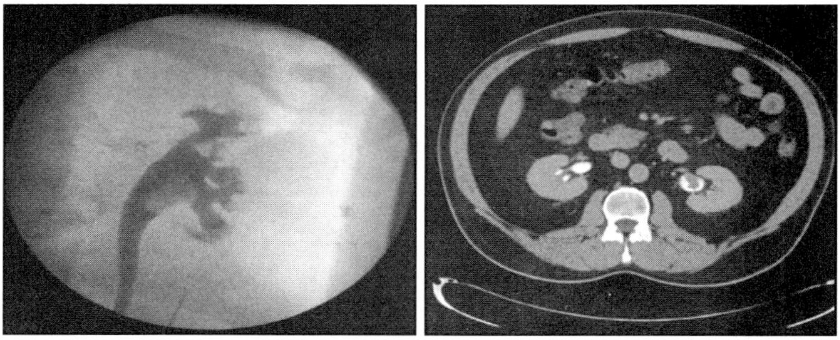

A 67-year-old man presented with macroscopic haematuria. Cystoscopy was normal.

1. **Describe the findings and likely diagnosis.**
2. **How would you manage this patient?**

Answer

1. RGP demonstrating a well-defined filling defect within the inferior aspect of the left renal pelvis. CT images demonstrate good contrast opacification of the renal collecting systems and confirm a mass-like filling defect within the left renal pelvis. There is no local infiltration.

The appearances are suspicious for transitional cell carcinoma

2. If this proves to be a localised tumour, with no contralateral upper tract tumour, then nephro-ureterectomy offers the best hope of cure. Endoscopic management may be used in selected patients with: smaller, low grade tumours; bilateral upper tract TCCs; a solitary kidney; chronic kidney disease.

12.16

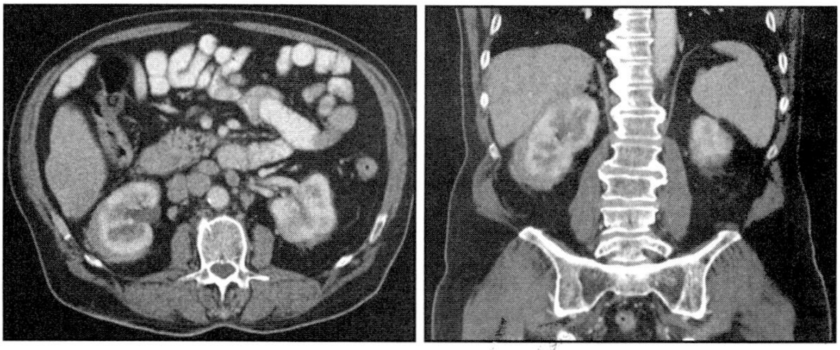

This patient presented with a history of flank discomfort and weight loss.

1. **Describe the findings on these CT images**
2. **What is the likely prognosis?**

Answer

1. CT images showing poorly-enhancing soft tissue encasing both kidneys without parenchymal compression. There are no distinct renal masses seen, but the parenchymal enhancement pattern is irregular. Enlarged para-aortic lymph nodes are also seen.
2. The diagnosis is lymphoma with a poor prognosis as renal involvement usually indicates disseminated disease.

12.17 (a) (b)

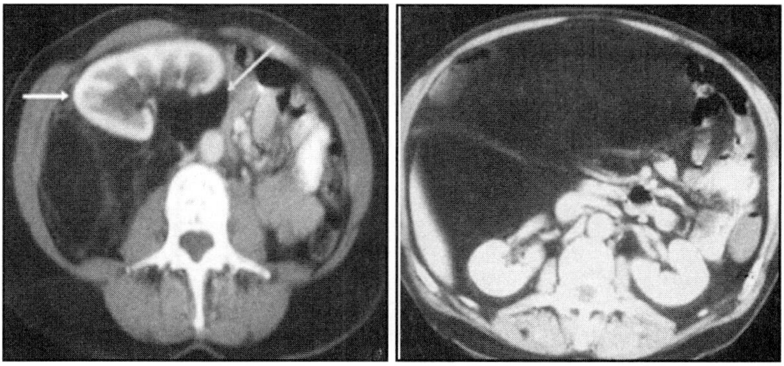

These CT images are from two separate patients

1. **What is the tumour shown in each case?**
2. **Which descriptive term has been given to this radiological appearance**

Answer

1. Figure shows a well-differentiated liposarcoma
2. Figure (a) shows the 'floating kidney sign' and signifies that the tumour does indeed arise from the retroperitoneum. Note that the right kidney is displaced rather than invaded. However, the envelopment of renal hilar structures (arrows) suggests that a nephrectomy will be required for a complete resection of the tumour.

13.1

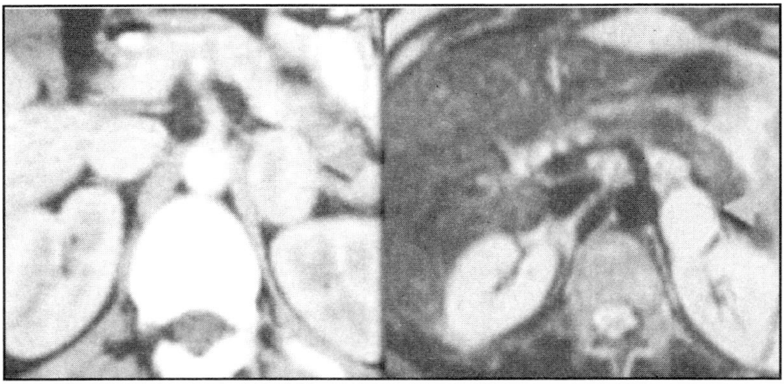

a) What does this specimen suggest?

b) Mention two hereditary form of disease?

Answer:

a) CECT scan & MRI showing left sided pheochromocytoma

b) MEN type I and II, VHL disease

13.2

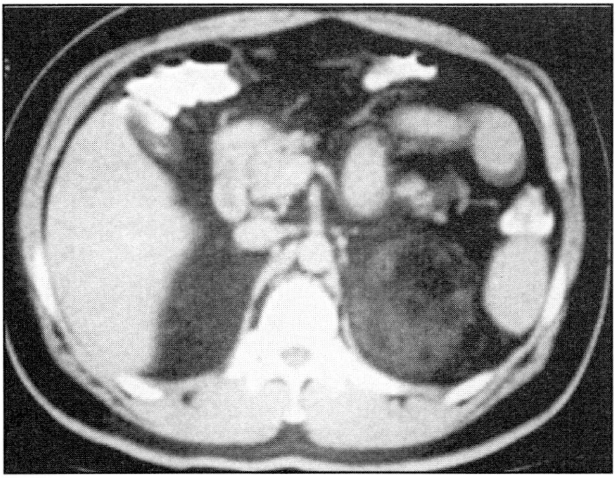

a) What is the diagnosis?

Answer:

a) Myelolipoma left adrenal

13.3

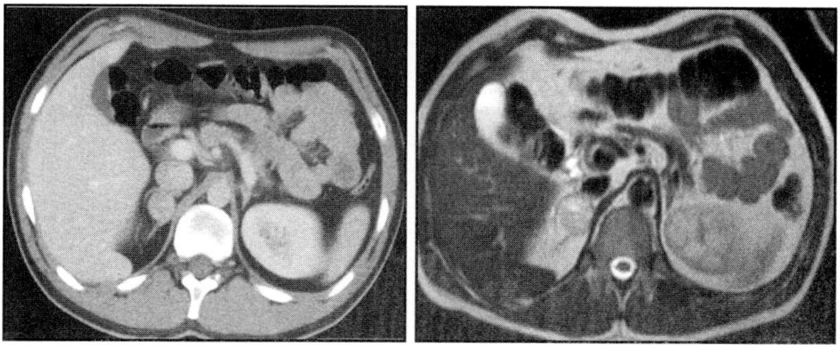

1. What are the different appearances of a phaeochromocytoma on CT and T2-weighted MRI?

Answer

1. Contrast-enhanced CT of a right-sided phaeochromocytoma. Phaechromocytomas do not contain lipid and enhance avidly after contrast on CT.
2. T2-weighted MR image demonstrating the most common appearance, with multiple 'pockets' of high T2 signal in a right-sided phaeochromocytoma. They may also appear 'classical' (the same signal as CSF), 'intermediate' (signal intensity between that of spleen and CSF) or 'marbled' (swirled areas of mixed intensity).

14.1

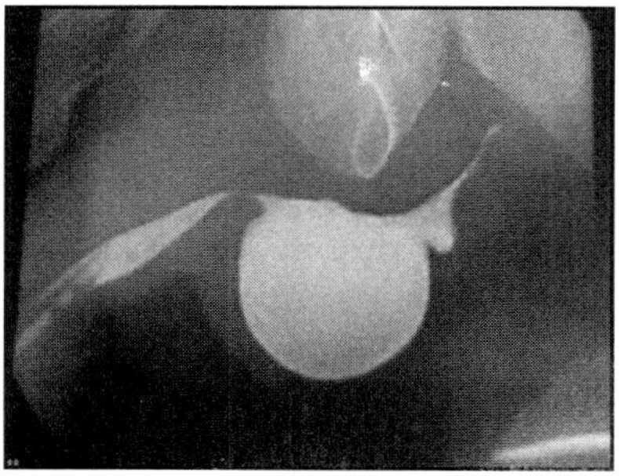

a) Name the study

b) Finding

Answer:

a) MCU

b) Formation of urethral diverticula following urethroplasty

14.2

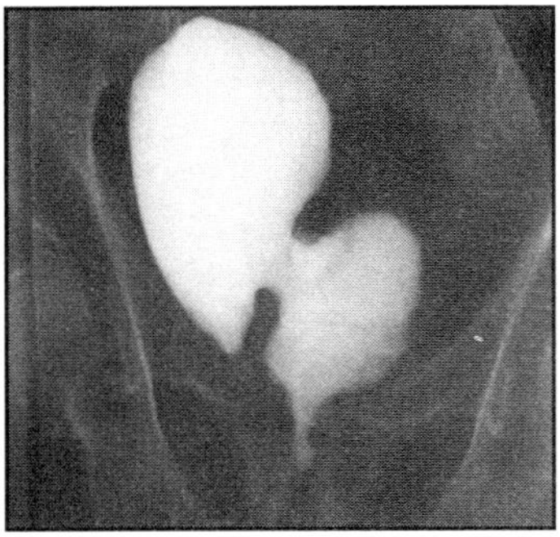

a) **Name the study**

b) **Finding**

Answer:

a) MCU

b) Bladder diverticula

14.3

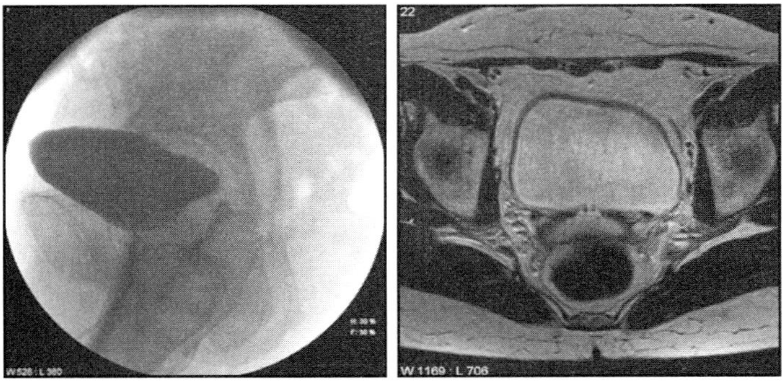

1. **Images from the radiographic investigation of a 50-yearold lady who presented with urine leakage per vagina, 1 week after an otherwise uneventful hysterectomy. What do the investigations show?**
2. **When should this lady be operated?**

Answer

1. Spot view from a cystogram. It shows a vesicovaginal fi stula with the vagina outlined with contrast (note the faint track of contrast outlining the vagina posteriorly).

It is an axial T2-weighted MRI in the same patient, and this better demonstrates the exact site of the posteriorly placed vesicovaginal fi stula.

2. This lady needs a speculum examination and a bladder catheter to divert the urine away from the fi stula.

   If repair is required this should be done early, within 14 days or delayed until after 3 months.

14.4

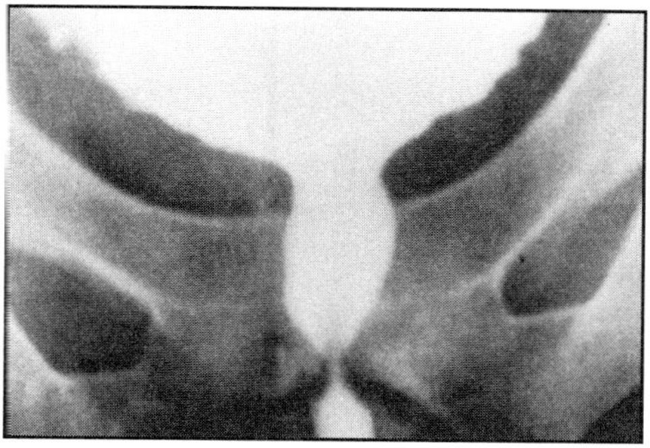

a) What are the findings shown in this MCU?

b) What is the treatment?

Answer:

a) Cystourethrographic configuration of DESD in a man during a bladder contraction

b) Most common approaches are (1) CIC , (2) Sphincterotomy, (3) Stent placement across the sphincter, (4) Injection of botulinum toxin into the sphincter, (5) Continuous catheterization

14.5

a) What does this CMG suggest?

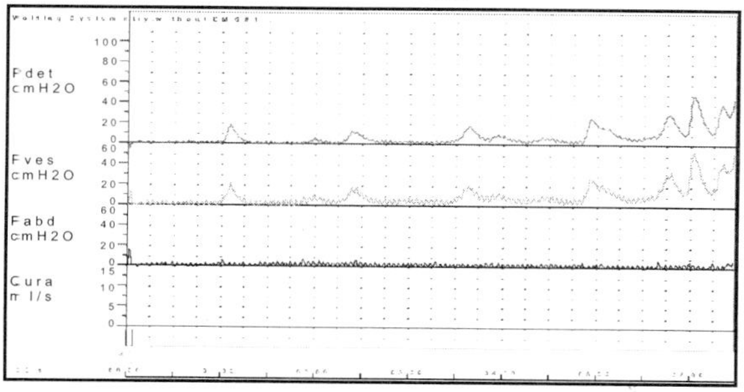

b) Best treatment option?

Answer :

a) Detrusor over activity

b) Bladder relaxants (anticholinergics)

14.6

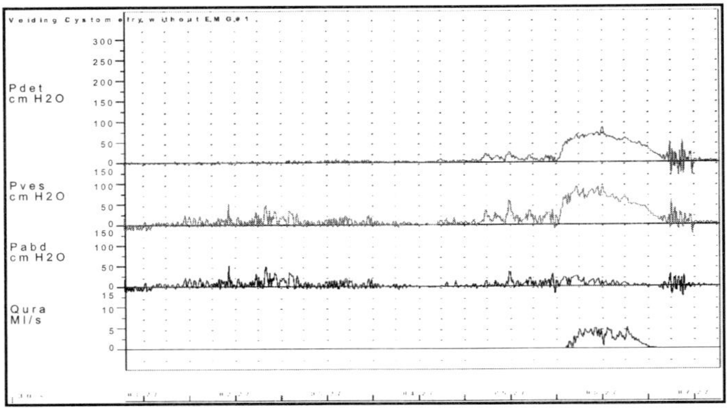

a) What does this CMG suggest?

b) Best treatment option?

Answer:

a) High pressure low flow study suggestive of BOO

b) Alpha blockers

14.7

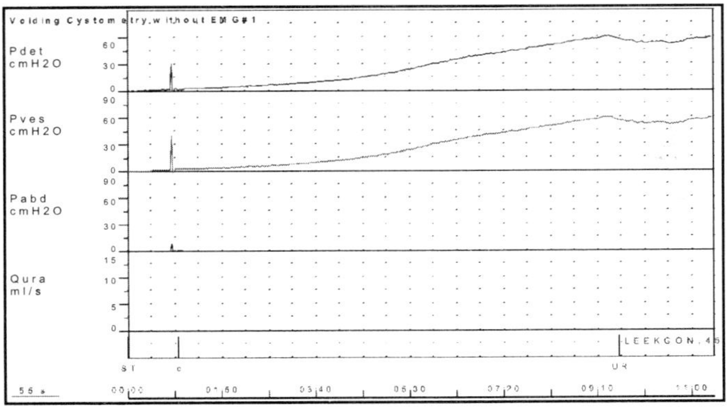

a) What does this CMG suggest?

b) Best treatment option?

Answer:

a) Poorly compliant bladder

b) Anticholinergics

14.8

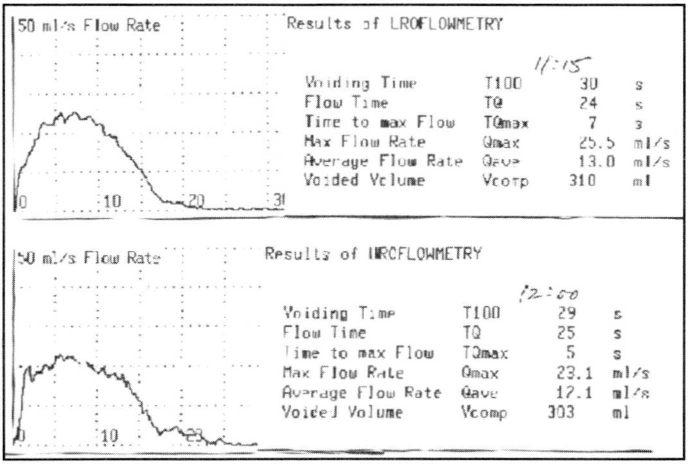

A 62-year-old man complains of lower urinary tract symptoms.

1. **What do the following two urofl ow studies demonstrate?**
2. **Are these normal studies?**

Answer

1. Both curves show a maximum fl ow rate of >20 ml/s for a voided volume of >300 ml. There is a steep rise in flow rate and the maximum flow rate is achieved within the first third of flow time. The flow time is also <30s in both cases.
2. These flow studies appear normal. The flow parameters are within normal limits and the curves are bell shaped. However, this does not necessarily exclude a urodynamic abnormality

14.9

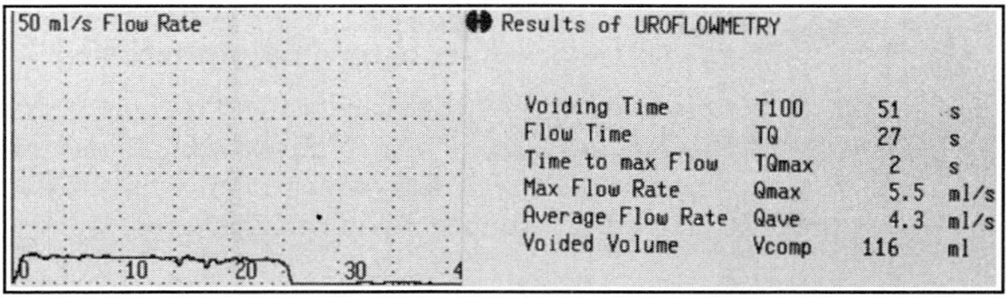

A 37-year-old man complains of long standing lower urinary tract symptoms

1. **Describe this fl ow rate.**
2. **What is the likely diagnosis?**

Answer

1. Fixed obstruction as the fl ow rate goes up and then plateaus.

   The maximum fl ow rate is very poor (5.5 ml/s). It has taken more than 20 s to pass only 116 ml.

2. This is the typical fl ow rate of a patient with urethral stricture

14.10

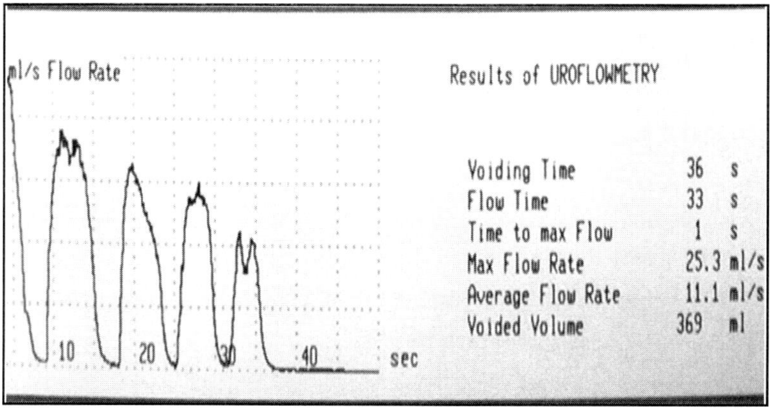

A 67-year-old man presented with mild lower urinary tract symptoms.

1. **What is this fl ow pattern?**
2. **Could this be an artefact?**

Answer

1. Flow pattern caused by abdominal straining. The patient may have obstruction or a hypocontractile detrusor.
2. Can be artefactual, created by the phenomenon of 'pinching'.

   This entails pinching and letting go of penis. Pinching creates a urinary jet that hits the rotating disc of the flow meter and a high flow rate is momentarily recorded, which rapidly tails off when the pinch is released, resulting in this unusual pattern.

14.11

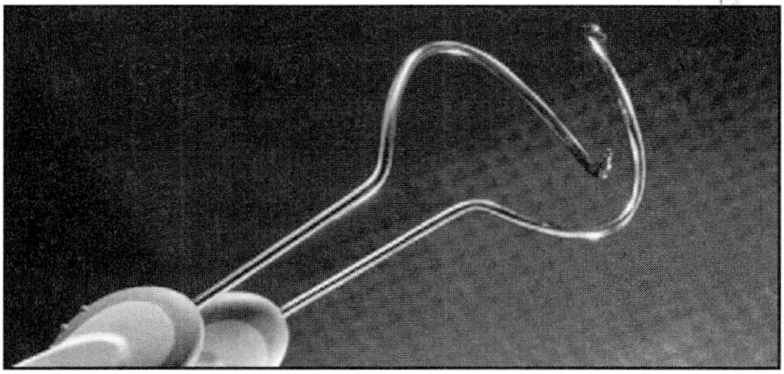

a) Name the device mentioned in the figure?

b) Indication of the device

Answer:

a) Monarch, it is midurethral device

b) It is the transobturator tape (TOT) outside in approach is used for the above tape

This is used for the management of stress urinary incontinence

15.1

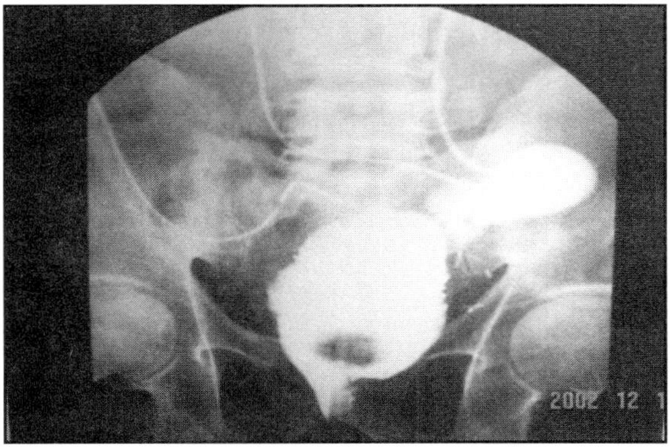

a) Name the study?

b) Finding

Answer:

a) MCU

b) Orthotopic neobladder (Studer). Bilateral ureter implanted in the afferent limb

15.2

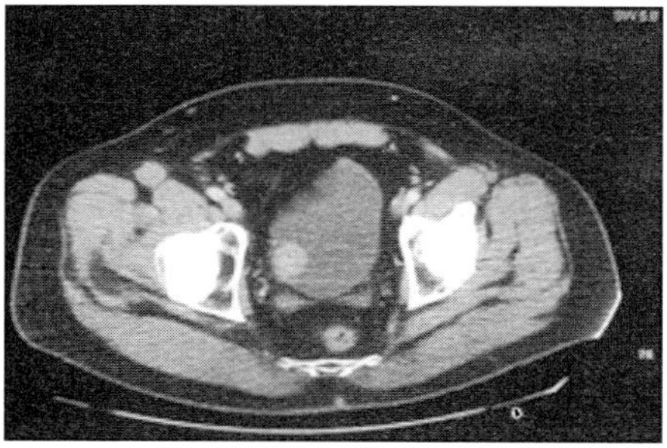

a) What is the diagnosis?

b) Best treatment option

Answer :

a) CECT Scan- bladder mass on right lateral wall

b) Best treatment option- TURBT and proceed according to biopsy report

15.3

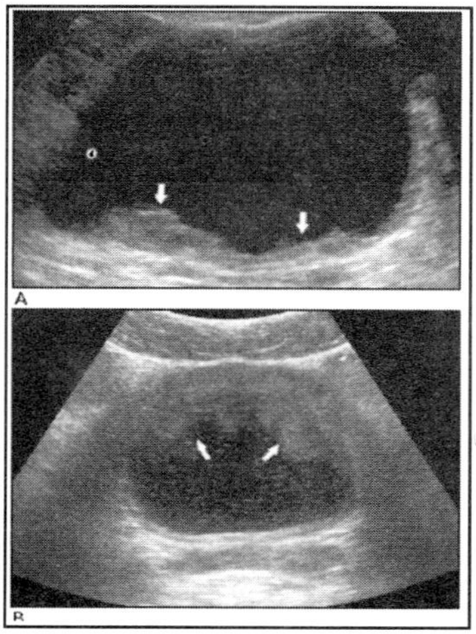

a) What is shown in the above figure?

b) What is the treatment?

Answer:

a) Bladder mass at base and anterior wall of bladder

b) TURBT and proceed according to biopsy report

15.4

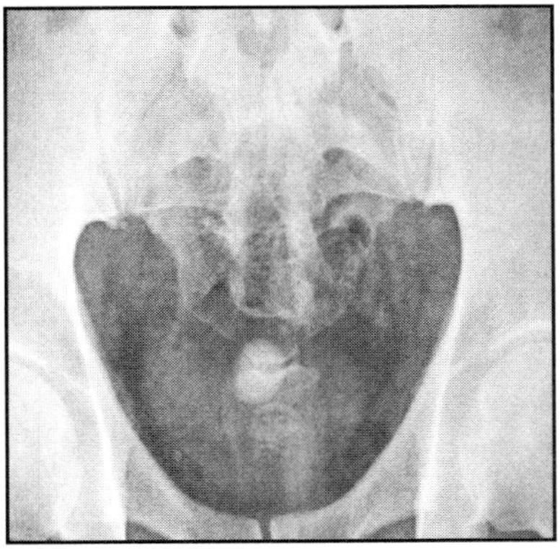

a) Identify the abnormality

b) Most accurate examination to confirm the diagnosis

c) Treatment modalities

Answer:

a) Bladder stone or phelobolith

b) Cystoscopy is the single most accurate examination to document the presence of a bladder calculus

c) Cystolithotomy and cystolitholapaxy

15.5

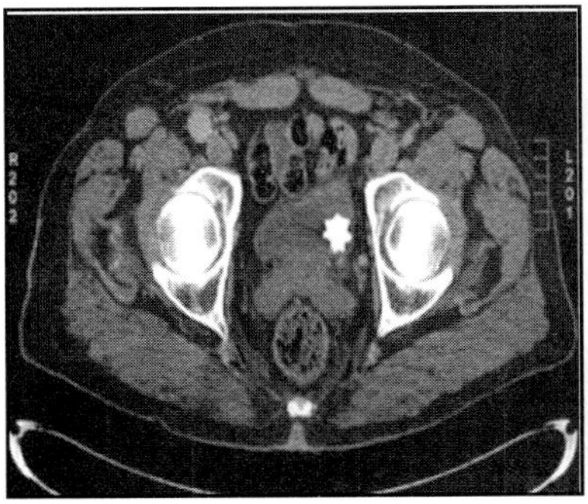

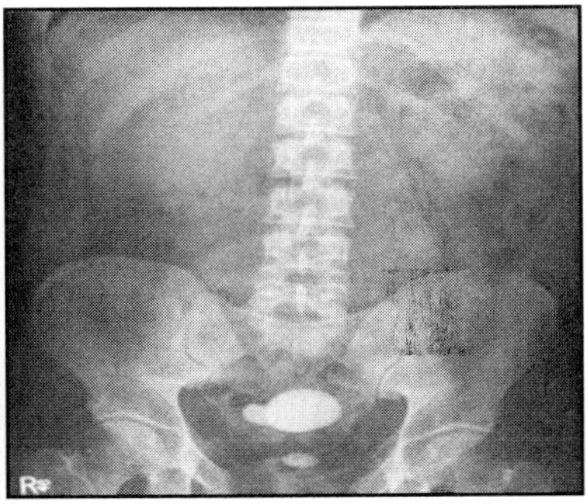

1. A 65-year-old man presents and haematuria and dysuria. To investigate this he had a CT scan. What is seen in Fig. (a) and what is the aetiology?

2. What two abnormalities can you see on the KUB X-ray in Fig. (b) ?

Answer

1. Figure (a) is a transverse CT scan showing a left-sided bladder calculus.

   Bladder stones occur in approximately 0.5% of men with BOO.

   Incomplete bladder emptying is believed to be the underlying cause.

2. Figure (b) is a KUB radiograph showing a patient with bladder exstrophy with at least three bladder stones; and widened pubic symphysis (diastasis).

15.6

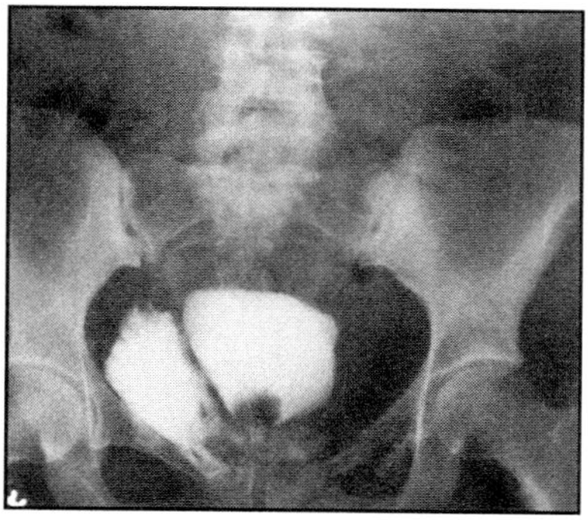

a) What is the diagnosis?

b) What is the management?

Answer:

a) Extraperitoneal rupture of bladder

b) The usual treatment of uncomplicated extraperitoneal bladder rupture, when conditions are ideal, is conservative management with urethral catheter drainage alone

16.1

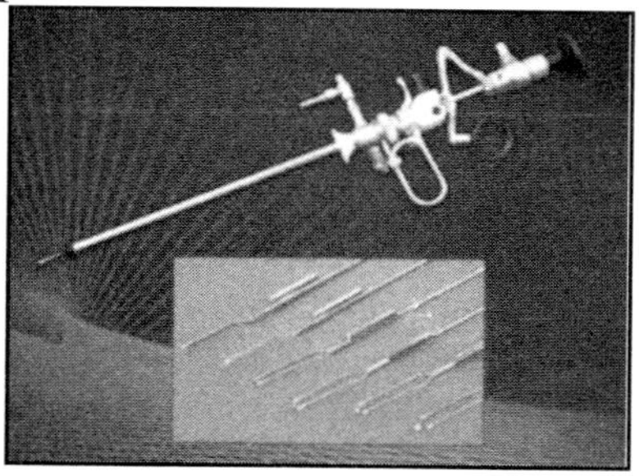

a) **Name the equipment?**

b) **What is the main use of this equipment?**

Answer:

a) Assembly of telescope, working element, outer and inner sheath and TUR loops (resectoscope)

b) Resectoscope is mainly used for transurethral resection of prostate

16.2

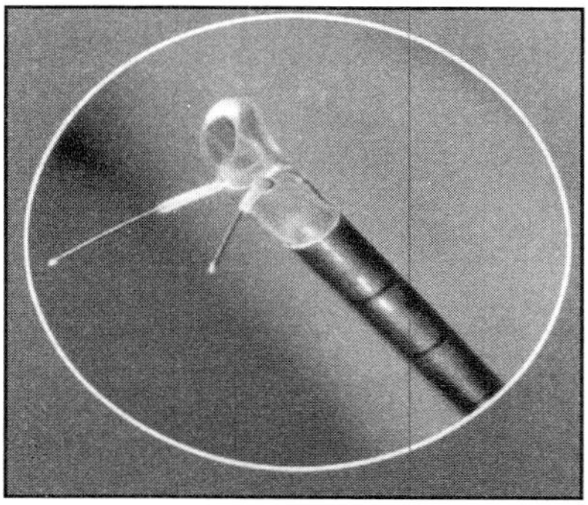

a) **What does this figure suggest?**

b) **What is the temperature generated?**

Answer:

a) The TUNA radiofrequency needles deployed

b) The generator produces low-level monopolar RF waves of about 490 kHz, which produce temperatures of about 100° C in the target area

16.3

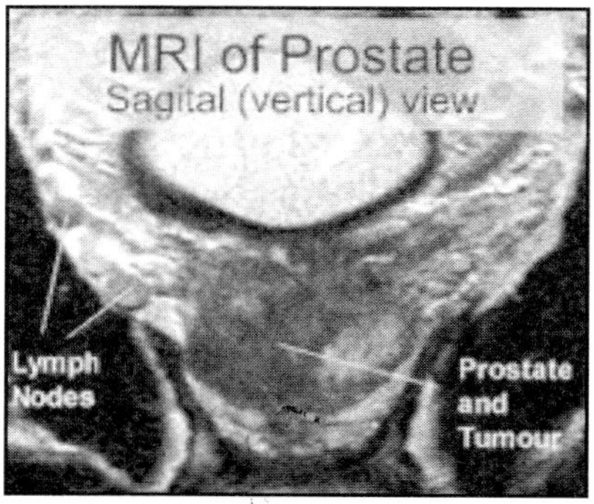

a) Mention stage 1 and 2 of prostate cancer

b) Which is the best management of localised carcinoma prostate

Answer:

a)

T1a	Tumor found in tissue removed at TUR; 5% or less is cancerous and histologic grade <7
T1b	Tumor found in tissue removed at TUR; >5% is cancerous or histologic grade >7
T1c	Tumor identified by prostate needle biopsy due to elevation in PSA
T2a	Tumor involves less than half of one lobe
T2b	Tumor involves more than half of a lobe but not both lobes
T2c	Tumor involves more than one lobe

a) Retropubic radical prostatectomy has best results for localised carcinoma prostate. It should be considered in patient with life expectancy >15 years

16.4

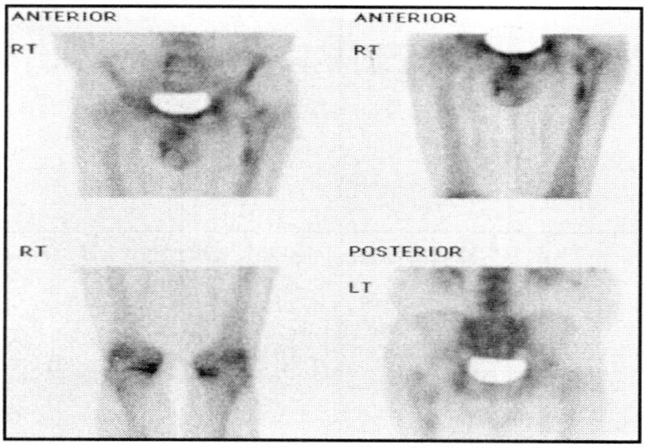

a) What is the investigation?

b) Name the findings seen in this investigation and condition associated with it.

Answer:

a) MDP Bone Scan

b) Increased uptake in vertebra, lower ends of femur and upper end of tibia. Condition associated with it is carcinoma prostate

17.1

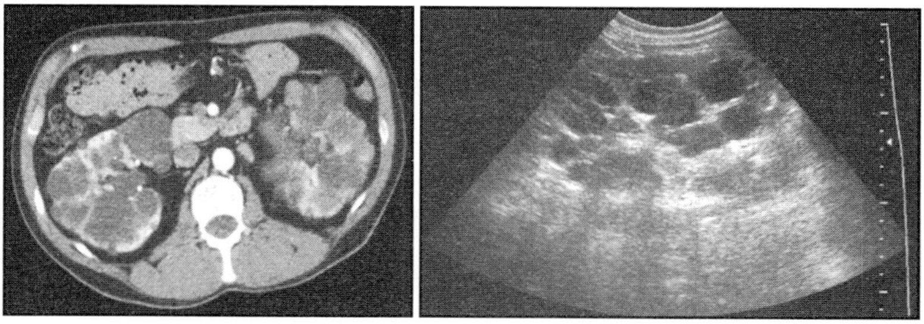

These studies are from a 20-year-old man with vague back pain.

1. **Describe these images and what is the likely diagnosis.**
2. **What is the differential diagnosis?**
3. **The patient reports that his father passed away from a sudden 'bleed in the brain'.**

   What is the most likely diagnosis?

Answer

1. Both the CT images show multiple bilateral renal cysts.
2. In an adult, the most common renal cystic syndromes are autosomal dominant polycystic kidney disease (ADPKD), von Hippel Lindau (VHL) disease, tuberous sclerosis (TS).
3. The family history of possible subarachnoid haemorrhage makes ADPKD most likely, as this is associated with intra-cerebral aneurysms. This condition is associated with at least two different genetic mutations: ADPKD1 on chromosome 16p, ADPKD2 on chromosome 4q

17.2

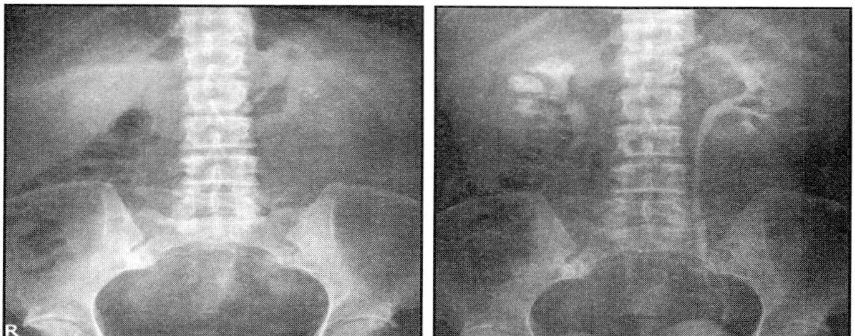

Presented with microscopic haematuria.

1. **Describe the findings**
2. **What is the differential diagnosis**

Answer

1. Plain radiograph showing multiple clusters of calcification in both kidneys. The IVU post contrast film demonstrates that although multiple calyceal calculi are possible, the calcification is relatively peripheral in location in the kidneys and likely to be parenchymal.
2. Nephrocalcinosis is a non-specific finding on plain radiography and the differential diagnosis includes hyperparathyroidism, renal tubular acidosis, medullary sponge kidney and, less commonly, primary hyperoxaluria and other causes for hypercalcaemia or hypercalciuria milk-alkali syndrome, sarcoidosis, hypervitaminosis D.

17.3

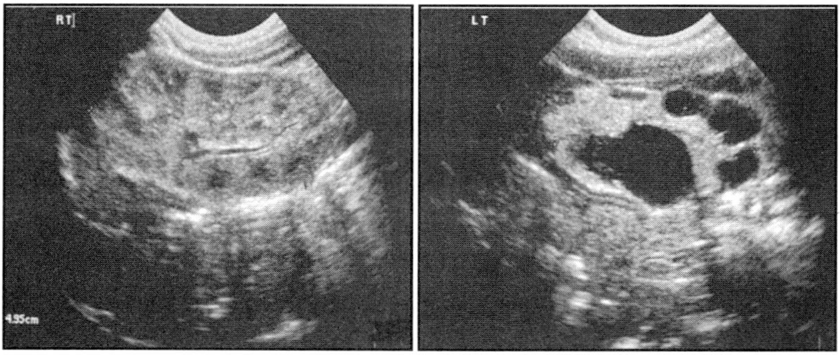

A male neonate has a left sided abdominal mass.

1. **What are the US findings and the likely diagnosis?**
2. **What further imaging test could be performed to differentiate between this condition and alternative possibilities?**

Answer

1. The ultrasound of the right kidney shows normal corticomedullary differentiation and no hydronephrosis. The left kidney demonstrates multiple hypoechoic cysts of variable shapes and size, with complete loss of corticomedullary differentiation. Cysts do not communicate. The appearances are suggestive of a multicystic dysplastic kidney.

2. Nuclear medicine studies (e.g. DMSA or MAG-3) are sensitive at detecting residual renal function in a hydronephrotic kidney in contrast to complete absence of function seen (MCDK).

17.4

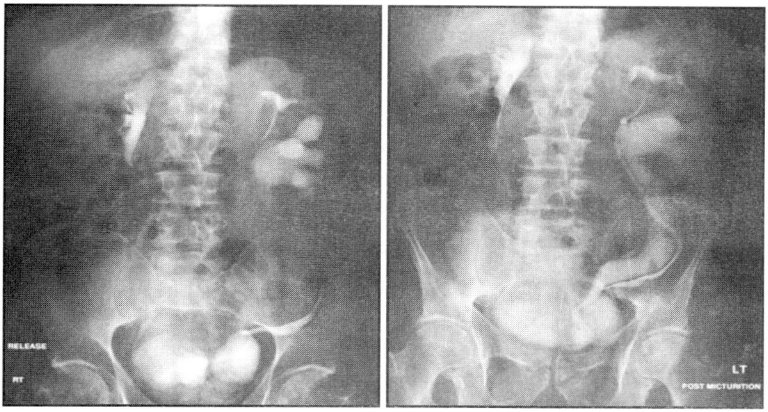

1. **Describe the congenital abnormalities on the left side of this patient.**
2. **There is a well-recognised general rule regarding the vesico-ureteric anatomy in this condition. What is the eponymous term for this rule and what does it state?**
3. **Describe the 'drooping lily' sign**

Answer

1. The left kidney is a complete duplex system, with completely separate ureteric insertions. There is also a Hutch diverticulum associated with the upper moiety ureter. The lower moiety pelvicalyceal system and ureter are distended.
2. The Weigert Meyer rule states that with a complete duplex system, the upper moiety ureter inserts more inferiorly and medially in the bladder than the lower moiety ureter. The lower moiety ureter is prone to refl ux. In comparison, the upper moiety ureter is prone to obstruction at the vesicoureteric junction and may be associated with an ureterocoele.
3. This is a characteristic appearance on IVU. The upper moiety obstructs and therefore does not opacify, but it does increase in size thereby pushing the lower moiety downwards. Therefore only the 'drooping' lower moiety is seen on IVU.

17.5

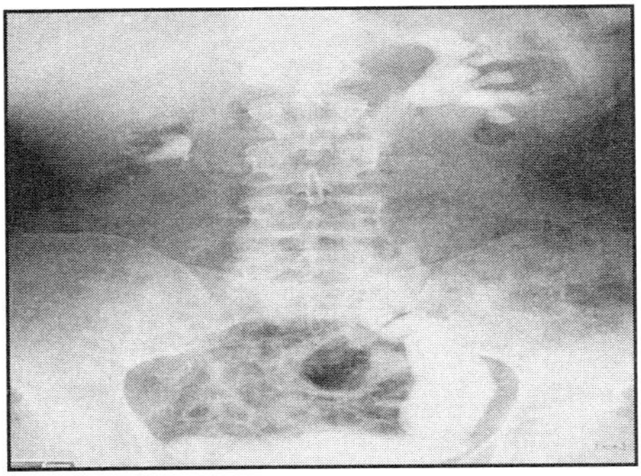

1. **Describe the images shown in this 23-year-old man with recurrent UTI and abdominal pains. What is the most likely diagnosis and what is the aetiology?**

Answer

1. Marked localised dilatation of the lower third of the left ureter, with mild prominence of the collecting system proximally. The differential diagnosis includes chronic ureteric obstruction, vesicoureteric reflux, diabetes insipidus, psychogenic polydipsia or primary megaureter.

   This is primary megaureter.

   The aetiology is abnormal muscle development within a segment of ureter near to the vesicoureteric junction.

17.6

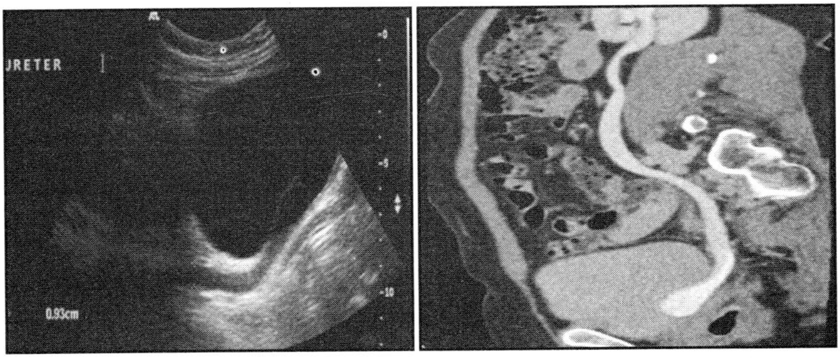

1. **A 25-year-old woman presented with a history of recurrent UTI and intermittent loin pain. She underwent an ultrasound examination followed by a CT scan. Describe the fi ndings.**

2. **What is the name of the radiological sign demonstrated in figure (b)?**

Answer

1. Ultrasound scan showing a thin-walled cystic structure. It is transonic and of water density internally, and therefore is not a soft tissue mass. True cysts of the bladder are excessively rare and the most likely diagnosis is an ureterocoele, especially in the context of the history. This was confi rmed by a CT urogram
2. Figure (b) demonstrates the 'Cobra head' sign. The head being the ureterocoele, and the tail is represented by the ureter, which may or may not be dilated.

17.7

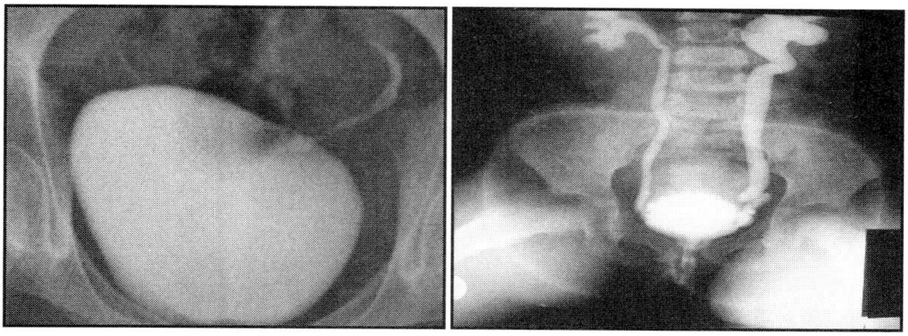

a) **Name the study in the above two slides**

b) **Diagnosis**

Answer:

a) **MCU**

b) **A) Left grade 1 VUR**

B) Bilateral grade 4 VUR

17.8

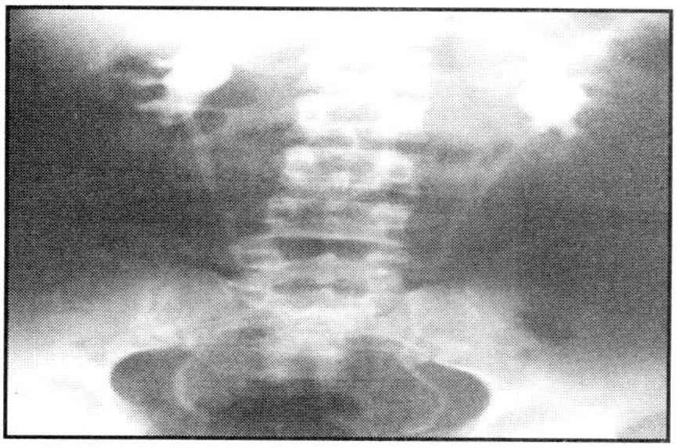

a) **Name the study**

b) Diagnosis

Answer:

a) IVU

b) Malrotated kidney

17.9

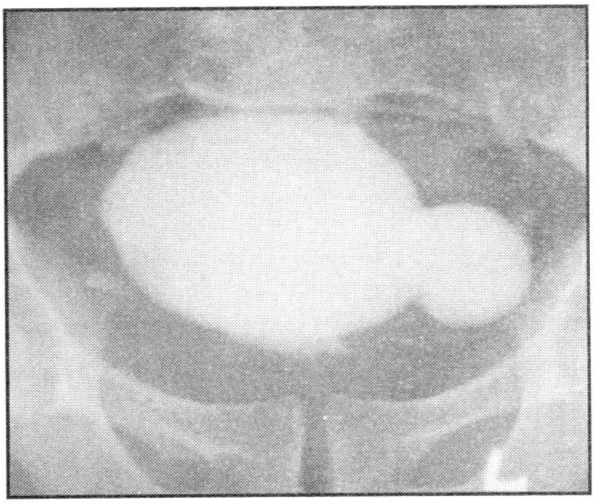

a) Name the study

b) Identify the diagnosis

Answer:

a) MCU

b) Bladder diverticulum

17.10

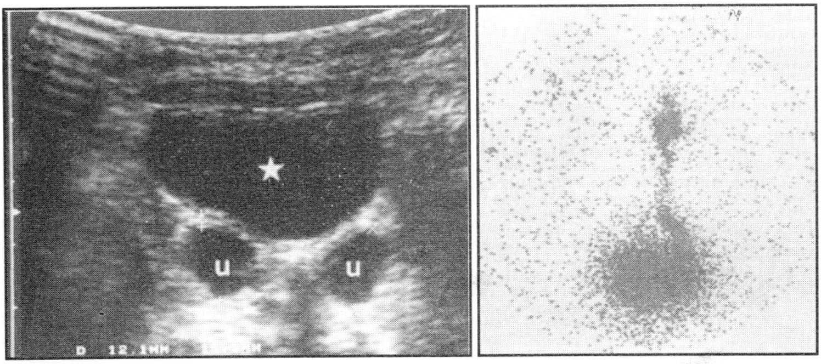

a) Name both the investigation?

b) Mention principle of management?

Answer:

a) USG and Nuclear scan showing VUR

b 1- Spontaneous resolution of reflux is very common

2-High grade reflux is less likely to resolve

3-Sterile reflux is benign

4-Extended use of prophylactic antibiotics is benign

5-Success rate with surgical correction is very high

17.11

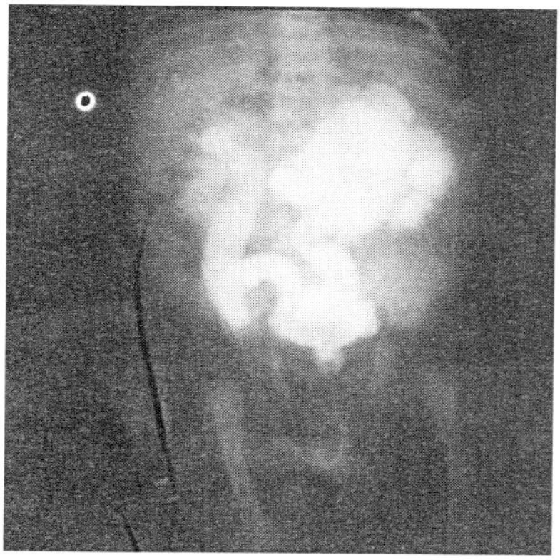

a) Name the study

b) Identify the diagnosis

Answer:

a) MCU

b) PUV with bilateral reflux

17.12

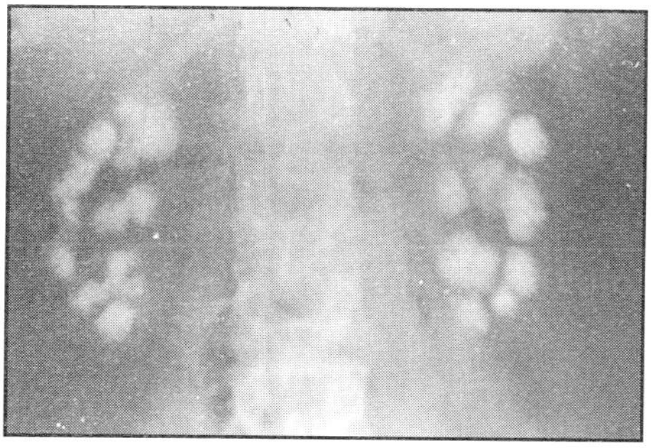

a) What is the diagnosis?

b) Condition associated with disease

Answer:

a) Nephrocalcinosis

b) Medullary sponge kidney is a disorder characterized by ectasia of the renal collecting ducts. Nephrocalcinosis and renal calculi are frequent complications of MSK

17.13

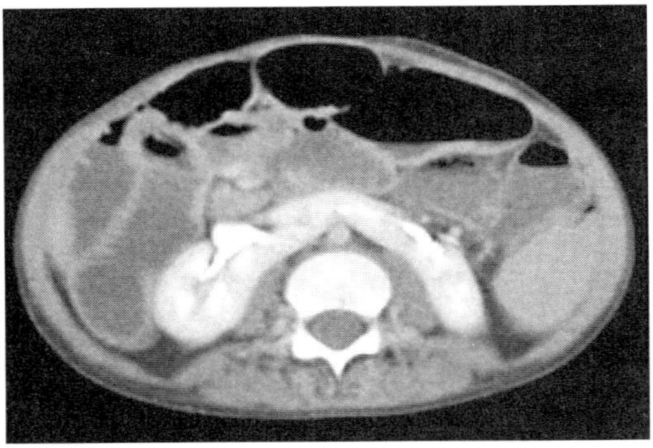

a) What is the diagnosis?

b) Which structure is the main culprit for this anomaly?

Answer:

a) CECT Scan- horse shoe kidney

b) Inferior mesenteric artery prevents full ascent of kidney by obstructing the movement of the isthmus

17.14

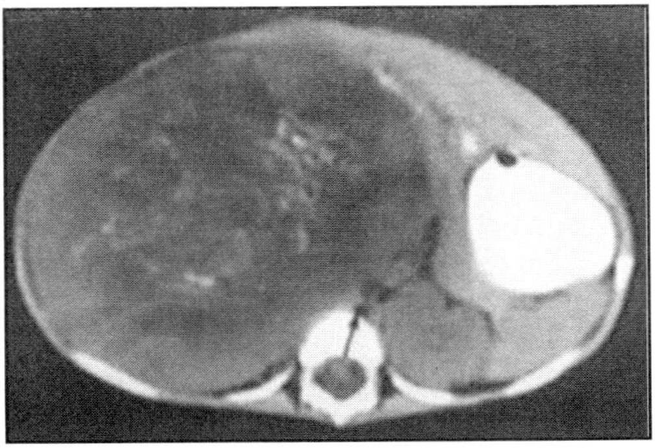

5 Years old boy presents with abdominal lump

a) What does this CT suggest?

b) Mention stage 1 and stage 2 of the above disease

Answer:

a) Wilms tumor

b)

Stage I	Tumor limited to the kidney and completely excised.
Stage II	Tumor beyond the kidney, but is completely resected.

17.15

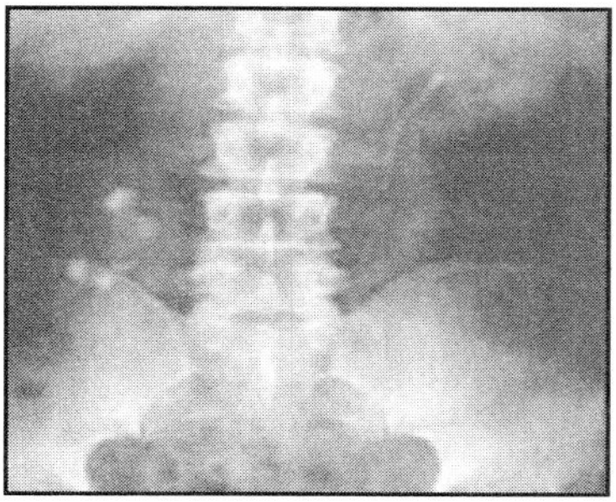

a) What does this IVU suggest

b) Differentiate this condition from renal ptosis

Answer:

a) Right ectopic kidney

b) It can be differentiated from renal ptosis, in which the kidney initially is located in its proper place but moves downward in relation to body position. The ectopic kidney never attains appropriate location.

17.16

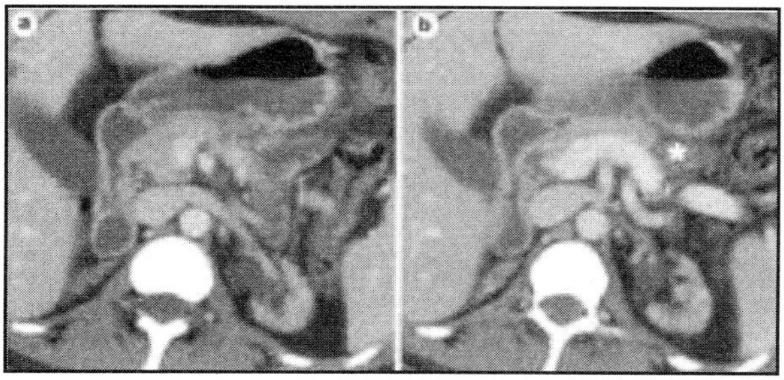

a) What does this CT suggest?

b) What is the embryological basis of this condition

Answer:

a) Agenesis of right kidney

b) The fault lies most probably with the ureteral bud. Complete absence of a bud or aborted ureteral development prevents maturation of the metanephric blastema into adult kidney tissue.

17.17

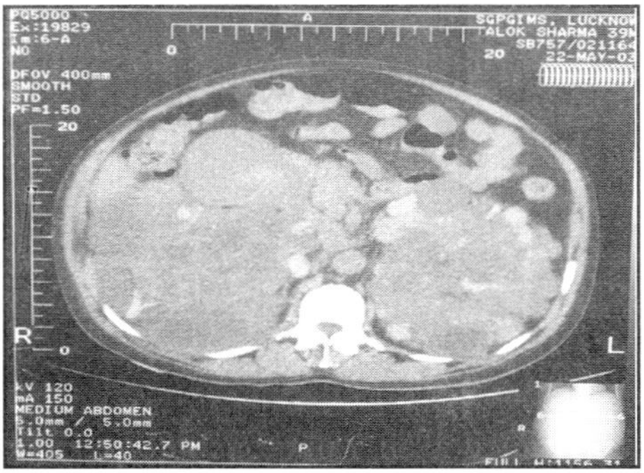

a) Name the finding?

b) Name the genes identified with this disease?

Answer:

a) ADPKD

b) Genes identified for ADPKD: (1) the polycystic kidney disease *(PKD1)* gene localized on the short arm of chromosome 16, and (2) the *PKD2* gene localized on chromosome 4

17.18

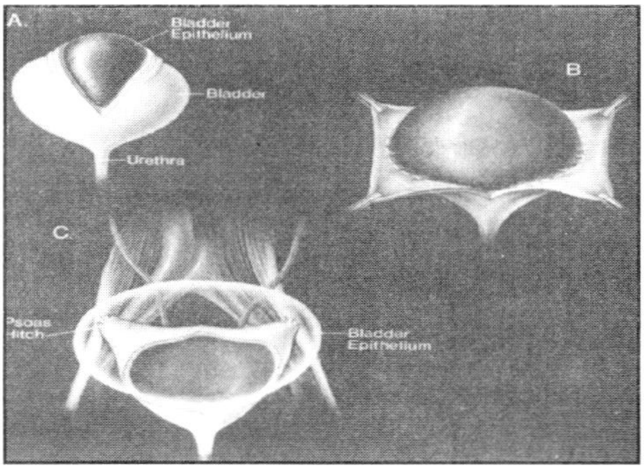

a) What is shown in the above figure?

b) What are the advantages?

Answer:

a) Autoaugmentation

b) Low morbidity and lack of side effects of bowel integration into the urinary tract are the definite advantages of these techniques.

17.19

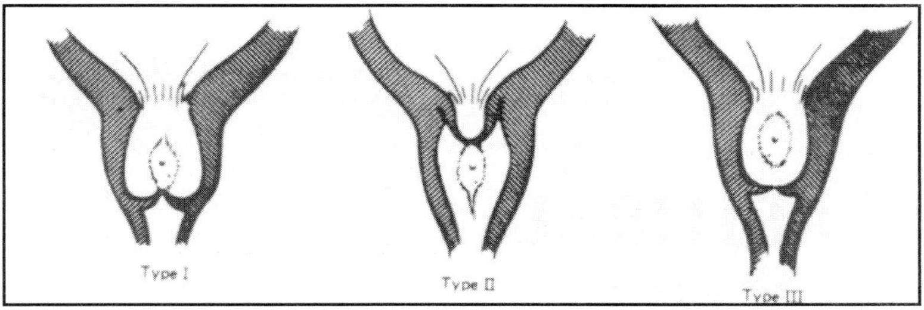

a) Name the classification system?

b) Which is the most common type?

Answer:

a) Young classification of PUV

b) Most common type is type 2

17.20

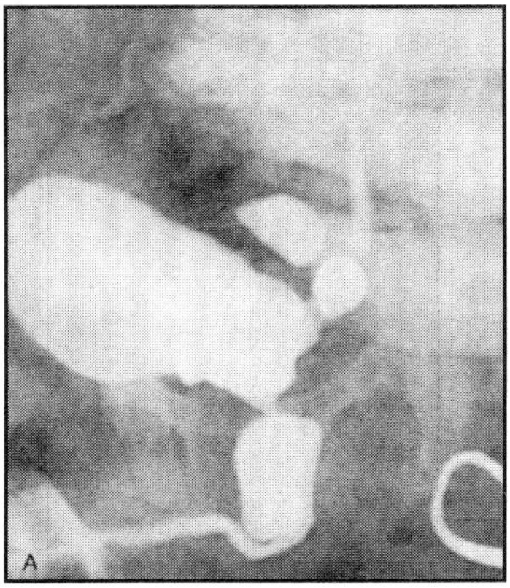

a) What are the findings?

b) What is the diagnosis?

Answer:

a) Dilated posterior urethra with severely trabeculated bladder

b) PUV

17.21

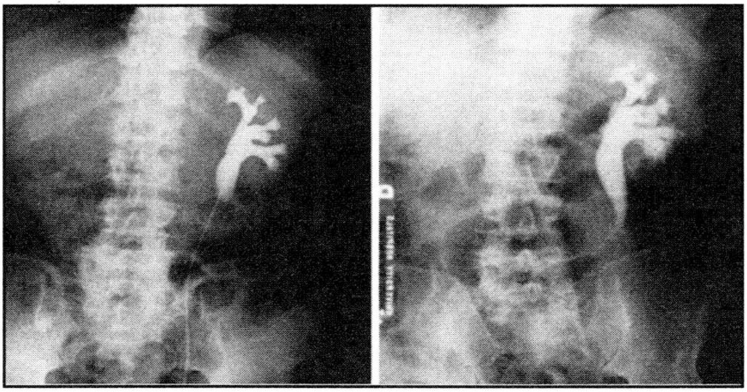

a) What are the findings?

b) What is the diagnosis?

Answer:

a) Pull-out radiograph demonstrates a HDN kidney with medial deviation of the ureter at the level of the fourth lumbar vertebra. There is presence of backflow that may be secondary to ureteral obstruction.

b) Horse shoe kidney

17.22

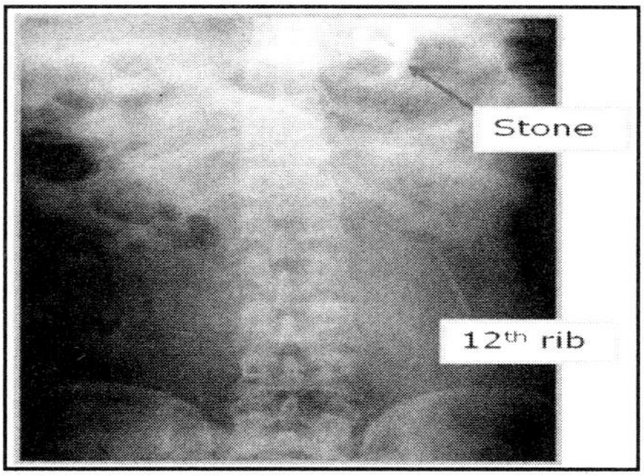

a) What are the findings?

b) What is the diagnosis?

c) Embryological basis?

Answer:

a) Left renal stone at 8th intercostal space

b) Thoracic kidney

c) Delayed closure of the diaphragmatic anlage allows for protracted renal ascent above the level of the future diaphragm or/and kidney overshoots its usual position because of accelerated ascent before normal diaphragmatic closure

17.23

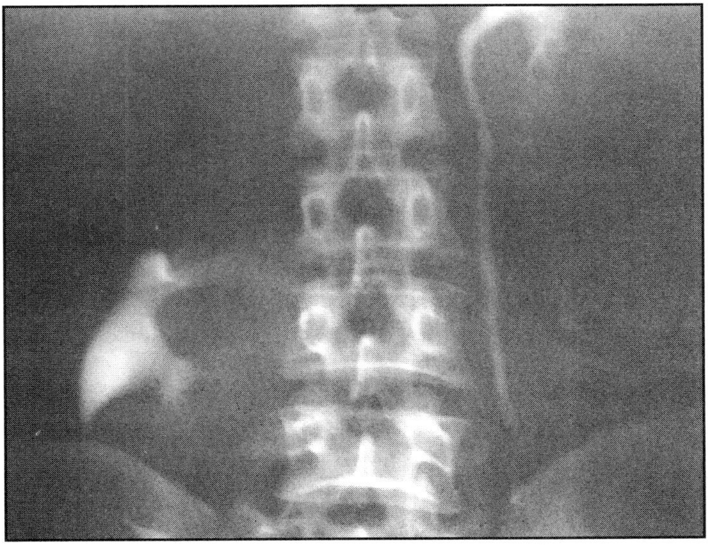

a) What are the findings?

b) What is the diagnosis?

c) Embryological basis?

Answer:

a) ROS in the region of pelvis

b) Pelvic ectopic kidney

c) Factors that may prevent the orderly movement of kidneys include ureteral bud maldevelopment , defective metanephric tissue that by itself fails to induce ascent , genetic abnormalities, and maternal illnesses

17.24

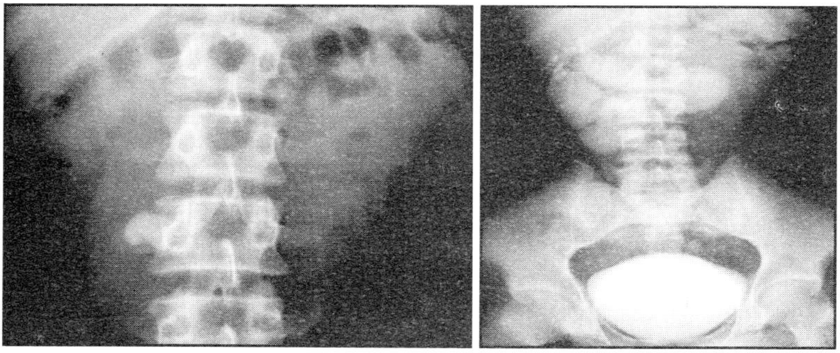

a) **What are the findings shown in this Xray-KUB and IVU?**

b) **What is the diagnosis?**

c) **Most common variety of this entity?**

Answer:

a) ROS in the region of pelvis

b) Cross fused ectopia

c) Unilaterally fused kidney with inferior ectopia is the most common variety

17.25

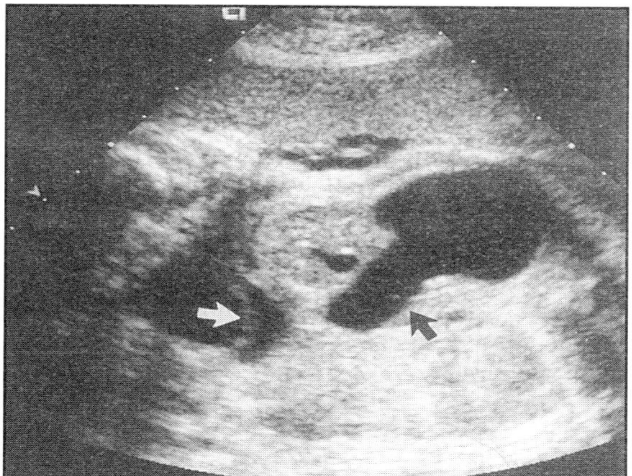

a) **What are the findings shown in this USG?**

b) **What is the diagnosis?**

Answer:

a) Marked upper pole hydronephrosis with a dilated ureter *(black arrow)* and a lower pole with mild pelvic dilation. The ureterocele *(white arrow)* is visible in the bladder.

b) Fetal ultrasound image showing a duplex system with an intravesical ureterocele

17.26

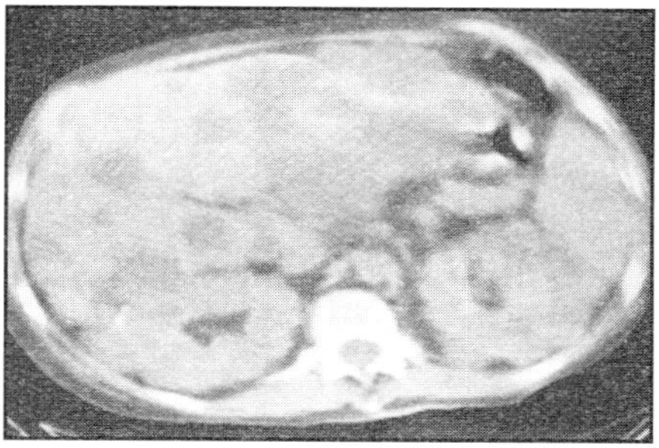

a) What are the findings shown in this CT?

b) What is the diagnosis?

Answer:

a) Bilateral renal cysts are seen in enlarged kidneys with calcification.

b) Computed tomographic scan of an adult male patient with autosomal dominant polycystic kidney disease.

17.27

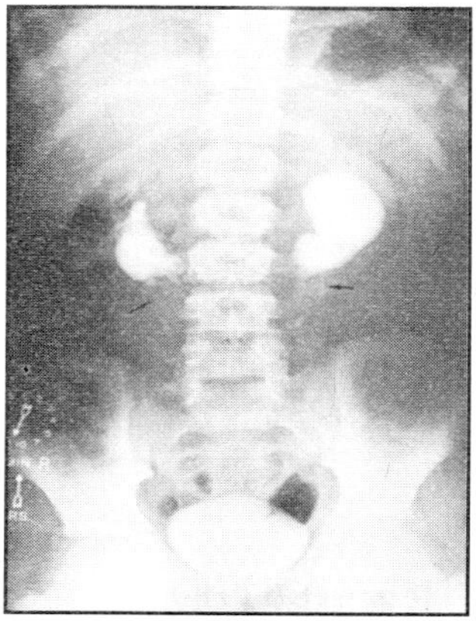

a) What is the finding in this IVU?

Answer:

a) IVU reveals a horseshoe kidney.

Findings are- Vertical renal axes and medial orientation of the collecting systems. The ureters (*arrows*) are laterally displaced and bow over the isthmus.

17.28 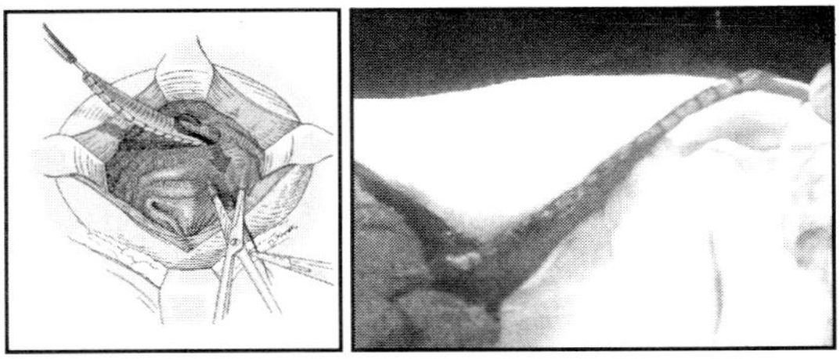

a) What is the procedure done in the above figure?

b) Name the indication.

Answer:

a) Excisional tapering is of ureter is done in the above figure

b) It is reserved for severely dilated ureter (1.75 cm) or a ureter that is markedly thickened, avoiding reimplantation of a bulky ureter

This is done in the management of megaureter

18.1 Name the present president, honorary secretary and treasurer of USI

Answer:

President- Dr P B Singh

Honorary secretary- Dr S K Singh

Treasurer-Dr Madhu S Agrawal

18.2 Name the present editorial committee of Indian journal of urology (IJU)

Answer:

Editor- Dr Nitin Kekre

Assistant-editor-Dr Anil Mandhani, Dr Rajeev Kumar, Dr Santosh Kumar and Dr J. Chandra Singh

Chairman-Dr Ganesh Gopalakrishnan

Treasurer- Dr Madhusudan Agrawal

18.3 Name the present chief editor of journal of urology

William D Steers.